Handbook
of
Basic
Pharmacokinetics
... including Clinical Applications
Sixth Edition

Handbook

of

Basic

Pharmacokinetics

... including Clinical Applications

Sixth Edition

Wolfgang A. Ritschel

Ph.D., M.D., Mr. Pharm., F.A.S.A., F.C.P.

Professor Emeritus of Pharmacokinetics
and Biopharmaceutics
College of Pharmacy
Professor of Pharmacology
and Cell Biophysics
College of Medicine
University of Cincinnati
Cincinnati, Ohio

Gregory L. Kearns

Pharm.D., Ph.D., F.C.P.

Marion Merrell Dow/Missouri Chair in Pediatric Pharmacology
Professor of Pediatrics and Pharmacology
University of Missouri—Kansas City
Chief, Division of Pediatric Pharmacology and Medical Toxicology
Director, Pediatric Pharmacology Research Unit
Children's Mercy Hospitals and Clinics
Kansas City, Missouri

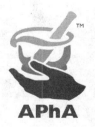

AMERICAN PHARMACISTS ASSOCIATION
WASHINGTON, D.C.

Acquiring Editor: Julian I. Graubart
Managing Editor: L. Luan Corrigan
Typography: Circle Graphics
Indexing: Lillian Rodberg

©2004 by the American Pharmacists Association
Published by the American Pharmacists Association, 2215 Constitution Avenue, NW, Washington, DC 20037-2985
APhA was founded in 1852 as the American Pharmaceutical Association.

To comment on this book via e-mail, send your message to the publisher at *aphabooks@aphanet.org*.

Library of Congress Cataloging-in-Publication Data

Ritschel, W. A. (Wolfgang A.)
  Handbook of basic pharmacokinetics— including clinical applications /
Wolfgang A. Ritschel, Gregory L. Kearns.— 6th ed.
    p. ; cm.
Includes bibliographical references and index.
  ISBN 1-58212-054-4
  1. Pharmacokinetics—Handbooks, manuals, etc. 2. Clinical
pharmacology—Handbooks, manuals, etc.
  [DNLM: 1. Pharmacokinetics—Handbooks. QV 39 R612h 2004] I. Kearns,
Gregory L. II. American Pharmaceutical Association. III. Title.

  RM301.5.R57 2004
  615.7—dc22

                                                      2003026662

How to Order This Book
Online: *www.pharmacist.com*
By phone: 800-878-0729 (from the United States and Canada)
VISA®, MasterCard®, and American Express® cards accepted

To my grandsons Felix, Florian,
Paul, and Paxton
—WAR

In loving memory of my
parents, Noel and Jacqueline
—GLK

Contents

Preface

First Edition 1976
Second Edition 1980
Third Edition 1986
Fourth Edition 1992
Fifth Edition 1999
Sixth Edition 2004

Pharmacokinetics, a comparatively young discipline among the health sciences, is interrelated with biopharmaceutics, pharmacology, and therapeutics. To a great extent, the foundation for pharmacokinetics, the study of change of drug concentrations, evolved in the fifties and sixties with the seventies bringing more mathematical refinement. During this latter period, pharmacokinetic applications may have been viewed by some as a "playground" for only the mathematically skilled researchers. Yet, at the same time, many started to apply pharmacokinetics clinically to the routine care of patients. In the eighties, the clinical use of pharmacokinetics became widely accepted in the form of therapeutic drug monitoring. It was also realized that the body is not just a one-, two-, or sophisticated higher compartment model, but a multimillion-compartment model. Although compartment models are valuable tools in research, the multicompartment models have limited use in clinical applications due in part to limitations in the number of blood samples which can be collected. Newer approaches such as Bayesian estimation and the use of compartment model-independent techniques enable both clinicians and basic scientists to obtain "robust" pharmacokinetic parameters which are most useful in characterizing drug disposition and/or the development of individualized drug dosing regimens.

The nineties brought a consolidation of pharmacokinetics in all areas of application: for drug monitoring and patient care in the clinical field, for clinical research in the area of drug product development, and for critical drug evaluation and the process of approval in the regulatory field. At the same time, there is increased interest in using pharmacokinetics for prediction of human pharmacokinetics from animal data (interspecies scaling) and for establishing correlations between pharmacokinetics and pharmacodynamics (PK/PD) or blood level profiles and clinical response and in vitro kinetics and pharmacokinetics (i.e., in vitro/in vivo), with the hope to eventually proceed from in vitro to clinical response correlation. Also pharmacokinetic evaluation has exceeded the rather traditional boundary of drug therapy to the evaluation of new biological products (e.g., recombinant hormones and hormone-releasing factors) and biological response modifiers (e.g., monoclonal antibodies, vaccines, immunoglobulins).

In the recent years we find on the horizon a fast growing interest in possible individualization of drug product design and individualized subcellular therapy as an outcome of the human genome project, already having resulted in new subdisciplines of pharmacogenetics and pharmacogenomics. A new look and classification of biotransformation pathways and processes and findings in the genetic basis of polypeptides and proteins in enzymatic and transport systems led to better understanding of drug absorption, distribution, and all kinds of interactions.

Pharmacokinetics has been viewed and is still considered by many as the field dealing with blood levels of a drug upon administration to the human or animal body. Lately, it seems that, in addition to the industrial and academic research interest in the area of modifying known compounds to obtain "better" conversion rates that produce the active moiety, increasing interest is mushrooming in the area of prodrugs. At this time, it seems that the pharmaceutical industry's major research interest is less in the area of synthesis of new compounds and more in the area of modifying known compounds to obtain conversion rates that produce the active moiety. The principle of new drug delivery systems, including prodrugs, microcapsules, nanocapsules, liposomes, osmotic pumps, pellets, matrices, lamellae, etc., is based on desired rates for conversion, release, or delivery. One can subdivide this approach from the conception of the principle to its clinical application according to the accompanying scheme.

This scheme shows that considerable overlap exists among the classical fields of pharmaceutics, biopharmaceutics, pharmacokinetics, and pharmacodynamics. Common to all, however, is the emphasis on RATE. Pharmacokinetics, derived from the Greek words, pharmakon (drug) and kinesis (motion, change of rate), therefore includes more than blood levels. To encompass the entire spectrum in the third edition, the author extended the previous ADME system (Absorption, Distribution, Metabolism, Elimination) to the LADMER system (Liberation, Absorption, Distribution, Metabolism, Elimination, Response) (see Chapter 2). As a direct result of the incorporation of important clinical aspects and material for design and adjustment of dosage regimens, beginning with the third edition the book title includes the term "Clinical." In the fourth edition, most of the chapters were revised or rewritten based upon many of the useful comments received from both clinicians and scientists who utilize the book. This edition included an attempt to further standardize the pharmacokinetic nomenclature used and to substantially increase the number of graphical illustrations to enhance the communication of concepts presented in the text.

Since the fifth edition, Dr. Gregory Kearns, an industrious, successful clinical scientist and former student of the principal author, became coauthor of the *Handbook*. The fifth edition was published by the American Pharmaceutical Association (APhA) after acquiring Drug Intelligence Publications, Inc. As before, the authors have relied heavily upon the recommendation made by their peers and colleagues in the fields of pharmacokinetics, biopharmaceutics, and clinical pharmacology to guide the most recent revision. In each instance where major revision has occurred, the authors have made a diligent attempt to include information which is both current and accurate and presented in a manner which fosters clinical application.

In summer of 2002 Mr. Julian Graubart of APhA suggested waiting no longer to update the *Handbook* to keep it current. The steadily growing amount of relevant scientific information has necessitated that the sixth edition have a new face and format. While it may no longer be easily kept in the pocket of a laboratory coat, it will provide a ready reference to be maintained close at hand (e.g., on the desktop) for practitioners who routinely rely upon pharmacokinetics to fulfill the demands of their profession.

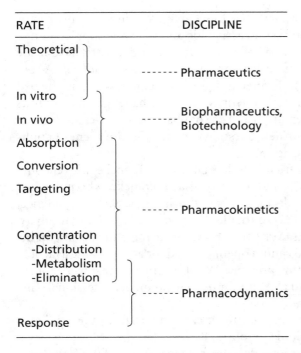

RATE	DISCIPLINE
Theoretical	
	Pharmaceutics
In vitro	
In vivo	Biopharmaceutics, Biotechnology
Absorption	
Conversion	
Targeting	
	Pharmacokinetics
Concentration	
-Distribution	
-Metabolism	
-Elimination	
	Pharmacodynamics
Response	

Our goal in preparing the sixth edition was to provide a focused update of the fifth edition. Accordingly, revisions have been made to the following chapters: 1 (Definitions and Glossary), 4 (Cell Membranes), 6 (Absorption/Transport Mechanisms), 10 (Biopharmaceutical Data of the Gastrointestinal Tract), 13 (Drug Biotransformation), 18 (Urinary and Biliary Recycling), 24 (Pediatric Pharmacokinetics), 27 (Drug Disposition in Pregnancy), 28 (Dosage Regimen Design), 30 (Physiological and Pathological Factors Influencing Drug Response), 36 (Bioavailability and Bioequivalence), and 38 (Extracorporeal Methods of Drug Removal). Additionally, the sixth edition contains a new chapter (Chapter 39), entitled Pharmacogenetics and Pharmacogenomics, created in recognition of the influence of genetic constitution on the enzymes and transporters that influence drug disposition and action. Significant contributions to Chapter 39 were made by J. Steven Leeder, Pharm.D., Ph.D. who currently is the Marion Merrell Dow Professor of Pediatric Pharmacogenomics and the chief of the Section of Developmental Pharmacology and Experimental Therapeutics at the Children's Mercy Hospitals and Clinics in Kansas City, Missouri. Finally, more than 220 drugs were added to the Appendix, now providing pharmacokinetic parameters of more than 640 drugs.

Despite its continued evolution, the *Handbook* is still intended to serve as a "user-friendly" consolidation of principles and useful techniques to a wide variety of individuals who find themselves either regularly or intermittently involved in the various applications of pharmacokinetics. These groups include:

a. the large group of practicing pharmacists, physicians, pharmacologists, and other health professionals who have had formal instruction in pharmacokinetics and need a review on and guide for pharmacokinetic problem solving for their professional work;

b. the clinical practitioner who needs quick information on the pharmacokinetic characteristics of specific drugs (Appendix), a readily accessible compilation of useful equations, and/or readily retrievable information on and effective summaries of specific topics;

c. undergraduate and graduate students studying for exams who would be aided by an effective "repetitorium";

d. the researcher in industry or academia who engages in preclinical and clinical studies, dosage form design and evaluation, the design of experimental protocols, and the analysis/interpretation of pharmacokinetic data.

The *Handbook of Basic Pharmacokinetics...including Clinical Applications* is not a textbook *per se* but rather an attempt to effectively distill the principles and facts which comprise the essence of the field. For these reasons, it remains as a widely used required or companion text in undergraduate and graduate teaching, giving the intuitive instructor great flexibility in lecturing where the book serves as a guide and welcome supplement.

The authors would like to thank all those colleagues who, over the years, have made constructive comments and recommendations for improvement of the *Handbook*. A special measure of gratitude is extended to our former and present mentors who have helped to equip us, to all of our present and former students who have challenged us and thus required us to think critically in our presentation and use of pharmacokinetics, and to our patients who present a constant source for new questions and the development of applications directed toward improving their existence.

Particular tribute is given to my dear friend, the late Dr. Don E. Francke, who encouraged the writing of the first edition in 1975, and to Dr. Gloria N. Francke, who published the second, third, and fourth editions; thanks for all her enthusiasm, publishing guidance, and friendship through the years. Our sincere thanks is given to Mr. Julian Graubart, Director of Books and Electronic Products, APhA, our Editor since the fifth edition, for his great interest in this book, his support and candid openness, and for always being available for ideas and discussions, and never exerting pressure. We also express our sincere appreciation to the professional publication staff at APhA for the outstanding, professional handling of this project from beginning to end.

Last but not least we would like to recognize the great secretarial support and give thanks to Ms. Donna Taylor and Ms. Meloni Clifton.

As we offer the sixth edition, a request is made to the reader and user of the *Handbook*: Nothing is perfect in the world but God. However, we all should try to do our best and seek to improve our world for the sake of mankind. Hence, the authors would very much appreciate receiving constructive criticism, especially suggestions of information on material to be included in or excluded from future editions. Finally, if the book is able to support the reader's and user's work and is able to benefit and help one single patient, it has fulfilled its purpose.

WOLFGANG A. RITSCHEL
GREGORY L. KEARNS

1

Definitions and Glossary

Absolute Bioavailability is the extent or fraction of drug absorbed upon extravascular administration in comparison to the dose size administered.

Absorption of drugs is the process of uptake of the compound from the site of administration into the systemic circulation. A prerequisite for absorption is that the drug be in aqueous solution. The only relatively rare exception is absorption by pinocytosis.

Accumulation is the increase of drug concentration in blood and tissue upon multiple dosing until steady state is reached.

Apparent Partition Coefficient is the ratio of the concentrations at equilibrium between a lipid phase (usually n-octanol) and an aqueous phase (usually buffer pH 7.4). The apparent partition coefficient is uncorrected for dissociation or association in either phase.

Area Under the Curve is the integral of drug blood level over time from zero to infinity and is a measure of quantity of drug absorbed and in the body.

Area Under First Statistical Moment Curve is mathematically defined by $AUMC = \int_0^\infty t \cdot C \cdot dt$, i.e., it is the area under the curve observed for the product of time and concentration versus time.

Biliary Recycling (Enterohepatic Recirculation) is the phenomenon that drugs emptied via bile into the small intestine can be reabsorbed from the intestinal lumen into systemic circulation.

Bioavailability is defined as both the relative amount of drug from an administered dosage form which enters the systemic circulation and the rate at which the drug appears in the bloodstream.

Bioequivalence of a drug product is achieved if its extent and rate of absorption are not statistically significantly different from those of the standard when administered at the same molar dose.

Bioequivalence Requirement is a requirement imposed by the Food and Drug Administration for in vitro and/or in vivo testing of specified drug products which must be satisfied as a condition of marketing.

Biological Half-Life (see Elimination Half-Life).

Biopharmaceutics deals with the physical and chemical properties of the drug substance, the dosage form, and the body and the biological effectiveness of a drug and/or drug product upon administration, i.e., the drug availability to the human or animal body from a given dosage form, considered as a drug delivery system. The time course of the drug in the body and the quantifying of the drug concentration pattern are explained by pharmacokinetics.

Biophase is the actual site of action of a drug in the body. It is the drug-receptor interaction on the molecular level or the effect of the presence of a drug on biopolymers. The biophase may be the surface of a cell or within the cell, i.e., one of the organelles.

Blood Flow Rate is the speed of blood perfusion in an organ, usually expressed in ml/100 g organ weight/min. Blood flow rates may differ several-fold between rest (or immobilization) and exercise.

Blood, Plasma, or Serum Levels demonstrate the concentration in blood, plasma, or serum upon administration of a dosage form by various routes of administration. Blood, plasma, or serum level curves are plots of drug concentration versus time on numeric or semilog graph paper. Blood, plasma, or serum levels are obtained from blood samples by venipuncture in certain time intervals after administration of the drug product and chemical or microbiological analysis of the drug in the biological fluid.

Central Compartment is the sum of all body regions (organs and tissue) in which the drug concentration is in instantaneous equilibrium with that in blood or plasma. The blood or plasma is always part of the central compartment.

Chronopharmacokinetics is the study of pharmacokinetic drug parameters as affected by circadian rhythm or diurnal variation.

Circadian Rhythm is the biological clock controlling rhythms of processes during a twenty-four hour cycle which is based on endogenous factors.

Clearance is the hypothetical volume of distribution in ml of the unmetabolized drug which is cleared per unit of time (ml/min or ml/h) by any pathway of drug removal (renal, hepatic, and other pathways of elimination).

Clinical Pharmacokinetics is the application of pharmacokinetic principles in the safe and effective treatment of individual patients and in the optimization of drug therapy.

A **Compartment** in pharmacokinetics is an entity which can be described by a definite volume and a concentration of drug contained in that volume. In pharmacokinetics, experimental data are explained by fitting them to compartment models.

Concentration Gradient is the difference in the concentration in two phases usually separated by a membrane.

Creatinine Clearance is the ratio of creatinine excreted in urine to the concentration of creatinine in plasma. The creatinine clearance decreases with renal impairment and with age.

Cumulative Urinary Excretion Curves are plots of the actual cumulative amounts of drug and/or its metabolites excreted into urine versus time after administration of a drug product by various routes of administration.

Depot Phase is that portion of a prolonged release dosage form which liberates the drug from the dosage form at a slower rate than its unrestricted absorption rate.

Diffusion Layer is the viscous layer of concentrated drug solution around a dissolving particle.

Disposition is the loss of drug from the central compartment due to transfer (distribution) into other compartments and/or elimination and metabolism.

Diurnal Variation is the biological clock controlling rhythms of processes during a twenty-four hour cycle which is based on external synchronizers (Zeitgeber).

Dosage Regimen or Dose Rate is the systematized dosage schedule for therapy, i.e., the proper dose sizes and proper dosing intervals required to produce clinical effectiveness or to maintain a therapeutic concentration in the body.

Dose Dependency refers to a change of one or more of the pharmacokinetic processes of absorption, distribution, metabolism, and excretion with increasing dose size.

Dose Dumping is a term used to describe the achievement of sustained drug concentration by simply increasing the dose size or by accidental fast release of drug from a sustained release dosage form.

Dose-Response Curve is the graphical presentation of the pharmacological or clinical effectiveness or toxicity (response) versus dose. A log dose-response curve is sigmoid with a straight-line middle section; a log dose-probability curve results in an entirely straight line.

Dose Size is the amount of drug in µg (= mcg), mg, units, or other dimensions to be administered.

Dosing Interval is the time period between administration of maintenance doses.

A **Drug** is a chemical compound of synthetic, semisynthetic, natural, or biological origin which interacts with human or animal cells. The interactions may be quantified, whereby these resulting actions are intended to prevent, to cure, or to reduce ill effects in the human or animal body, or to detect disease-causing manifestations.

A **Drug Product** or **Dosage Form** is the gross pharmaceutical form containing the active ingredient(s) [drug(s)] and vehicle substances necessary in formulating a medicament of desired dosage, desired volume, and desired application form, ready for administration.

Drug-Receptor Interaction is the combining of a drug molecule with the receptor for which it has affinity and the initiation of a pharmacologic response by its intrinsic activity.

Drug Release or **Liberation** is the delivery of the active ingredient from a dosage form into solution. The dissolution medium is either a biological fluid or an artificial test fluid (in vitro). Drug release is characterized by the speed (liberation rate constant) and the amount of drug appearing in solution.

A **Drug Specialty** or **Brand Product** is a drug product, usually of unvarying composition, labeled with a registered trademark of a single company.

Elimination Half-Life of a drug is the time in hours necessary to reduce the drug concentration in the blood, plasma, or serum to one-half after equilibrium is reached. The elimination half-life may be influenced by: dose size, variation in urinary excretion (pH), intersubject variation, age, protein binding, other drugs, and diseases (especially renal and liver diseases).

Loss of drug from the body, as described by the elimination half-life, means the elimination of the administered parent drug molecule (not its metabolites) by urinary excretion, metabolism, or other pathways of elimination (lung, skin, etc.).

Enterohepatic Recirculation (Biliary Recycling) is the phenomenon in which drugs emptied via bile into the small intestine can be reabsorbed from the intestinal lumen into systemic circulation.

Enzyme Induction is the increase in enzyme content or rate of enzymatic processes resulting in faster metabolism of a compound. If a drug stimulates its own metabolism, it is called auto-induction, and, if it is caused by other compounds, it is called foreign-induction.

Enzyme Inhibition is the decrease in rate of metabolism of a compound usually by competition for an enzyme system.

Excretion of drugs is the final elimination from the body's systemic circulation via the kidney into urine, via bile and saliva into intestines and into feces, via sweat, via skin, and via milk.

Extravascular Administration refers to all routes of administration except those where the drug is directly introduced into the bloodstream. Extravascular routes are: IM, SC, PO, Oral, Rectal, IP, Topical, etc.

Feathering refers to a graphical method for the separation of exponents such as separating the absorption rate constant from the elimination rate constant, or the α-slope from the β-slope, or the absorption rate constant from the α-rate constant. The term **Residual Method** is synonymous with feathering.

First-Pass Effect describes the phenomenon whereby drugs may be *metabolized* (not chemically degraded) following absorption but before reaching systemic circulation. Hepatic first-pass effect may occur following PO and deep rectal administration. It may be avoided by using sublingual and buccal routes of administration. Pulmonary first-pass effect cannot be avoided by intravenous, buccal, or sublingual routes.

Flip-Flop Model is the phenomenon observed if the rate of absorption is slower than the rate of elimination, or if one of the distribution rates is slower than the rate of elimination.

The **Gastrointestinal Tract** is a part of the alimentary canal comprising stomach, small intestine, and large intestine.

A **Generic Product** is a drug product marketed under the nonproprietary or common name of the drug(s).

Hepatic Clearance is the hypothetical volume of distribution in ml of the unmetabolized drug which is cleared in one minute via the liver.

Homeostasis is the maintenance of a steady state which characterizes the internal environment of the healthy organism. An important function of homeostasis is the regulation of the fluid medium and volume of the cell.

Hybrid Rate Constants are composite rate constants consisting of two or more microconstants. α and β are hybrid rate constants.

Initial Phase is that portion of a prolonged release dosage form which is immediately available for absorption.

Intravascular Administration refers to all routes of administration where the drug is directly introduced into the bloodstream, i.e., IV, Intra-arterial, and Intracardiac; bioavailability = 100 percent, f = 1.

Intrinsic Clearance is the theoretical unrestricted maximum clearance of unbound drug by an eliminating organ.

IV Bolus is a physiologic nonsense and poor use (misuse) of language. A bolus (Greek: bolos) is a bite, something solid which is swallowed and is then absorbed from the intestines. The correct term would be **IV Push.**

The LADMER System deals with the complex dynamic processes of liberation of an active ingredient from the dosage form, its absorption into systemic circulation, its distribution and metabolism in the body, the excretion of the drug from the body, and the achievement of response.

Lag Time is the period of time which elapses between the time of administration and the time a measurable drug concentration is found in blood. Lag times are often found upon PO administration due to slow disintegration and dissolution of tablets or capsules.

Lean Body Weight is a patient's body weight minus the fat mass. Drugs of low lipid solubility should be dosed in obese patients according to the lean body weight.

Loading Dose, Priming Dose, or **Initial Dose** is the dose size used in initiating therapy so as to yield therapeutic concentrations which will result in clinical effectiveness.

Local Effect is obtained when the drug product is administered at the site where the pharmacological response is desired and when the drug released from the product acts by adsorption to the skin or mucosa or penetrates into the skin or mucosa but does not enter the systemic blood circulation or lymphatic stream.

Maintenance Dose is the dose size required to maintain the clinical effectiveness or therapeutic concentration according to the dosage regimen.

Mean Transit or **Residence Time** is the time when 63.2 percent of an intravenous dose has been eliminated from the pharmacokinetic system.

Metabolism is the sum of all the chemical reactions for biotransformation of endogenous and exogenous substances which take place in the living cell.

Metabonomics is the study of changes in the global pool of intermediary metabolites present in the target tissues or biological fluids following pathophysiologic stimuli.

Michaelis-Menten Kinetics uses equations to characterize certain phenomena such as protein binding, adsorption, and nonlinear or saturation processes often observed with increasing dose sizes.

Microconstants are those constants which are part of the hybrid constants. Examples of microconstants are k_{12}, k_{21}, k_{13}.

Monitoring is the determination and recording of drug concentrations during the course of therapy in order to adjust, if necessary, the dosage regimen.

Multiple Dose Administration is when a drug is given repeatedly at intervals shorter than those required to completely eliminate the drug of the previously given dose.

Nonlinear Kinetics or **Saturation Kinetics** refers to a change of one or more of the pharmacokinetic parameters during absorption, distribution, metabolism, and excretion by saturation or overloading of processes due to increased dose sizes.

Oral Administration includes buccal, sublingual, and perlingual administration routes where the drug is absorbed from the mouth cavity (no first-pass effect).

Peripheral Compartment is the sum of all body regions (i.e., organs, tissues, or parts of it) to which a drug eventually distributes, but is not in instantaneous equilibrium. The peripheral compartment is sometimes further subdivided into a **Shallow** and a **Deep Compartment.**

Peroral Administration indicates that the dosage form is swallowed and the drug is absorbed from the GI-tract (first-pass effect possible).

Pharmaceutical Alternatives are drug products that contain the identical therapeutic moiety, or its precursor, but not necessarily in the same amount or dosage form or as the same salt or ester.

Pharmaceutical Equivalents are drug products that contain identical amounts of the identical active drug ingredient, i.e., the same salt or ester of the same therapeutic moiety, in identical dosage forms, but not necessarily containing the same inactive ingredients.

Pharmacogenetics deals with interindividual variation in DNA sequence related to drug absorption and distribution (pharmacokinetics) or drug action (pharmacodynamics).

Pharmacogenomics is the application of genomic principles and technologies in drug discovery to pharmacological function, disposition, and therapeutic response.

Pharmacokinetics deals with the changes of drug concentration in the drug product and changes of concentration of a drug and/or its metabolite(s) in the human or animal body following administration, i.e., the changes of drug concentration in the different body fluids and tissues in the dynamic system of liberation, absorption, distribution, body storage, binding, metabolism, and excretion.

Protein Binding is the phenomenon which occurs when a drug combines with plasma protein (particularly albumin) or tissue protein to form a reversible complex. Protein binding is usually nonspecific and depends on the drug's affinity to the protein molecule, the number of protein binding sites, and protein and drug concentrations. Drugs can be displaced from protein binding sites by other compounds having higher affinity for the binding sites.

Rate-Limiting Step is the process with the slowest rate constant in a system of simultaneous kinetic processes.

A Receptor is a site in the biophase to which drug molecules can be bound. A receptor (= substrate) is usually a protein or proteinaceous material.

Relative Bioavailability is the extent of drug absorbed upon extravascular administration in comparison to the dose size of a standard administered by the same route.

Renal Clearance is the hypothetical plasma volume in ml (volume of distribution) of the unmetabolized drug which is cleared in one minute via the kidney.

Single Dose Administration occurs when the next dose of the same drug is administered only after the drug of the previously given dose is completely eliminated from the body.

Sorption Promoters or **Permeation Enhancers** are defined as substances that have no pharmacological properties of their own in the amount used, but which can improve the penetration of drugs into the skin or their permeation through skin or mucosa by reducing the barrier resistance.

Steady State is a level of drug accumulation in blood and tissue upon multiple dosing when input and output are at equilibrium. The steady state drug concentrations fluctuate (oscillate) between a maximum and a minimum steady state concentration within each of the dosing intervals.

Structural Nonspecific Drugs are those whose pharmacological action is not directly dependent on chemical structure. They have no functional groups, are highly lipophilic, and do not react easily. They act by physicochemical processes. Examples include ether, nitrous oxide, halothane, phenol, ethyl alcohol, octyl alcohol, and acetone.

Structural Specific Drugs are those whose pharmacological action results primarily from their chemical structure. They have functional groups and combine to the three-dimensional structure of receptors in the biophase. Examples include antibiotics, sulfonamides, glycosides, alkaloids, etc.

Sustained Release is the property of prolonged release dosage forms where the liberation (drug release) rate constant is smaller than the unrestricted absorption rate constant.

Systemic Effect is obtained when the drug released from the drug product enters the bloodstream and/or lymphatic stream and is distributed within the body—or at least in several organs—regardless of the site and route of administration.

Total Clearance describes the clearance of the hypothetical plasma volume in ml (volume of distribution) of a drug per unit time due to excretion via kidney, liver, lung, skin, etc., and metabolism.

A Unit Membrane is the physical barrier to transport in the body. It is lipoidal in nature and consists of a double row of phospholipids sandwiched between one layer each of protein.

Urinary Recycling is the phenomenon that occurs when drugs filtered through the glomeruli are reabsorbed from the tubuli into systemic circulation.

A **Vehicle** is the carrier of the drug in the drug product. It is composed of all necessary vehicle substances.

Vehicle Substances are additives which are necessary in formulating a dosage form from the drug. The vehicle substances should be chemically inert and should not have any pharmacological effect in the dose used. Vehicle substances are used to produce, from a relatively small amount of drug, a dosage form of the desired strength, volume, and form or consistency suitable for administration.

Volume of Distribution is not a "real" volume but an artifact—a hypothetical volume of body fluid that would be required to dissolve the total amount of drug at the same concentration as that found in the blood. It is a proportionality constant relating the amount of drug in the body to the measured concentration in biological fluid (blood, plasma, or serum).

New Nomenclature

Nearly every textbook and article on pharmacokinetics uses its own nomenclature and symbols. Unless well defined (which consumes printing space), the use of two or more symbols for the same parameter or expression is often confusing and time-consuming for the reader. The American College of Clinical Pharmacology (ACCP) developed a nomenclature in hope that this would simplify reading of pharmacokinetic publications and would make superfluous the printing of symbols in each publication. Unfortunately, the ACCP nomenclature has not received the attention hoped for; hence, the new nomenclature was not fully adopted for the present edition of this *Handbook*. Nevertheless, the reader should become familiar with the most important aspects of the ACCP nomenclature.

Drug concentrations in blood, plasma, or serum are symbolized by C, followed by a number in parentheses indicating the time after administration, i.e., $C(3)$ is the concentration 3 hours after drug administration. $C(0)$ is the "fictitious" zero time drug concentration. The intercept of the back-extrapolated terminal phase with the ordinate is C_z (previously termed B), the other intercepts are C_1, C_2, etc., starting with the intercept of the steepest monoexponential line, i.e., $C_1 = A$, $C_2 = C$, etc. The terminal rate constant is λ_z (lambda z), i.e., β (beta). The largest (fastest) rate constant is λ_1, the next is λ_2, etc. The volume of distribution during the terminal phase is V_z (i.e., $V_{d\beta}$); the others are V_c and V_{ss}.

The expression AUC denotes the total area under the curve. Truncated areas have a qualifier, such as AUC(0–12) for zero to 12 hours. The AUC during a dosing interval at steady state is AUC_τ^{ss}. The fraction of drug absorbed (absolute bioavailability) is f, and the fraction of unchanged drug excreted into urine is f_e. D is any dose size. DL and DM are loading dose and maintenance dose, respectively. The total clearance is expressed by CL. CL_{int}, CL_{NR}, CL_R, CL_H, and CL_{CR} are intrinsic, nonrenal, renal, hepatic, and creatinine clearance. t_{lag}, t_{max}, t_{mp}, t_{pi}, and T are lag time, peak time, midpoint time, postinfusion time, and duration of infusion, respectively.

The general blood level equations for the one-, two-, and three-compartment models after IV administration:

$$C = C_p^0 \cdot e^{-k_{el} \cdot t}$$

$$C = A \cdot e^{-\alpha \cdot t} + B \cdot e^{-\beta \cdot t}$$

$$C = P \cdot e^{-\pi \cdot t} + A \cdot e^{\alpha \cdot t} + B \cdot e^{-\beta \cdot t}$$

are written according to the ACCP nomenclature as:

$$C(t) = \sum_{i=1}^{n} C_i \cdot e^{-\lambda_i \cdot t}$$

For a listing of symbols and equations, the reader is referred to the literature: Allen, L., Kimura, K., MacKichan, J., and Ritschel, W. A.: Manual of Symbols, Equations, and Definitions in Pharmacokinetics, *J. Clin. Pharmacol. 22*:S1 (1982).

2

The LADMER System
Liberation, Absorption, Distribution, Metabolism, Elimination, and Response

In the relationship between dose and effectiveness or dose response, not only the amount of drug administered and the pharmacological effect of the drug are of importance but many other factors are responsible for the entrance of a drug into the body. These factors are based on the physical and chemical properties of the drug substance and of the drug product. What happens to the active ingredient in the body after administration of a drug product in its various dosage forms? This entire cycle of processes is termed *fate of drugs*. Whether a blood level curve will reach its peak rapidly or slowly depends on the route of administration; the dosage form; the liberation rate of the drug from the dosage form; diffusion, penetration, and permeation of the drug; its distribution within the body fluids and tissues; the type, amount, and rate of biotransformation; recycling processes; and elimination. In addition to these factors there are also others, depending on the individual disposition, diseases, etc.

The fate of drugs is described in the leading literature on biopharmaceutics and pharmacokinetics by the LADMER system showing that liberation, absorption, distribution, metabolism, and elimination are involved to elicit the response.

Liberation is the first step which determines onset of action, rate of absorption, availability, etc., which is true for all drug products by all routes of administration, except intravenous (IV) and the peroral use of true solutions. Liberation is controlled by the characteristics of the drug product.

Figure 2-1 gives a schematic diagram of the LADMER system. On both sides of the diagram are the five processes, liberation, absorption, metabolism, elimination, and response (underlined). A drug administered in a dosage form by any route of administration must be released from the dosage form (except IV, and true solutions for other routes). In order that a drug can be absorbed it must be present in the form of solution; therefore dissolution becomes the first and sometimes rate-limiting step. Upon administration of suspensions, capsules, tablets, suppositories, implants, and intramuscular (IM) suspensions, we find drug particles in the gastrointestinal (GI) tract, in body cavities, or in tissue. After dissolution, the drug diffuses to the site of absorption, i.e., buccal, sublingual, gastrointestinal, percutaneous, subcutaneous, intramuscular, intraperitoneal, intracutaneous, ocular, nasal,

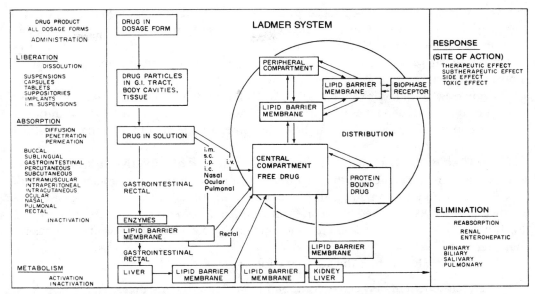

Figure 2-1. Diagram of LADMER System showing the complex interrelationships among drug, drug product, and body.

pulmonal, rectal, etc. Some of the drug will already be inactivated before it can be absorbed. Only drugs administered intravenously in solution enter the circulatory system immediately. With all other routes of administration, the drugs must pass membranes which act as lipid barriers. Different transport mechanisms are employed to penetrate into and to permeate through these membranes. Most of the drugs are absorbed or transported by passive diffusion, which depends on the pK_a value of the drug, the pH of the solution, and the lipid solubility of the unionized form.

Drugs passing through the lipid barrier may directly enter the central compartment, i.e., after intramuscular, subcutaneous, intraperitoneal, intracutaneous, nasal, ocular, pulmonal, and, partly, after rectal administration. Drugs administered perorally and some of the drugs administered rectally are confronted with enzymes as they pass through the liver with the blood flow. In the liver, the main place of metabolism, some drugs are inactivated and metabolized during the first pass; other drugs are activated here. Most drugs are at least partially bound to protein in the bloodstream. Only the free, unbound form of the drug is available for action. The protein-bound fraction is not permanently trapped but is in equilibrium and will be released from the protein as the free drug is eliminated from the plasma.

The drug may enter the peripheral compartment by again passing a lipid barrier until it finally reaches the biophase (process of distribution, characterized by the circle in Figure 2-1). This is a cell, or even a cell component, where the final interaction between drug and receptor takes place. After releasing the drug from its receptor binding, the drug again passes through a lipid barrier and enters the central compartment, from which the drug, by again passing a lipid barrier, is metabolized in the liver or kidney or in the tissue or plasma. It then passes either via biliary excretion into the intestines, or passes through the kidney where it will be either reabsorbed or finally excreted into urine. Elimination is not only by urinary and biliary means but also through the salivary glands, the milk glands, the sweat glands, and through the lungs. Reabsorption takes place not only in the kidney by tubular reabsorption but also in the intestine after enterohepatic cycling if the drug or its metabolite is in absorbable form. All these factors are involved in determining whether the drug administered will produce a therapeutic effect or yield only a subtherapeutic effect or even show toxic effects.

Knowledge and understanding of the LADMER system enable the scientist to design a drug product controlling these factors. Onset of action, intensity of effect, and duration of effect are controllable. The sum of all these phenomena is the quantitative characteristic of a drug product's effect.

For most of the drug products a relatively rapid and quantitative absorption and a slow elimination are required, thus maintaining a therapeutic drug concentration for a long period of time. In some cases this goal may easily be achieved if the drug is soluble, highly unionized, is absorbed by passive diffusion, and has a long elimination half-life. If this is not the case many manipulations are necessary to create a drug product of desired characteristics.

The LADMER system is the key to the following tasks:

- Development of new active compounds, analogs, or derivatives;
- Development of dosage forms with desired release characteristics;
- Determination of pharmacokinetic parameters and pharmacokinetic drug product profiles;
- Determination and evaluation of bioavailability;
- Selection of the most appropriate route of administration;
- Determination of effective dose sizes; and
- Adjustment of dosage regimen to achieve a desired therapeutic concentration of drug in the body based on physiologic (body weight, age, sex, etc.) and pathologic factors (renal, hepatic, or heart failure, obesity, malnutrition, etc.).

3

Organs, Tissues, Cells, and Organelles

The human body is composed of organs, tissues, and cells organized in a manner similar to that shown in Table 3-1.

Tissue

The different types of tissue perform different functions and accordingly show different vascularization. Hence, distribution of drugs will differ. Some drugs are more or less evenly distributed in all tissues, e.g., ethanol, urea, amidopyrine. Highly lipid soluble drugs are distributed predominantly in fat and nervous tissue. A survey of types of tissues, their main locations, and functions is given in Table 3-2.

The Cell

A cell is the smallest functional unit of life whose parts are in dynamic equilibrium exhibiting the manifestations of life which include metabolism, reproduction, and response to stimuli.

A schematic diagram of a liver parenchymal cell and its organelles, their function, and localization of enzymes is given in Figure 3-1.

The cell or its membrane is the site of drug-receptor interaction; the biophase is where pharmacologic action takes place.

Cells are connected in tissue by means of their cell coats. If hyaluronidase is given (IM, SC), hyaluronic acid is hydrolyzed and intercellular cement dissolves. Drugs can then penetrate between the cells. Absorption is faster since a larger tissue area is exposed to the drug solution. Pain at the injection site is reduced since less pressure per unit area is exerted.

TABLE 3-1. Organization of the Human Body

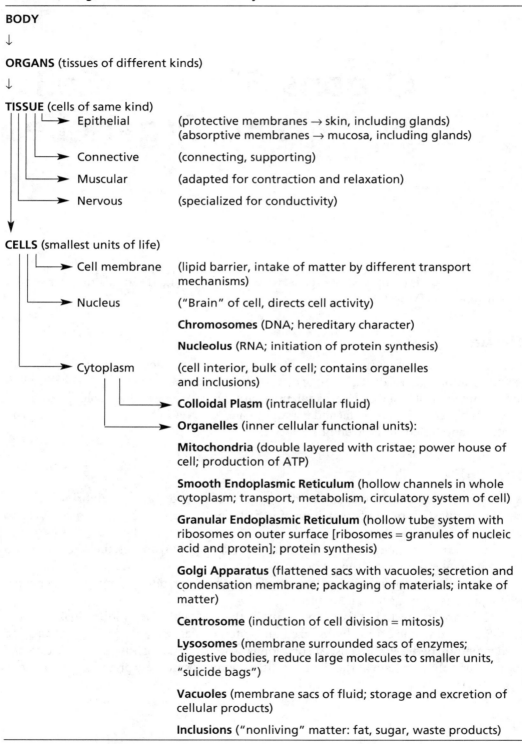

BODY

↓

ORGANS (tissues of different kinds)

↓

TISSUE (cells of same kind)

Epithelial — (protective membranes → skin, including glands)
(absorptive membranes → mucosa, including glands)

Connective — (connecting, supporting)

Muscular — (adapted for contraction and relaxation)

Nervous — (specialized for conductivity)

CELLS (smallest units of life)

Cell membrane — (lipid barrier, intake of matter by different transport mechanisms)

Nucleus — ("Brain" of cell, directs cell activity)

Chromosomes (DNA; hereditary character)

Nucleolus (RNA; initiation of protein synthesis)

Cytoplasm — (cell interior, bulk of cell; contains organelles and inclusions)

Colloidal Plasm (intracellular fluid)

Organelles (inner cellular functional units):

Mitochondria (double layered with cristae; power house of cell; production of ATP)

Smooth Endoplasmic Reticulum (hollow channels in whole cytoplasm; transport, metabolism, circulatory system of cell)

Granular Endoplasmic Reticulum (hollow tube system with ribosomes on outer surface [ribosomes = granules of nucleic acid and protein]; protein synthesis)

Golgi Apparatus (flattened sacs with vacuoles; secretion and condensation membrane; packaging of materials; intake of matter)

Centrosome (induction of cell division = mitosis)

Lysosomes (membrane surrounded sacs of enzymes; digestive bodies, reduce large molecules to smaller units, "suicide bags")

Vacuoles (membrane sacs of fluid; storage and excretion of cellular products)

Inclusions ("nonliving" matter: fat, sugar, waste products)

Table 3-2. Survey of Tissues, Their Main Locations, and Functions

TISSUES	MAIN LOCATIONS	FUNCTIONS
1. Epithelial		
a. Simple squamous (single layer flat cells)	1. Alveoli of lungs	1. Diffusion of gases between air and blood
	2. Cover of GI membrane	2. Absorption, secretion
	3. Endothelium	3. Lining of blood vessels
	4. Glomerular capsule and loop of Henle	4. Exchange, diffusion of solutes
b. Simple columnar (one row tall cells)	1. Secreting cells of glands	1. Secretion and absorption, border
	2. Respiratory tract (bronchioles)	
	3. Reproductive organs (uterus)	Border
	4. GI tract	
	5. Gallbladder	
c. Stratified squamous (several layers of cells, top layer flattened)	1. Outer layer of skin (epidermis)	1. Protection
	2. Mouth	
	3. Esophagus	Border
	4. Pharynx	
	5. Corneal surface	
d. Stratified columnar (several layers of cells, top layer columnar)	1. Vagina	
	2. Nose	
	3. Larynx	Border
	4. Trachea	
	5. Larger bronchi	
2. Muscle		
a. Skeletal (voluntary or striated)	1. Attached to bones	1. Movement of bones
	2. Extrinsic eyeball muscles	2. Eye movements
	3. Upper one-third of esophagus	3. First part of swallowing
b. Visceral (involuntary or smooth)	1. Walls of tubular viscera	1. Movement of substances along tubes
	2. In walls of blood vessels and large lymphatics	2. Changes in size of blood vessels
	3. In ducts of glands	3. Movement of substances along ducts

(Continued)

Table 3-2. Survey of Tissues, Their Main Locations, and Functions *(Continued)*

TISSUES	MAIN LOCATIONS	FUNCTIONS
	4. Intrinsic eye muscle (iris and ciliary body)	4. Changes in size of pupils and in shape of lens
	5. Arrector muscle of hairs	5. Erection of hairs (gooseflesh)
c. Cardiac (branching)	1. Wall of heart	1. Contraction of heart
3. Connective (most widely distributed of all tissues)		
a. Areolar (loose connective tissue)	1. Between other tissues 2. Between organs 3. Superficial fascia	1. Cements various parts of body together
b. Adipose (fat)	1. Subcutaneously 2. Padding at various points	1. Protection 2. Insulation 3. Support 4. Reserve food
c. Dense fibrous	1. Tendons 2. Ligaments 3. Aponeuroses 4. Deep fascia 5. Scars 6. Capsule of kidney, etc.	1. Furnish flexible but strong connection
d. Hemopoietic		
(1) Myeloid	1. Bone marrow	1. Forms red blood cells, granular leukocytes, (neutrophils, eosinophils, basophils), and platelets
(2) Lymphatic or lymphoid	1. Lymph nodes	1. Form nongranular white blood cells (lymphocytes and monocytes) and plasma cells; filter lymph
	2. Spleen	2. Forms lymphocytes, monocytes, and plasma cells; filters blood
	3. Thymus gland	3. Forms lymphocytes
	4. Tonsils and adenoids	4. Form lymphocytes and plasma cells

(Continued)

Table 3-2. Survey of Tissues, Their Main Locations, and Functions *(Continued)*

TISSUES	MAIN LOCATIONS	FUNCTIONS
e. Bone	1. Skeleton	1. Support
		2. Protection
f. Cartilage		
(1) Hyaline	1. Part of nasal septum	1. Furnishes firm but flexible support
	2. Covering articular surfaces of bones	
	3. Larynx	
	4. Rings in trachea and bronchi	
(2) Fibrocartilage	1. Discs between vertebrae	
	2. Symphysis pubis	
(3) Elastic	1. External ear	
	2. Eustachian (auditory) tube	
4. Nervous	1. Brain	1. Receives and transmits stimuli
	2. Spinal cord	
	3. Nerves	
5. Blood (vascular)	1. Blood	1. Transportation
		2. Protection against microorganisms

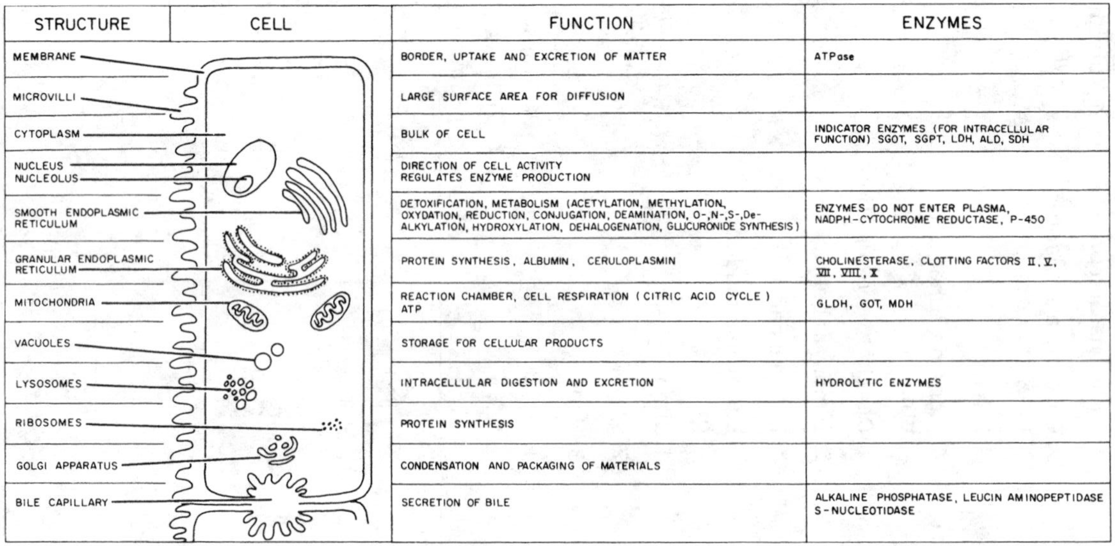

STRUCTURE	CELL	FUNCTION	ENZYMES
MEMBRANE		BORDER, UPTAKE AND EXCRETION OF MATTER	ATPase
MICROVILLI		LARGE SURFACE AREA FOR DIFFUSION	
CYTOPLASM		BULK OF CELL	INDICATOR ENZYMES (FOR INTRACELLULAR FUNCTION) SGOT, SGPT, LDH, ALD, SDH
NUCLEUS / NUCLEOLUS		DIRECTION OF CELL ACTIVITY / REGULATES ENZYME PRODUCTION	
SMOOTH ENDOPLASMIC RETICULUM		DETOXIFICATION, METABOLISM (ACETYLATION, METHYLATION, OXIDATION, REDUCTION, CONJUGATION, DEAMINATION, O-,N-,S-,DE-ALKYLATION, HYDROXYLATION, DEHALOGENATION, GLUCURONIDE SYNTHESIS)	ENZYMES DO NOT ENTER PLASMA, NADPH-CYTOCHROME REDUCTASE, P-450
GRANULAR ENDOPLASMIC RETICULUM		PROTEIN SYNTHESIS, ALBUMIN, CERULOPLASMIN	CHOLINESTERASE, CLOTTING FACTORS II, V, VII, VIII, X
MITOCHONDRIA		REACTION CHAMBER, CELL RESPIRATION (CITRIC ACID CYCLE) ATP	GLDH, GOT, MDH
VACUOLES		STORAGE FOR CELLULAR PRODUCTS	
LYSOSOMES		INTRACELLULAR DIGESTION AND EXCRETION	HYDROLYTIC ENZYMES
RIBOSOMES		PROTEIN SYNTHESIS	
GOLGI APPARATUS		CONDENSATION AND PACKAGING OF MATERIALS	
BILE CAPILLARY		SECRETION OF BILE	ALKALINE PHOSPHATASE, LEUCIN AMINOPEPTIDASE, 5-NUCLEOTIDASE

Figure 3-1. Overview of the organelles of the liver cell, their functions, and location of enzymes.

Selected References

1. Brachet, J.: The Living Cell, *Sci. Am. 205*:3 (1961).
2. Dyson, R. D., *Cell Biology,* Allyn & Bacon, Inc., Boston 1974.
3. Novikoff, A. B. and Holtzman, E.: *Cells and Organelles,* 2nd Ed., Holt, Rinehart and Winston, New York 1976.

4

Cell Membranes

Membranes are boundary surfaces which divide and connect. In biology, membranes are barriers between morphological and functional units. They form a continuum with the interior of the cell and are not separated distinctly from it. Membranes are responsible for uptake of liquid and solid material, for extrusion of endogenous and waste material, and for permeation and transport mechanisms. Membranes are lipid in nature.

Table 4-1 presents the structure and function of membranes while Table 4-2 depicts their properties.

A schematic diagram of a membrane structure is given in Figure 4-1.

Although the unit membrane model helps in understanding some of the mechanisms involved in the transport of substances across the cell boundary, it is probably a gross oversimplification.

A modern concept is the *fluid mosaic model*. The fluid mosaic model views the membrane as being composed of a fluid (nonrigid) lipid matrix with which are associated relatively mobile protein masses (protein "icebergs" floating in an "oily sea"). The proteins may penetrate wholly or partially through the fluid lipid layer. Others are associated with either only the inside or the outside membrane surface. The protein may move in vertical or horizontal direction.

The lipid matrix is fluid because a considerable proportion of the fatty acid tails are unsaturated and the melting temperature for the bilayer is below normal body temperature.

All plasma membranes are similar in composition of lipids, proteins, and carbohydrates, the proportions of these components exhibiting considerable variation. For instance, the ratios of membrane proteins to phospholipids are 0.23, 0.83, 1.11, and 1.5 in the membranes of myelin, hepatocytes, erythrocytes, and leucocytes, respectively. Membrane lipids are classified into two groups: polar (phospholipids and glycolipids) and neutral (sterols and mono-, di-, and triglycerides).

Phospholipids, the major lipid components of all biological membranes, comprise a glycerol skeleton esterified by two chains of fatty acids, while the third alcohol group carries the polar group (phosphate, phosphatidylcholine, phosphatidylethanolamine, phospho-

Table 4-1. Structure and Function of Membranes

ANATOMY	COMPOSITION	FUNCTION	THICKNESS
Cell coat	Chondroitin sulfuric acid Hyaluronic acid Collagen Elastin Sialic acid	Principal component of connective tissue Adsorption of compounds	?
Cell membrane	Protein	Hydrophilic layer	20–25 Å
	Triglycerides Steroids (cholesterol) Phospholipids (lecithin)	Lipophilic layer, bimolecular (barrier)	25–35 Å
	Protein	Hydrophilic layer	20–25 Å

inositol, phosphatidylserine, and phosphoglycerol). Other phospholipids are derived from sphingosine (sphingomyelin), which is also the source of glycolipids and cerebrosides.

When placed in an aqueous medium, phospholipids spontaneously form double layers, orienting the polar groups outwards and their acyl chains inwards, the whole assembly being stabilized by hydrophobic (mainly Van der Waals) and hydrophilic forces (electrostatic bonds and hydrogen bridges). This structure is identical in cell membranes, but the phospholipids are distributed throughout in an asymmetric but nonabsolute manner.

The Singer-Nelson fluid mosaic model differs fundamentally from the simple lipid bilayer model (see Figure 4-1) in that there are no "unfolded" globular proteins spread all over the surface.

Table 4-2. Properties of Membranes

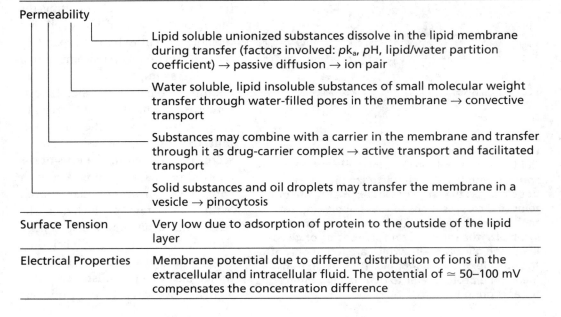

Permeability

— Lipid soluble unionized substances dissolve in the lipid membrane during transfer (factors involved: pk_a, pH, lipid/water partition coefficient) → passive diffusion → ion pair

— Water soluble, lipid insoluble substances of small molecular weight transfer through water-filled pores in the membrane → convective transport

— Substances may combine with a carrier in the membrane and transfer through it as drug-carrier complex → active transport and facilitated transport

— Solid substances and oil droplets may transfer the membrane in a vesicle → pinocytosis

Surface Tension	Very low due to adsorption of protein to the outside of the lipid layer
Electrical Properties	Membrane potential due to different distribution of ions in the extracellular and intracellular fluid. The potential of $\simeq$ 50–100 mV compensates the concentration difference

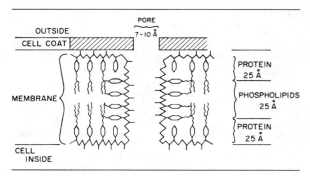

Figure 4-1. Schematic diagram of the membrane structure having a pore.

Later studies by Chapman confirmed and expanded the Singer-Nelson model to the *modified fluid mosaic* model, emphasizing several kinds of transmembrane protein structures for the intercalation and translocation across membranes. A recent emphasis is given to peripheral proteins which either form or interact with a two-dimensional filamentous network under the bilayer of the plasma membrane. This network gives structural integrity for the membrane and permits motility and morphological changes.

The modified Singer-Nelson fluid mosaic model is highly adaptable and not only applies to the plasma membrane, but also to other membranes, such as those of organelles.

A schematic diagram of the ultrastructure of the modified Singer-Nelson fluid mosaic membrane is given in Figure 4-2. It consists of a basic bimolecular lipid layer with protein molecules nested in it. Linear arrays constitute the hydrophobic region, globular structures present the hydrophilic region of the bilayer. Proteins are either spanning the entire bilayer or are only partially embedded. Carbohydrate chains are bound to lipids and proteins present on the surface. On the inner side are cytoplasmic, peripheral proteins, in part embedded within the lipid matrix. Within the proteins are areas containing hydrophilic amino acids which interact with and bind to lipids, thus anchoring these proteins within the membrane.

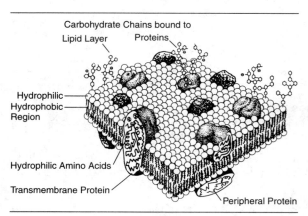

Figure 4-2. Schematic diagram of the modified fluid mosaic membrane model (Singer-Nelson). The spheres with the tails characterize the phospholipid double layer; the large bodies exemplify the proteins (the cross sections of these bodies indicate their internal structure); the hexagonal structures symbolize the carbohydrate side chains of glycolipids and glycoproteins which are found only at the outside of the membrane. The dots in transmembrane protein refer to hydrophilic amino acids for anchoring to lipids.

A membrane in common parlance in pharmacokinetics refers not only to the structure separating the media outside and inside a cell, but includes the entire barrier separating the two functional or anatomic units.

An example of a functional, anatomic barrier is the blood-cerebrospinal fluid (CSF) barriers to drug transport into the brain. As reflected by Figure 4-3, CSF is secreted by the epithelial cells of the choroid plexus which are in contact with the brain ventricular spaces. Within the brain parenchyma, the cells comprising the vascular endothelium are connected by occluding zonulae of "tight junctions." Thus, low molecular weight substances such as drugs delivered to the brain via the circulatory system cannot readily permeate the **blood-brain barrier** by translocation across intercellular channels (e.g., pores) between endothelial cells but rather must either passively diffuse or be actively transported across the cell. Thus, drugs whose physicochemical characteristics do not favor passive diffusion have limited access across the blood-brain barrier. In contrast, the CSF is separated from brain tissue by epithelial cells lining the ventricles (i.e., ependymal cells). These cells are not connected by occluding zonulae and hence the CSF-brain barrier is extremely permeable, offering unrestricted passage of drug molecules between the CSF and brain cells. This is especially true for drugs which can be directly delivered to the CSF (i.e., via intrathecal or intraventricular administration).

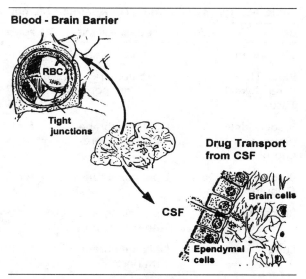

Figure 4-3. Schematic diagram of the blood-brain and blood-CSF barriers (adapted with permission from Seeman and Kalant, 1998).

In addition to physicochemical factors that alter drug transport across the blood-brain barrier, transport proteins can also influence drug disposition in the central nervous system. P-Glycoprotein (P-gp) is a 170 kDa membrane-bound protein that has been implicated as a primary cause of multidrug resistance in tumors, hence its initial designation as *mdr*. The responsible gene, MDR1, has recently been reclassified as part of the ABCB subfamily of the ATP-binding cassette transporters; in humans, it is polymorphically expressed with differences in activity between allelic variants. In addition to the brain, P-gp is found in the small intestine, liver, kidneys, and gonads where it functions as an ATP-dependent efflux transporter. Because of its predominant expression in the luminal membrane of brain endothelial cells, P-gp appears to have a greater impact on limiting cellular uptake of drugs from the circulation to the brain than enhancing the excretion of drugs out of neural cells. Therefore, when considering the pharmacokinetics of drug transport across the blood-brain barrier and/or penetration into the brain, it is important to consider the rate/extent of influx diffusion, the rate of P-gp efflux transport, and the nonspecific binding of drug to neural cells/tissues. The most common types of functional or anatomic membranes and their permeability characteristics are listed in Table 4-3.

Sorption Promoters or Permeation Enhancers

Sorption promoters or permeation enhancers are substances that have no pharmacological properties of their own in the amount/concentration used, but which can improve the penetration of drugs into the skin or mucosa, or their permeation through (across) skin or mucosa by reducing the barrier resistance. Sorption promotion applies to passive transport by simple diffusion (through lipid layer), aqueous channel diffusion, or facilitated diffusion involving carrier mediated transport proteins.

Table 4-3. Types of Functional or Anatomic Membranes and Their Permeability for Drugs

ORGAN	TYPE OF MEMBRANE	PERMEABILITY
Blood/Brain	Lipid membrane	for lipophilic drugs only
Blood/Liver Parenchymal Tissue	Lipid membrane with large pores	for both lipophilic and hydrophilic drugs
Blood/Kidney (Bowman's Capsule)	Lipid membrane with large pores	for both lipophilic and hydrophilic drugs
Blood/Kidney (Tubuli)	Lipid membrane	for lipophilic drugs only
Blood/Placenta	Lipid membrane with many pores	for both lipophilic and hydrophilic drugs
Lung	Lipid membrane with pores	for both lipophilic and hydrophilic drugs
Stomach	Lipid membrane with few pores	for lipophilic, nonionized acidic drugs, less for small molecular size nonelectrolytes
Small Intestine	Lipid membrane with few pores	for lipophilic drugs (acidic and basic), less for hydrophilic drugs

The application of absorption enhancers is one of the few possibilities left to increase the absorption of unchanged drug before turning to the chemical derivatization of original compounds. Various compounds may be used to enhance absorption of drugs via the trans- and/or para-cellular route. Various mechanisms have been proposed for the action of absorption enhancers, some of which are listed below:

- Increased membrane fluidity;
- Reduced glutathione levels in the cell;
- Inhibition of cyclooxygenase;
- Binding of mucosal Ca^{+2};
- Binding of intracellular Ca^{+2};
- Surfactant action;
- Antagonism of calmodulin-dependent processes; and
- Alterations of the action of protein-kinase C.

Generally, the application of absorption enhancers has been limited to medications administered by the transdermal (e.g., azone and derivatives, DMSO) and rectal routes. Very potent enhancers (e.g., acylcarnitine, sodium taurodihydrofusidate) have

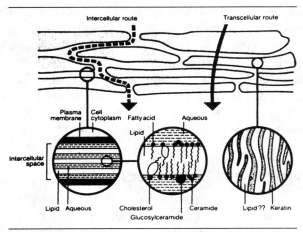

Figure 4-4. Schematic diagram of the stratum corneum and the intercellular and transcellular pathway for penetration/permeation (With permission of author and publisher).

been applied to enhance the intranasal absorption of peptides (e.g., arginine vasopressin, growth hormone releasing peptide). Finally, physical procedures (e.g., iontophoresis) have been used to enhance the systemic absorption of several drugs (e.g., peptides, corticosteroids) as it can enhance the dermal translocation of ionic compounds into the capillary circulation of the epidermis.

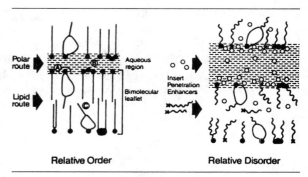

Figure 4-5. Schematic diagram of mechanism of sorption promotion for the intercellular route by creating a relative disorder in the polar or lipid layers (or both) of the intercellular matrix (With permission of author and publisher).

The penetration/permeation of skin according to the postulate of Elias is either by the intercellular or the transcellular route as shown in Figure 4-4. The intercellular matrix is formed by alternate layers of lipid and aqueous material. The intercellular pathway seems to be the one most affected by sorption promoters. Sorption promoters disturb the relative order of either the lipid or aqueous layers, or both, resulting in either expansion of the layer(s), reduction in viscosity (increasing in fluidity), or chelating of matrix groups. A schematic view of sorption promoter action is given in Figure 4-5.

Selected References

1. Barry, B. W.: *Dermatological Formulations: Percutaneous Absorption,* Marcel Dekker, New York, NY, 1983.

2. Barry, B. W.: Penetration Enhancers. In: *Skin Pharmacokinetics.* B. Shroot and H. Schaefer, Editors, S. Karger, Basel, Switzerland, 1987, pp. 121–137.

3. Brown, F. and Danielli, J. F.: In: Bourne, G. H., Editor, *Cytology and Cell Physiology,* 3rd Ed. Academic Press, New York, 1964, p. 239.

4. Bungenberg de Jong, H. G. and Bonner, J.: Phosphatide Autocomplex Coacervates as Ionic Systems and Their Relation to the Protoplasmic Membrane, *Proc. Acad. Sci., Amsterdam, 38*:797 (1935).

5. Capaldi, R. A.: A Dynamic Model of Cell Membranes, *Sci. Am. 230*:27 (1974).

6. Chapman, D.: Biomembrane Structure and Function: Recent Studies and New Techniques, *Parasitology 96*(Suppl): 11 (1988).

7. Davson, H. and Danielli, J. F.: *The Permeability of Natural Membranes,* Cambridge University Press, 1952, p. 64.

8. de Boer, A. G., van Hoogdalem, E. J. and Breimer, D. D.: Improvement of Drug Absorption Through Enhancers, *Eur. J. Drug Metab. Pharmacokinet. 15*:155–157 (1990).

9. Deleers, M. and El Tamer, A.: Role and Function of Membrane Phospholipids, *Essentialia Ucb 17(2)*:11–16 (1988).

10. Elias, P. M.: Lipids and the Epidermal Permeability Barrier, *Arch. Dermatol. Res. 270*:95–117 (1981).

11. Fox, C. F.: The Structure of Cell Membranes, *Sci. Am. 226*:31 (1972).

12. Hober, R.: *Physical Chemistry of Cells and Tissues,* The Blakiston Company, Philadelphia 1945, pp. 1–676.

13. Kim, R. B.: MDRI Single Nucleotide Polymorphisms: Multiplicity of Haplotypes and Functional Consequences. *Pharmacogenetics 12*:425–427 (2002).

14. Lin, J. H. and Yamazaki, M.: Role of P-Glycoprotein in Pharmacokinetics: Clinical Implications. *Clin. Pharmacokinet. 42*:59–98 (2003).

15. Nicolson, G. L.: Transmembrane Control of the Receptors of Normal and Tumor Cells. I. Cytoplasmic Influence on Cell Surface Components, *Biochim. Biophys. Acta 57*:37 (1976).

16. Ritschel, W. A. and Sprockel, O. L.: Sorption Promoters for Topically Applied Substances, *Drugs of Today* 24:613–628 (1988).

17. Robertson, D. J. and Locke, M.: *Cellular Membrane in Development I,* Academic Press, New York, N.Y. 1964.

18. Robertson, D. J.: The Membrane of the Living Cell, *Sci. Am. 206*:4 (1962).

19. Seeman, P. and Kalant, H.: Drug Solubility, Absorption and Movement Across Body Membranes, In *Principles of Medical Pharmacology,* 6th Ed., Kalant, H. and Roschlau, W. H. (editors), Oxford University Press, New York, N.Y., pp. 11–27, (1998).

20. Singer, S. J. and Nicolson, G. L.: The Fluid Mosaic Model of the Structure of Cell Membranes, *Science 175*:720 (1972).

5

Drug-Receptor Interactions

Structural Nonspecific Drugs are those in which the pharmacological action is not directly dependent on the chemical structure of the drug, except that structure affects physicochemical properties. Structural nonspecific drugs act by physicochemical processes.

The pharmacologic action depends directly on thermodynamic activity, which is high in most of the cases (large doses needed).

The chemical structure may be very much different, yet the pharmacological actions are similar.

A slight modification in chemical structure does not produce a dramatic change in pharmacological action.

Structural Specific Drugs are those in which the pharmacological action depends directly on the chemical structure of the drug, which attaches itself to a three-dimensional structure of a receptor in the biophase. Prerequisites of the binding of a drug to a receptor are: chemical reactivity, presence of functional groups, electronic distribution, and topographic mirror-like image of the receptor.

The pharmacologic action is not solely dependent on thermodynamic activity, which is low in most cases (small doses needed).

Drugs of similar pharmacological action have usually some common structural characteristics with functional groups in similar spatial direction.

A slight modification in chemical structure may produce dramatic change in pharmacological action (from increased activity to antagonism).

Receptors are all specific molecules, molecule-complexes, or parts of these, which bind the drug chemically, and this complex exerts a pharmacological action.

Drug-Receptor Interactions in the biophase may initiate responses by altering the permeability of membranes, by interfering with transport mechanisms, by modifying templates, or by acting on enzymes.

At present day, there are particularly two receptor types of importance: enzyme-linked receptors (e.g., insulin, epidermal growth factor, platelet-derived growth factor) and channel-linked receptors (e.g., nicotinic, $5HT_3$, NMDA, GABA).

Enzyme-Linked Receptors mediate signals from a group of endogenous compounds. A hormone or drug, the *first messenger,* binds to the cell via a receptor. The occupied receptor activates a translation unit, the *transducer.* This protein is called a *G-protein* because it may also bind guanosine triphosphate (GTP) which, in turn, activates *adenylate cyclase.* This enzyme produces a new cyclic nucleotide from ATP intracellularly, cyclic adenosine monophosphate (c-AMP), which acts as the second messenger and is responsible for the induction of hormonal action within the cell. In the cell wall there are both stimulatory and inhibitory receptors, each having separate G-proteins (G_i or G_s) capable of modulating activity. Currently, four families of mammalian G-proteins are known (i.e., G_s, G_i, G_q, and G_{12}) and collectively represent a total of 15 different G-proteins. The family of G-proteins that transduce signals from membrane receptors to effector enzymes and ion channels are known as the heterotrimeric G-proteins. Each of these proteins is composed of three distinct subunits, termed α, β, and γ in order of decreasing molecular weight. The α subunit of the trimer binds guanine nucleotides and is the major mediator of the G-protein's actions on its effector. Table 5-1 provides examples of several drugs whose action is modulated by G-protein-coupled adenylate cyclase receptors.

Channel-Linked Receptors are more complicated in their structure than enzyme-linked receptors. For example, the nicotinic acetylcholine receptor is activated only if both α subunits are occupied by acetylcholine. Consequently, the membrane channel opens for 1 to 2 milliseconds enabling the rapid influx of approximately 6000 sodium ions per millisecond for drugs such as muscle relaxants. The muscarinic acetylcholine receptor opens the channel for the flux of potassium ions (for parasympathomimetic drugs). Other receptors (e.g., voltage dependent calcium channels) contain compound-specific binding sites which regulate the transmembrane flux of calcium ions upon interaction with certain drugs (e.g., calcium channel blockers such as nifedipine, diltiazem, verapamil). Finally, the benzodiazepine class of sedative, anxiolytic agents exerts pharmacologic activity via a chloride channel utilizing the inhibitory neurotransmitter, GABA.

Effect of Drugs on Receptors

Drugs that act on a specific receptor can be classified by their effect on the receptor. *Agonists* are drugs or chemicals that mimic the effect of the endogenous ligands

Table 5-1. Examples of Drugs Whose Action is Modulated by Adenylate Cyclase-Linked Receptors

LINKAGE	RECEPTORS	AGONISTS	ANTAGONISTS
Stimulation	β	Fenoterol	Propranolol
	H_2	Histamine	Cimetidine
Inhibition	α_2	Clonidine	Yohimbine
	Dopamine	Levodopa	Haloperidol
	Opioid	Morphine	Naloxone

and evoke a response when bound to the receptor (e.g., morphine). Agonists are generally classified as *full agonists* (i.e., able to elicit a maximal response) or *partial agonists* (i.e., those that cannot elicit maximal response even at high concentrations). The efficacy of a drug should not be confused with *potency* which is the relationship between the concentration of the drug and its ability to elicit an effect. Inhibition of the actions of endogenous ligands is frequently produced with the administration of antagonists. *Antagonists* bind to the receptor but do not activate it. Thus they do not elicit a response but rather block the response elicited by endogenous agonists (e.g., naloxone, antihistamines). In some instances where a compound can interact with multiple types of receptors, it can serve as both an antagonist and a partial agonist (e.g., nalbuphine).

Drug-Receptor Theories

Hypothesis of Clark. The pharmacological effect depends on the percentage of receptors occupied. The drug must have affinity for the receptor. If all receptors are occupied maximum effect is obtained. Chemical binding follows law of mass action. (See Figure 5-1.)

Hypothesis of Ariëns and Stephenson. In addition to affinity, another constant, "intrinsic activity" or "efficacy," must be present. There are many homologous substances which have various degrees of affinity for the receptor. Yet some possess high effectiveness, some have low effectiveness, and others are not effective. Still, the ineffective substance may block or inhibit the receptor. Effectiveness lasts as long as the receptor is occupied. **(Occupation Theory).**

Hypothesis of Paton. Effectiveness does not depend upon actual occupation of the receptor by the drug, but upon obtaining the proper stimulus only. The stimulus occurs at the moment the drug attaches itself to the receptor. This is known also as the **Rate Theory.**

Lock and Key Hypothesis. The drug molecule must "fit into a receptor" like a "key fits into a lock" (intrinsic activity). (See Figure 5-2.)

Affinity is the combination of drug molecule with a receptor. If a drug has affinity and generates an impulse which activates the biologi-

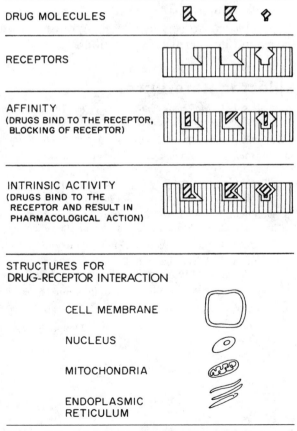

Figure 5-1. Schematic, simplified view of drug-receptor interaction.

AFFINITY

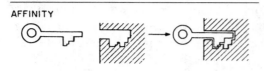

THE KEY FITS INTO THE LOCK, HOWEVER THE KEY DOES NOT UNLOCK IT. THE KEY (DRUG) HAS AFFINITY FOR THE LOCK (RECEPTOR).

AFFINITY AND INTRINSIC ACTIVITY

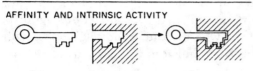

THE KEY FITS INTO THE LOCK AND UNLOCKS IT. THE KEY (DRUG) HAS AFFINITY FOR THE LOCK (RECEPTOR) AND INTRINSIC ACTIVITY.

Figure 5-2. Characterization of "lock and key" hypothesis for drug-receptor interaction.

cal effector system, the drug has intrinsic activity.

If a drug has affinity, but does not have intrinsic activity and does not result in pharmacologic response, the drug *inhibits* the system (antagonism).

Types of Antagonism

Chemical Antagonism. Interaction of drug (agonist) with another chemical (antagonist) outside of receptor to form an inactive complex.

Competitive Antagonism. Drug (agonist) is displaced from drug-receptor binding by another chemical (antagonist). Competitive antagonism is reversible and depends on actual drug and antagonist concentration in the biophase (**law of mass action**).

Partial Antagonism. Antagonist has high affinity but low intrinsic activity.

Nonequilibrium Antagonism. Antagonist forms irreversible receptor binding.

Noncompetitive Antagonism. Agonist and antagonist bind to different receptors and have opposite pharmacologic actions.

Selected References

1. Ariëns, E. J.: *Molecular Pharmacology; The Mode of Action of Biologically Active Compounds,* Academic Press, New York, Vol. 1, 1979.

2. Ariëns, E. J.: Receptors: From Fiction to Fact, *Trends in Pharmacol. Sci. 1*:11–15 (1979).

3. Bourne, H. R., Sanders, D. A. and McCormick, F.: The GTPase Superfamily: Conserved Structure and Molecular Mechanism, *Nature 349*:117–127 (1991).

4. Clark, A. J.: In Heffter, A. and Heubner, H., editors: *Handbuch der Experimentellen Pharmakologie,* Springer Verlag, Vienna, Vol. 4, 1937.

5. Dohlman, H. G., Thorner, J., Caron, M. G. and Lefkowitz, R. J.: Model Systems for the Study of Seven Transmembrane Segment Receptors, *Ann. Rev. Biochem. 60*:653–688 (1991).

6. Hulme, E. C. (ed.): Receptor-Ligand Interactions: A Practical Approach, IRL Press, Oxford (1990).

7. Paton, W. D. M.: A Theory of Drug Action Based on the Rate of Drug-Receptor Combinations, *Proc. R. Soc. Med. 154*:21 (1961).

8. Stephenson, R. P.: A Modification of Receptor Theory, *Br. J. Pharmacol. 11*:379 (1956).

9. Tang, W. J. and Gilman A. G.: Adenylyl Cyclases, *Cell 70*:869–872 (1992).

10. Unwin, N.: Neurotransmitter Action: Opening of Ligand-Gated Ion Channels, *Neuron 10*(Suppl):31–41 (1993).

6
Absorption/Transport Mechanisms

The predominant route of administration is extravascular, such as orally, perorally, intramuscularly, subcutaneously, intrathecally, intradermally, rectally, or topically. In all these cases the drug must be absorbed in order to enter the systemic circulation. At times, drugs are introduced directly into the circulation. This is the case with IV injection, IV infusions, and intracardial injections (intravascular route of administration).

A prerequisite of absorption is that the drug be released from the dosage form. Drug release or liberation depends on physicochemical factors of the drug, of the dosage form, and of the environment in the human (or animal) body at the site of administration or absorption. Formulation of the dosage form (pharmacotechnical factors) is the most important factor in obtaining proper drug release.

A released drug, however, is not necessarily absorbed. If the drug molecule is bound to the surface of the skin or mucosa by ion-binding, hydrogen-binding, or van der Waals forces, we call it **adsorption.** If the drug reaches deeper layers of the skin, yet does not reach blood capillaries, we call it **penetration.** Only if the drug permeates through the capillary walls and enters the bloodstream, do we call it **absorption.**

The two terms—penetration and permeation—comprise the collective term *sorption.*

A prerequisite for absorption is that the drug must be present in aqueous (true) solution at the absorption site. This is valid for all mechanisms of absorption but one, pinocytosis.

In the lumen of the gastrointestinal tract, for example, more than one membrane must be permeated before a drug molecule passes from the outside into a capillary; however, only the rate of permeating through the epithelium cells seems to be rate-controlling. Other factors are definitely the vascularity and the rate of blood flow at the absorption site. This is usually true following oral, peroral, rectal, and topical administration.

The mechanisms of absorption of drugs are, in order of their importance: (1) passive diffusion, (2) convective transport, (3) active transport, (4) facilitated transport, (5) ion-pair transport, and (6) endocytosis (pinocytosis).

Among the active transporters are the ion pumps (P-gp) for both influx and efflux processes across a number of tissues, such as intestine, kidney, liver, and central nervous system. Secondary active transporters use voltage and ion gradients generated by the primary active transporters. Among the facilitative transporters are organic anion transporting polypeptides (OATP) which operate energy independent and do not require ATP for energy production.

The mechanisms described here for absorption of drugs are unequivocally applicable to the transport within the body and are responsible for distribution of drug within the body such as leaving the capillaries and entering interstitial space, entering cells, permeating tissue, crossing the blood/brain barrier, entering the hepatocyte, entering bile, crossing the urinary tubular endothelium, etc.

Typical Absorption Profiles

Peroral absorption is a complex process since the various segments of the gastrointestinal tract differ in histology, anatomy, physiology, secretion, tonus, movement, sphincter activity, etc.

First-Order Absorption is the most widely found process of peroral drug uptake. The absorption rate constant k_a can easily be determined by employing simple compartmental modeling and analysis. In most cases, input (absorption) is much faster than output (elimination), i.e., $k_a \gg k_{el}$. However, there are cases when $k_a < k_{el}$, which is termed the "flip-flop" model.

Zero-Order Absorption is found with some drugs such as ethanol, erythromycin, griseofulvin, and sulfisoxazole and for drugs with modified (zero-order) release characteristics.

Atypical Absorption Profiles

Some drugs show double or multiple peaks because of parallel absorption either by different processes or different speed from different segments. Such drugs are said to have *Parallel First-Order Absorption. Mixed Zero-/First-Order Absorption* refers to processes that simultaneously exhibit first- and zero-order kinetics.

An *Absorption Window* refers to an uptake of drug from a limited portion of the gastrointestinal tract such as from the stomach only, stomach and duodenum, or small intestine.

Absorbing Surface Area

Topical absorption is limited due to the anatomical structure of the skin. The skin is much less permeable than mucosa (lining of mouth and nose cavity, gastrointestinal tract, rectum, lung). Moreover, the surface area of the skin is only 1.73 m^2 (Caucasian adult) whereas the absorbing surface area of the lung is about 70 m^2. The large surface area of about 120–200 m^2 of the gastrointestinal tract is due to the presence of macrovilli and microvilli in the small intestine (see Figure 6-1).

Passive Diffusion

Passive diffusion is transport through a semipermeable membrane. The drug must be in aqueous (true) solution at the absorption site. In passing through the membrane, the drug

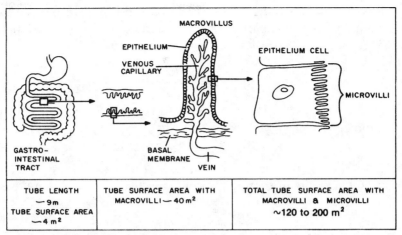

Figure 6-1. Anatomical explanation for magnitude of intestinal surface area.

molecule dissolves in the lipid material of the membrane according to its lipid solubility and lipid/water partition coefficient. The drug molecule then leaves the lipid membrane and dissolves again in an aqueous medium, this time at the inside of the membrane according to the concentration gradient. Since ions usually have no lipid solubility they cannot permeate. However, most drugs are electrolytes, either weak acids or weak bases. The unionized moiety is usually lipid soluble. Therefore, the pK_a of the drug and the pH at the absorption site will determine the degree of drug being unionized and absorbable. Passive diffusion follows Fick's first law of diffusion and absorption should, therefore, proceed until equilibrium is obtained on both sides of the membrane. *In situ* we do not obtain equilibrium, since the drug which permeates through the membrane is carried away by the bloodstream, thus maintaining the concentration gradient, and the drug can be more or less quantitatively absorbed.

As seen from Figure 6-2 the transport stream of the drug from the outside compartment through the membrane to the inside compartment can be quantified according to Equation 6.1:

$$q = -D \cdot \frac{A}{h} \cdot K \cdot (C_o - C_i) \qquad (1)$$

A = surface area

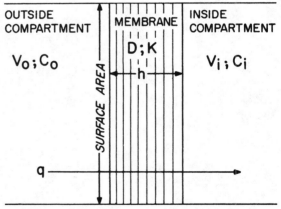

Figure 6-2. Schematic diagram characterizing transport of a drug in solution across a membrane by passive diffusion.
V_o = volume of outside compartment
V_i = volume of inside compartment
C_o = drug concentration in outside compartment
C_i = drug concentration in inside compartment
D = diffusion constant of drug in lipid material
K = partition coefficient
h = membrane thickness
q = transport stream [mass of solute diffused per unit time across the membrane]

Under the assumption that the transport is unidirectional since the drug is constantly carried away from the inside compartment, thus maintaining the concentration gradient, one can use Fick's first law of diffusion, as given in Equation 6.2:

$$dq = -D \cdot A \cdot \frac{dc}{dx} \cdot dt \tag{2}$$

$\dfrac{dc}{dx}$ = concentration gradient

Since $C_o \gg C_i$, the latter one can be assumed zero. By combining D, A, h, and K to give a new constant k, the first-order permeation rate constant, we obtain Equation 6.3:

$$\frac{dC_o}{dt} = -k \cdot C_o \tag{3}$$

$\dfrac{dC_o}{dt}$ = concentration of drug diffusing from the outside compartment to the inside compartment per unit time

C_o = concentration in outside compartment

k = permeation rate constant

After integration with the limits of drug concentration C_o^0 at time t_o (at the beginning) and C_o at time t (any later time) and logarithmic transformation of ln in log we obtain the permeation rate constant k (Equations 6.4–6.8):

$$\int_{C_o^0}^{C_o} \frac{dC_o}{\pi C_o^0} = -k \cdot \int_{t_o}^{t} dt \tag{4}$$

$$\ln C_o - \ln C_o^0 = -k \cdot (t - t_o) \tag{5}$$

$$\ln C_o - \ln C_o^0 = -k \cdot t \tag{6}$$

$$\log C_o - \log C_o^0 = -\frac{k \cdot t}{2.303} \tag{7}$$

$$k = \frac{2.303}{t} \cdot \log \frac{C_o^0}{C_o} \tag{8}$$

The characteristics of passive diffusion and examples of drugs transported by passive diffusion are summarized in Table 6-1.

Convective Transport

In convective transport, drug molecules dissolved in the aqueous medium at the absorption site move along with the solvent (shifting of solvent) through the pore. Ions (if they have the opposite charge of the pore lining), as well as neutral molecules, may pass through the pore. Since the cylindrical water-filled pores have a diameter of 7–10 Å, only molecules

Table 6-1. Absorption Mechanisms

ABSORPTION MECHANISM	CHARACTERISTICS	EXAMPLES
Passive Diffusion	pk_a of substance Lipid/water partition coefficient pH outside and inside of membrane Concentration gradient Surface area and membrane thickness Diffusion coefficient	Weak organic acids; Weak organic bases; Organic nonelectrolytes: alcohol, urea, amidopyrine; Cardiac glycosides in part
Convective Absorption	Pore diameter $\simeq 7$ Å Shifting of solvent Hydrostatic pressure difference Surface area and membrane thickness Number of pores Specific resistance (viscosity) Electrical charge	Inorganic and organic electrolytes up to 150 to 400 MW; Ions of opposite charge of pore lining; Ionized sulfonamides
Active Transport	Carrier Against concentration gradient Against electrochemical potential Saturation of transport Specificity Competitive inhibition Poisoning of carrier	Na^+, K^+, I^-, hexoses, monosaccharides, amino acids, strong organic acids and bases (phenol red), organic phosphates Cardiac glycosides, Pyrimidine bases, B-vitamins, testosterone estradiol, 5-fluorouracil, Fe^{++}, Ca^{++} P-gp: See Table 6-2
Facilitated Transport	Carrier Specificity Competitive inhibition Poisoning of carrier Saturation of transport With concentration gradient	Vitamin B_{11} OATP: Fexofenadine, fluoroquinolones (some), nonsteroidal antiinflammatory drugs, statins OCTP: Epinephrine, choline, dopamine, guanidine, antiarrhythmics, some antihistamines
Ion Pair	Complex of organic anion of substance with cation of medium or membrane	Quaternary ammonium compounds, Sulfonic acids
Endocytosis/ Pinocytosis	Engulfing vesicles	Fats, glycerin, starch, Parasite eggs, Vitamins A, D, E, and K, Plastic particles, hairs and yeast cells; Ferritin and insulin

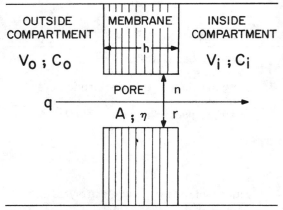

Figure 6-3. Schematic diagram characterizing transfer of a drug in solution across a membrane by the process of convective transport.
V_o = volume of outside compartment
V_i = volume of inside compartment
C_o = drug concentration in outside compartment
C_i = drug concentration in inside compartment
n = number of pores
h = thickness of membrane
r = radius of pore
A = surface area of pore
η = viscosity of fluid in pore
q = transport stream [mass of solute diffusing per unit time across the membrane]

with smaller diameters can pass. In general, spherical compounds up to a molecular weight of 150 and chain-like compounds up to a molecular weight of 400 have been found to be absorbed by convective transport.

As seen from Figure 6-3, the transport stream of the drug from the outside compartment through the water-filled pores to the inside compartment can be quantified according to Equation 6.9 by diffusion:

$$q = D' \cdot \frac{n \cdot r^2 \cdot A}{h} \cdot (C_o - C_i) \qquad (9)$$

where D' is mobility of drug in solution, or by bulk flow, expressed by Equation 6.10:

$$q = \frac{n \cdot r^4 \cdot \pi}{8\eta} \cdot \Delta p \cdot C \qquad (10)$$

where $\Delta p \cdot C$ characterizes both a hydrostatic pressure and a concentration gradient.

In the case of electrically charged pore lining for the absorption of ions a modified model, as given in Figure 6-4, can be used.

The characteristics of convective transport are summarized in Table 6-1.

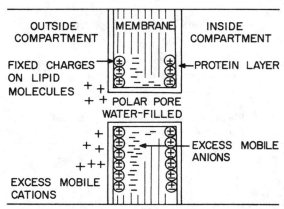

Figure 6-4. Schematic diagram characterizing transfer of small ions across a membrane by convective transport.

Active Transport

For active transport, the drug molecule must be in aqueous solution at the absorption site. The transport is mediated by means of carriers under expenditure of energy (utilization of ATP). Each drug or group of drugs needs a specific carrier. The binding of a drug molecule to the carrier follows the drug-receptor theory. Drugs with higher affinity to the carrier displace drugs of lower affinity from the carrier (competitive inhibition). The carriers seem to be enzymes or at least proteinaceous material.

Substances which interfere with cell metabolism (CN^-, F^-, iodine acetate) inhibit the active transport noncompetitively. Absorption proceeds against a concentration gradient and, in the case of ions, against an electrochemical potential. The active transport becomes saturated if there are more drug molecules present than carriers available. The carriers are located on the external surface of the membrane. They form a complex with the drug molecule which moves across the membrane utilizing energy provided by ATP. At the inside of the membrane, the drug molecule dissociates from the carrier and the carrier

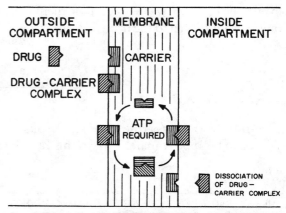

Figure 6-5. Schematic diagram characterizing transport of a drug in solution across a membrane by active transport.

returns to the outside of the membrane. A schematic drawing of active transport is given in Figure 6-5.

A special type of active transport is the so-called sodium pump, which does not use a carrier but a wave of electrons and the actual transport occurs through a pore as seen in Figure 6-6.

ATP is broken down in the membrane by the enzyme ATPase into ADP and phosphate ion releasing 3 electronegative charges per molecule of ATP. The electrons travel along the inner membrane surface to the pore and to the outer membrane surface. Each wave consisting of 3 electrons lets 3 Na^+ travel through the pore simultaneously. Then, the K^+ ions, having a smaller diameter than the Na^+ in the hydrated form, do pass through the pores into the cell.

To quantify the absorption process by active transport, enzyme kinetics is used in the form of a modified Michaelis-Menten Equation 6.11.

$$-\frac{dc}{dt} = \frac{\frac{dc}{dt}max \cdot [S]}{K_c + [S]} \qquad (11)$$

dc/dt = rate of absorption
dc/dt max = maximal rate of absorption at high drug concentration
[S] = drug concentration
K_c = affinity constant of the drug for the carrier

If $K_c >>> [S]$, then $K_c + [S]$ can be considered as K_c. Since $\frac{dc}{dt}$ max and K_c are constant for a given defined substrate

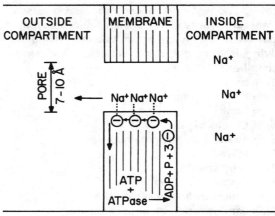

Figure 6-6. Schematic diagram of the "sodium pump" (active transport of ions through a pore).

in enzyme reaction, we may combine them to a new constant K. In this case the absorption rate is proportional to the drug concentration as seen in Equation 6.12.

$$-\frac{dc}{dt} = \frac{\frac{dc}{dt}\max \cdot [S]}{K_c} = K \cdot [S] \tag{12}$$

If $[S] >>> K_c$, as is the case in high substrate concentration, then $K_c + [S]$ can be considered to be approximately $[S]$. In this case the absorption proceeds at constant speed.

Active transport occurs unidirectional across the membrane. In the case of the intestine it proceeds from the mucosa to the serosa side. For testing of active transport the guinea pig ileum sac and the everted guinea pig ileum sac (Wilson-Wiseman test) are used. The normal ileum bag tied on both sides and filled with a drug solution is immersed into an oxygenated, thermostatically controlled Ringer's solution. In the case of passive diffusion, the drug will diffuse into the outside liquid (C_s = concentration at serosa side) until equilibrium is obtained. In the case of active transport, more or less all of the drug will be transported to the outside solution. If the everted ileum bag is used (serosa is inside, mucosa is outside), passive diffusion will commence as before; however, the drug transported by active transport will stay in the bag. A schematic diagram of the procedure and the differentiation curves between passive diffusion and active transport are given in Figure 6-7.

The characteristics of active transport are summarized in Table 6-1, with examples.

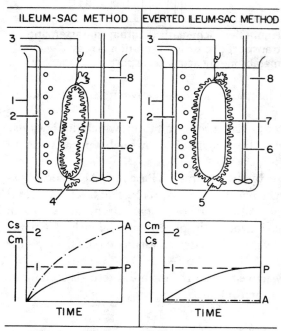

Figure 6-7. Schematic diagram of experimental set-up and resulting concentration ratio versus time curve for testing transport mechanism by passive diffusion and active transport using the living, isolated guinea pig ileum in a perfusion chamber.
1 = beaker
2 = oxygen supply
3 = hook
4 = Guinea pig ileum sac
5 = everted Guinea pig ileum sac
6 = stirrer
7 = drug solution
8 = Ringer's solution
C_s = concentration at serosa side
C_m = concentration at mucosa side
P = passive diffusion
A = active transport

Facilitated Transport

For facilitated transport, drug molecules must be in aqueous solution at the absorption site. In principle, the mechanism is the same as for active transport with the only difference that the transport does *not* proceed against a concentration gradient.

For this reason facilitated transport is sometimes considered as a subgroup of active transport.

The classical example of facilitated transport is the absorption of vitamin B_{12}. The vitamin B_{12} molecules form a complex with the intrinsic factor produced by the stomach wall. The B_{12}-intrinsic factor complex then combines with a carrier for transport, as seen in Figure 6-8.

Up to approximately 1.5 µg of vitamin B_{12} are absorbed by facilitated transport. If relatively large amounts of vitamin B_{12} are present in the intestine (>3000 µg), passive diffusion also seems to occur. Through this mechanism about 0.1 percent of the drug is absorbed.

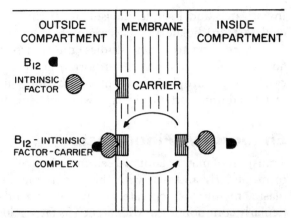

Figure 6-8. Schematic diagram characterizing transfer of a drug in solution across a membrane by facilitated transport.

Also, other carrier mechanisms may be considered as facilitated transport such as lipophilic counterions in presence of a pH or alkali ion gradient (see also under Ion-Pair Transport).

The characteristics of facilitated transport are summarized in Table 6-1.

Ion-Pair Transport

The absorption of some highly ionized compounds at physiological pH cannot be explained by simple or passive diffusion or any other existing hypothesis of absorption. Higuchi found that some highly ionized compounds, such as quaternary ammonium compounds and sulfonic acids, form electrochemically neutral complexes with cations. It is assumed that these drugs form ion-pairs with endogenous substances of the gastrointestinal tract, such as mucin, and that these neutral ion-pair complexes are then absorbed by passive diffusion, since the complex is water soluble as well as lipid soluble. A schematic diagram of ion-pair absorption is given in Figure 6-9. Characteristics of ion-pair absorption and examples are listed in Table 6-1.

Drugs for which ion-pair transport has been shown *in vivo* and *in vitro* include ampicillin, atenolol, bretylium bromide, chloramphenicol succinate, doxorubicin, metoprolol tartrate, oxprenolol HCl, pholedrine sulfate, propranolol HCl, quinine HCl, timolol maleate, and tropsium HCl. Counterions, other than endogenous substances, have been

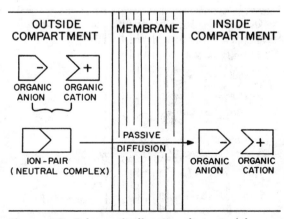

Figure 6-9. Schematic diagram characterizing transfer of a drug in solution across a membrane by ion-pair transport.

investigated and include alkylsulfate, trichloracetate, alkylcarboxylates, cholate, deoxycholate, taurocholate, hexylsalicylate, etc.

According to recent studies, the transport of ion pairs across lipid membranes appears to follow a specific transport mechanism, with the lipophilic counterions acting as carriers for hydrophilic molecules. Thus, ion-pair transport can be considered as a type of facilitated transport, particularly when pH and alkali ion gradients are established.

Endocytosis-Pinocytosis

Transport of material out of a cell and into a cell involving vesicles which are either formed intracellularly and fuse with the plasma membrane (exocytosis) or are formed by the plasma membrane, separate, and fuse intracellularly with lysosomes (endocytosis) is particularly common for nutrients such as fatty acids, fats, amino acids, peptides, hormones, proteins, and the oil soluble vitamins A, D, E, and K. Also particulate matter such as parasite eggs, starch, plastic particles, etc., may enter systemic circulation by this route. A schematic diagram is given in Figure 6-10.

In exocytosis which is a ubiquitous cell function to transport material out of a cell, cytoplasmic vesicles or granules fuse with the plasma membrane. Two pathways have been postulated: constitutive and regulated exocytosis. Constitutive exocytosis is independent of extracellular stimuli and proceeds at a steady rate. It supplies the plasma membrane with proteins for insertion and facilitates secretion of the extracellular matrix component. Regulated exocytosis is triggered by extracellular stimuli and is responsible for secretion of hormones, neurotransmitters, digestive enzymes, etc., and the insertion of membrane transport proteins.

Endocytosis is the uptake of extracellular material, exogenous molecules, or macromolecules into a cell by invagination of the plasmalemma and vesicle formation. Endocytosis is subdivided into phagocytosis (cell eating) to describe internalization of particulate matter visible under the light microscope and pinocytosis (cell drinking) to describe uptake of very small solid particles (not visible under the light microscope), solutes, and fluid. The vesicles internally fuse with lysosomes releasing the entrapped content.

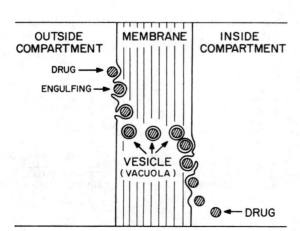

Figure 6-10. **Schematic diagram characterizing transfer of particulate matter or oil droplets across a membrane by endocytosis.**

A special type of endocytosis is the *Receptor-Mediated Endocytosis,* where the cells synthesize receptors which have an important function in the plasma membrane to recognize, concentrate, and internalize substances by endocytosis. More than 25 different macromolecules or complexes thereof are taken up by this mechanism. They include insulin, α_2-macroglobulin, epidermal growth factor, melanocyte stimulating hormone, luteinizing hormone, prolactin, interferon, thyroid hormones, transferrin, polymeric IgA, maternal IgG, lysosomal enzymes, glycoproteins, toxins, and viruses. A schematic diagram of phagocytosis, pinocytosis, and receptor-mediated endocytosis is given in Figure 6-11.

Endo- and exocytosis are apparently closely related to membrane fluidity, loci of amphiphilic lipids (phospholipids, glycolipids), where fusion or vesiculation occurs. Membrane fluidity can be modulated by physical means (temperature, pressure, membrane potential, pH), chemical means (chain length, polarity, unsaturation, proteins, detergents, fatty acids), hormones, metabolic processes, neoplasia, etc.

Endocytosis is the only transport mechanism in which a drug or compound does not have to be in aqueous solution in order to be absorbed. In case of absorption of small oil or fat droplets and of solid particles, pinocytosis is also referred to as corpuscular or particulate absorption.

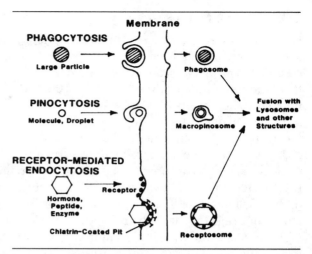

Figure 6-11. Schematic diagram of endocytosis by phagocytosis, forming a phagosome, pinocytosis, forming a macropinosome, and receptor-mediated endocytosis, forming a receptosome, all of which fuse intracellularly with structures, usually lysosomes.

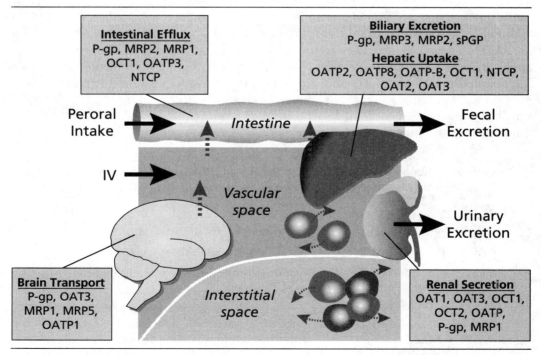

Figure 6-12. Schematic diagram of important human transport proteins and their known locations in humans. Spheres correspond to drug molecules (adapted from Ayrton and Morgan 2001).

Transport Proteins

Drug transporters are expressed in various tissues (intestine, brain, liver, kidney, Figure 6-12) and play key roles in the absorption, distribution, and excretion of drugs. Transporters are classified as primary, secondary, or tertiary, all of which utilize ATP as an energy source and therefore are considered to be "active." Furthermore, each gene family of transporters is composed of a multiplicity of members.

Several of the major drug transporters shown to be of significance from a pharmacokinetic perspective are described in Table 6-2.

At present, the most well-studied drug transporter with respect to human pharmacokinetics is P-glycoprotein (P-gp/MDR1). As reflected by Figure 6-13, P-gp is an efflux transporter which, in the intestine, can actively pump absorbed drug back into the lumen of the small intestine. This, in turn, may contribute to the presystemic clearance (first-pass effect) of drugs that are substrates for P-gp. As illustrated in Figure 6-13, both P-gp and CYP3A4/5 are colocated in the enterocyte and can play a cooperative and coordinate role to alter the extent of systemic exposure for drugs that are substrates for these proteins. The resultant increase in first-pass effect (presystemic clearance) occurs when P-gp limits the availability of a CYP3A4/5 substrate to enzyme by transporting it back into the lumen of the small intestine. Accordingly, P-gp activity can be a major determinant of the bioavailability of drugs that are substrates for this transporter and, in particular, for compounds that also are substrates for CYP3A4/5.

As might be predicted from the coordinate relationship between P-gp and CYP3A4/5, many drugs that are substrates for one of these proteins are also substrates of the other. This produces the potential for drug-drug interactions by compounds that can induce or inhibit either P-gp or CYP3A4/5 as reflected by the examples contained in Table 6-3. In addition, potentially significant transporter interactions can occur such as the inhibition of OATP by furanocoumarins and bioflavonoids contained in grapefruit, orange, and apple juice as exemplified by recent data demonstrating a concentration-dependent increase in the AUC of fexofenadine in humans after concomitant administration of these juices. These particular interactions could conceivably be of clinical significance in young infants living in developed countries who are often given a substantial amount of their daily fluid intake as fruit juice.

Table 6-2. Human Drug Transporters That Have Pharmacokinetic Significance (adapted from Mizuno and Sugiyama 2002)

ABBREVIATION	FULL DESIGNATION
MDR1/P-gp	Multidrug resistant gene/P-glycoprotein
BSEP/SPGP	Bile salt export pump/sister P-glycoprotein
MRP1, MRP2, MRP3	Multidrug resistance associated proteins
NTCP	Sodium taurocholate co-transporting peptide
PEPT1, 2	Oligopeptide transporter 1
OATP1, OATP2	Organic anion transporting peptide
OCT1, OCT2	Organic cation transporter
OAT1, OAT2, OAT3	Organic anion transporter

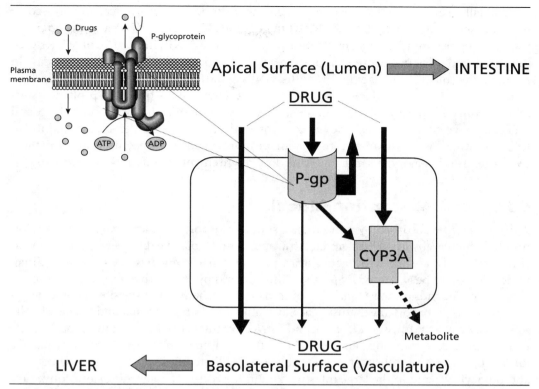

Figure 6-13. Schematic diagram of the action of P-glycoprotein (P-gp) in the small intestine. As illustrated, P-gp is colocated with cytochrome P450 3A (CYP3A) in the enterocyte and in a cooperative fashion can increase the first-pass effect (presystemic clearance) of drugs that are substrates for these proteins by extrusion of the drug back into the intestinal lumen (by the efflux transporter P-gp) and/or biotransformation in the enterocyte by CYP3A.

Table 6-3. Examples of P-gp Interactions with Drugs and Natural Products (adapted from Mizuno and Sugiyama 2002)

COMPOUND	INHIBITOR OR INDUCER	REPORTED INTERACTIONS
Atorvastatin	Inhibitor	Digoxin ($\uparrow$ AUC by 15%)
Cyclosporine	Inhibitor	Docetaxel, Paclitaxel ($\uparrow$ bioavailability 8–11-fold)
Erythromycin	Inhibitor	Atorvastatin, Cyclosporine, Fexofenadine, Saquinavir ($\uparrow$ Cmax and AUC by 32–115%)
Grapefruit juice	Inhibitor	Paclitaxel ($\uparrow$ bioavailability by 7-fold)
Ketoconazole	Inhibitor	Fexofenadine, Saquinavir, Tacrolimus ($\uparrow$ AUC by 1.6–2-fold)
Rifampin	Inducer	Digoxin, Fexofenadine, Saquinavir, Tacrolimus, Talinolol ($\downarrow$ AUC by 37–70%)
Ritonavir	Inhibitor	Saquinavir ($\uparrow$ AUC)
St. John's wort	Inducer	Digoxin ($\downarrow$ AUC)
Verapamil	Inhibitor	Talinolol ($\uparrow$ clearance by 29–56%)

Finally, several transporters have been shown to be polymorphically expressed in humans including MDR1, MRP1, MRP2, OATP1, and OCTN2 (novel organic cation transporter 2). For example, a single nucleotide polymorphism (SNP) in exon 26 of MDR1 produces reduced intestinal expression of P-gp, which has been associated with an increase in the oral bioavailability of digoxin. Two other SNPs in the P-gp gene (one in exon 12 and the other in exon 26) are linked and produce enhanced activity of the transport protein, resulting in reduced bioavailability of fexofenadine. Also, polymorphisms in both P-gp and CYP3A5 have recently been shown to cooperatively influence the bioavailability of tacrolimus, and, as a consequence, the haplotype represented by the polymorphisms in these two proteins is a major determinant of the dose requirement for this antirejection drug.

Combined Absorption Models

A drug might be absorbed by more than just one transport mechanism, such as the vitamin B_{12} which is absorbed by facilitated transport and by passive diffusion. Cardiac glycosides are partly absorbed by active transport and partly by passive diffusion. Small molecules might be absorbed by passive diffusion and by convective transport. However, absorption depends on the availability of transport mechanisms at the site of contact.

Various transport mechanisms are available in different organs and tissues. In the mouth cavity we find passive diffusion and convective transport; in the stomach passive diffusion, convective transport, and probably active transport; in the small intestine passive diffusion, convective transport, active transport, facilitated transport, ion-pair transport, and pinocytosis; and in the large intestine and in the rectum passive diffusion, convective transport, and pinocytosis. Absorption through the skin is only by passive diffusion and convective transport.

The intestinal uptake of a drug by both active transport and passive diffusion may be described by flux, J, as shown in Equation 6.13:

$$J = [(J_{max} \cdot C_i/(K_m + C_i)] + k_d \cdot C_i \tag{13}$$

where J_{max} is the maximal flux, K_m is the Michaelis-Menten constant, C_i is the mean lumenal concentration, and k_d is the passive permeability constant.

Absorption-Distribution Transport Model

A drug being absorbed upon extravascular administration has to first cross a barrier which might be an epithelium cell (intestine), or cells (buccal), or even multiple layers of keratinized cells and epithelial cells (skin) before reaching interstitial space, and then to cross the endothelial structure of blood or lymph capillaries. A drug entering a blood capillary is directly taken up into the systemic circulation, whereas a drug entering a lymphatic capillary will eventually reach the systemic circulation by lymph emptying into the bloodstream (indirect pathway).

The opposite of entering the capillaries for absorption is the leaving of the drug from the capillaries for distribution into the tissue. The clearance of the tissue again is by reentry of drug into capillaries to be carried to site(s) of metabolism and excretion, where again the drug leaves the capillaries. During the entire system of pharmacokinetic phases, i.e., absorption, distribution, metabolism, and elimination, there is a constant crossing of endothelial cells and other cell membranes.

Blood and lymph capillary walls are formed by a unicellular layer of flattened cells, the endothelium, rolled up to form a tube. Tight junctions hold the cells together. The tight junctions are formed by fusion of glycocalyx layers of two adjacent cells. Usually, the tight junctions in capillaries are impermeable to molecules larger than 1.8 to 2 nm in diameter, whereas those in postcapillary venules may be permeable for molecules up to 6 nm in diameter. In lymph nodes, liver, spleen, and bone marrow a sinusoidal type of capillaries is found, i.e., absence of basal membrane and absence of tight junctions, thus permitting free exchange with interstitial fluid.

The crossing of compounds across the endothelium in both directions occurs via different pathways.

It is only in recent years that we gained more understanding on the transport of larger molecules such as peptides. This process involves transport of plasmalemmal vesicles which are formed by endocytosis on the outside of the membrane and, after travelling across the cell, are discharged on the opposite side by exocytosis. The transport vesicles have a diameter of about 70 nm. The transport occurs in both directions. Several vesicles may fuse together. If the fusion occurs from vesicles on both sides of the flattened cell, temporary transendothelial channels may be formed which are like large pores, so that macromolecules may freely pass across the endothelial cell. The flux transfer of solutes through gaps in intercellular junctions and through transendothelial channels is forced by hydrostatic pressure, whereas the vesicle transport is probably diffusion controlled.

Capillaries in the brain lack pores, have impermeable tight junctions, and have very few vesicles (blood-brain barrier). Macromolecules introduced directly into cerebrospinal fluid are rapidly cleared by pinocytosis of specialized cells.

Selected References

1. Agnes, L. and Burckart, G. J.: P-glycoprotein and Drug Therapy in Organ Transplantation. *J. Clin. Pharmacol.* 39:995–1005 (1999).

2. Alberts, B., Bray, D., Lewis, J., Raff, M., Roberts, K. and Watson, J. D., Editors: *Molecular Biology of the Cell.* Garland Publishing Inc., New York, London 1983, p. 302ff.

3. Alpers, D. H.: Uptake and Fate of Absorbed Amino Acids and Peptides in the Mammalian Intestine, *Fed. Proc.* 45:2261–2266 (1986).

4. Ayrton, A. and Morgan, P.: Role of Transport Proteins in Drug Absorption, Distribution and Excretion. *Xenobiotica* 31:469–497 (2001).

5. Cordon-Cardo, C., O'Brien, J. P., Boccia, J., Casals, D., Bertino, J. R. and Melamed, M. R.: Expression of the Multidrug Resistance Gene Product (P-glycoprotein) in Human Normal and Tumor Tissues. *J. Histochem. Cytochem.* 38:1277–1287 (1990).

6. Dresser, G. K., Bailey, D. G., Leake, B. F., Schwarz, U. I., Dawson, P. A., Freeman, D. J. and Kim, R. B.: Fruit Juices Inhibit Organic Anion Transporting Polypeptide-Mediated Drug Uptake to Decrease the Oral Availability of Fexofenadine. *Clin. Pharmacol. Ther.* 71:11–20 (2002).

7. Du Buske, L. M.: Drug Transport Systems. Pharmacy Perspectives 3, Supplement, *U.S. Pharmacist,* Dec. 2001.

8. Elden, I. and Speiser, P.: Endocytosis and Intracellular Drug Delivery, *Acta Pharm. Technol.* 35:109–115 (1989).

9. Fordtran, J. S. and Dietschy, J. M.: Water and Electrolyte Movement in the Intestine, *Gastroenterol.* 50:263 (1966).

10. Gardner, M. L. G.: Evidence For, and Implications of Passage of Intact Peptides Across the Intestinal Mucosa. *Biochem. Soc. Trans.* 2:810–812 (1983).

11. Hogben, C. A. M., Tocco, D. J., Brodie, B. B. and Schanker, L. S.: On the Mechanism of Intestinal Absorption of Drugs. *J. Pharmacol. Exp. Ther. 125*:275 (1959).

12. Kim, R. B.: MDR1 Single Nucleotide Polymorphisms: Multiplicity of Haplotypes and Functional Consequences. *Pharmacogenetics 12*:425–427 (2002).

13. Lan, L.-B., Dalton, J. T. and Scheutz, E. G.: Mdr1 Limits CYP3A Metabolism in Vivo. *Mol. Pharmacol. 28*:863–869 (2000).

14. Lifson, H. and Hakim, A. A.: Simple Diffusive-Convective Model for Intestinal Absorption of a Non-Electrolyte (Urea), *Am. J. Physiol. 211*:1137 (1966).

15. Lin, J. H. and Yamazaki, M.: Role of P-Glycoprotein in Pharmacokinetics. Clinical Implications. *Clin. Pharmacokinet. 42*:59–98 (2003).

16. Martel, F., Grundemann, D., Calhau, C. and Schomig, E.: Typical Uptake of Organic Cations by Human Intestinal Caco-2 Cells; Putative Involvement of ASF Transporters. *Naunyn-Schmiedeberg's Arch. Pharmacol. 363*:40–49 (2001).

17. Martinez, M. N. and Amidon, G. L.: A Mechanistic Approach to Understanding the Factors Affecting Drug Absorption: A Review of Fundamentals. *J. Clin. Pharmacol. 42*:620–643 (2002).

18. Mathews, D. M.: Intestinal Absorption of Peptides. *Biochem. Soc. Trans. 2*:808–810 (1983).

19. Mizuno, N. and Sugiyama, Y.: Drug Transporters: Their Role and Importance in the Selection and Development of New Drugs. *Drug Metab. Pharmacokin. 17*:93–108 (2002).

20. Neubert, R.: Ion Pair Transport Across Membranes, *Pharmacol. Res. 6*:743–747 (1989).

21. Neubert, R., Amlacher, R. and Hartl, A.: Ion Pair Approach of Bretylium, *Drugs Made in Germany 35*:125–127 (1992).

22. Ritschel, W. A.: Absorption of Drugs, *Pharm. Internat. 1*:30 (1974).

23. Schanker, L. S.: On the Mechanism of Absorption of Drugs from the Gastrointestinal Tract, *J. Med. Pharm. Chem. 2*:343 (1960).

24. Schanker, L. S. and Jeffrey, J. J.: Active Transport of Foreign Pyrimidines Across the Intestinal Epithelium, *Nature 190*:727 (1961).

25. Shore, P. A., Brodie, B. B. and Hogben, C. A. M.: The Gastric Secretion of Drugs: A pH Partition Hypothesis, *J. Pharmacol. Exp. Ther. 119*:361 (1957).

26. Volkheimer, G., Schulz, F. H., Aurich, I., Strauch, S., Beuthin, K. and Wendlandt, H.: Persorption of Particles, *Digestion 1*:78 (1968).

27. Wagner, J. G.: Biopharmaceutics: Gastrointestinal Absorption Aspects, *Antibiot. Chemother., Adv. 12*:53 (1964).

28. Wilson, T. H.: *Intestinal Absorption,* W. B. Saunders Co., Philadelphia, 1962.

29. Zhou, H.: Pharmacokinetic Strategies in Deciphering Atypical Drug Absorption Profiles. *J. Clin. Pharmacol. 43*:211–227 (2003).

7

pK$_a$ and Degree of Ionization

Drugs may be classified into three categories according to their physical behavior in aqueous solution: (1) they may exist entirely as ions, such as K^+, Cl^-, or NH_4^+ (strong electrolytes); (2) they may be undissociated, as with the steroids and the sugars (non-electrolytes); or (3) they may be partially dissociated and exist in both an ionic and a molecular form, the relative concentrations of which will depend on the pK$_a$ of the agent and the pH of the medium (weak electrolytes).

Most of the drugs are either weak acids or weak bases. And because of the fact that most drugs are absorbed by passive diffusion of the *nonionized* moiety, the extent to which a drug is in its ionized and nonionized forms at a certain pH is of great importance. But pH, or to be more precise, hydrogen ion concentration, influences the physical and chemical properties associated with absorption, such as solubility of the drug, lipid/water partition coefficient, electrical membrane potential, permeability of the membrane, and chemical reactivity.

At a certain pH, the relative concentration of the ionic and the molecular moieties of a drug are given by the Henderson-Hasselbalch equation. For a weak acid HA, which ionizes according to Equation 7.1:

$$HA + H_2O = H_3O^+ + A^- \tag{1}$$

the dissociation constant is given in Equation 7.2:

$$K_a = \frac{[H_3O^+] \cdot [A^-]}{[HA]} \tag{2}$$

K$_a$ = dissociation constant
A$^-$ = molar concentration of the acidic anion
H$_3$O$^+$ = molar concentration of the hydronium ion
HA = molar concentration of the undissociated acid

The Henderson-Hasselbalch equation for weak acids is calculated from Equation 7.2 by taking the logarithm of both sides of the equation and multiplying both sides of the resultant equation by minus one. The relation as given in Equation 7.3 is obtained:

$$pH = \log \frac{[A^-]}{[HA]} + pK_a \qquad (3)$$

As seen from Equation 7.3, the concentration of the ionic moiety of weak acids increases with increasing pH of the aqueous solution.

Acids are substances donating hydrogen ions, and bases are substances accepting hydrogen ions. If the acid BH$^+$, which is a conjugate of a weak base with a hydrogen ion, is in contact with water, an ionization or dissociation constant K$_a$ can be obtained for the weak base, too:

$$BH^+ + H_2O = H_3O^+ + B \qquad (4)$$

The Henderson-Hasselbalch equation for a weak base is therefore as follows:

$$pH = \log \frac{[B]}{[BH^+]} + pK_a \qquad (5)$$

As seen from Equation 7.5, the concentration of the molecular (undissociated) moiety of a weak base increases with increasing pH of an aqueous solution.

Analogous to the pH (negative logarithm of hydrogen ion concentration) the ionization constant K$_a$ is expressed as pK$_a$:

$$pK_a = -\log K_a \qquad (6)$$

It is easily recognized that for acidic drugs the lower the pK$_a$ the stronger the acid, while for basic drugs the higher the pK$_a$ the stronger the base.

Using the Henderson-Hasselbalch equation, one can calculate the percentage of ionization (Table 7-1) of a monobasic weak acid or monoacidic weak base from the ratio of the concentration of the drug present in the ionic moiety to the total concentration of the drug present in the ionic and in the undissociated moiety, multiplied by 100:

$$\text{percent ionization} = \frac{I \cdot 100}{I + N} \qquad (7)$$

I = ionized moiety
N = nonionized moiety

On rearrangement we obtain:

$$\frac{N}{I} = \text{antilog } (pK_a - pH) \qquad (8)$$

Table 7-1. Percent of Ionization of Weak Electrolytes

	PERCENT IONIZED	
pK$_a$ − pH	IF ANION (WEAK ACID)	IF CATION (WEAK BASE)
−4	99.99	0.01
−3	99.94	0.06
−2	99.01	0.99
−1	90.91	9.09
−0.9	88.81	11.19
−0.8	86.30	13.70
−0.7	83.37	16.63
−0.6	79.93	20.07
−0.5	75.97	24.03
−0.4	71.53	28.47
−0.3	66.61	33.39
−0.2	61.32	38.68
−0.1	55.73	44.27
0	50.00	50.00
+0.1	44.27	55.73
+0.2	38.68	61.32
+0.3	33.39	66.61
+0.4	28.47	71.53
+0.5	24.03	75.97
+0.6	20.07	79.93
+0.7	16.63	83.37
+0.8	13.70	86.30
+0.9	11.19	88.81
+1	9.09	90.91
+2	0.99	99.01
+3	0.06	99.94
+4	0.01	99.99

which can be solved for N:

$$N = I \cdot antilog\,(pK_a - pH) \tag{9}$$

Upon substitution of Equation 7.9 into Equation 7.7 we obtain the percentage of ionization for a weak acid:

$$percent\ ionization\ (acid) = \frac{100}{1 + antilog\,(pK_a - pH)} \tag{10}$$

For a weak base the following Equation 7.11 is derived:

$$percent\ ionization\ (base) = \frac{100}{1 + antilog\,(pH - pK_a)} \tag{11}$$

It follows, further, from the Henderson-Hasselbalch equation, that when a substance is half ionized and half nonionized at a certain pH, its pK$_a$ is equal to this pH. Or, in other words, at that pH which is equal to the pK$_a$ value, half of the molecules of a drug are in ionized and half are in nonionized form. The relation between ionization and pH is not linear, but sigmoidal.

A small change in pH will, therefore, have a great change in ionization, if pH and pK$_a$ values are close together.

Knowing the pK$_a$ value of a drug the theoretical equilibrium ratio can be calculated as follows:

for weak acids:

$$R_a = \frac{C_x}{C_p} = \frac{1 + 10^{(pH_x - pK_a)}}{1 + 10^{(pH_p - pK_a)}} \tag{12}$$

or

$$R_a = \frac{1 + antilog\,(pH_x - pK_a)}{1 + antilog\,(pH_p - pK_a)} \tag{13}$$

for weak bases:

$$R_b = \frac{C_x}{C_p} = \frac{1 + 10^{(pK_a - pH_x)}}{1 + 10^{(pK_a - pH_p)}} \tag{14}$$

or

$$R_b = \frac{1 + antilog\,(pK_a - pH_x)}{1 + antilog\,(pK_a - pH_p)} \tag{15}$$

R_a = concentration ratio between gut, or any other compartment, and plasma for weak acids

R_b = concentration ratio between gut, or any other compartment, and plasma for weak bases

C_x = concentration in the extravascular compartment (milk, cerebrospinal fluid, sweat, rectal fluid, stomach fluid, intestinal fluid)

C_p = concentration in the plasma

pH_x = pH of extravascular compartment (milk, cerebrospinal fluid, sweat, rectal fluid, stomach fluid, intestinal fluid)

pH_p = pH of plasma = 7.4

Hogben has shown, furthermore, that the pH at the site of absorption in the jejunum is not necessarily identical with the pH of the intestinal content in the lumen. He calculated a "virtual" pH of 5.3 for the site of absorption at the intestinal membrane surface. However, the true existence of such a virtual pH is highly doubtful and is probably an artifact due to the experimental procedure.

If we consider two compartments separated by a membrane, we may find some ions in the solution on one side of the membrane which cannot cross to the other side. Such a situation results in the *Donnan distribution*. This is the case with erythrocytes, where the presence of hemoglobin anions affects the distribution of normally diffusible ions such as chloride. We find in this case a cell to plasma ratio of about 0.7 instead of 1.0. The distribution ratio of a cation would then be the reciprocal of the chloride ratio, namely 1.4.

This phenomenon must be distinguished from *unequal equilibrium distribution*. If we consider two liquid compartments with different pH values, separated by a membrane, selectively permeable to the nonionized form, we may find different drug concentrations in the

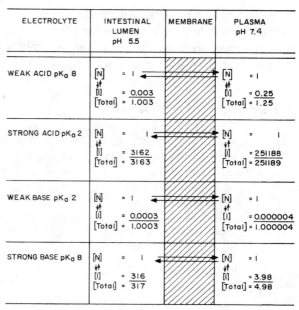

Figure 7-1. Distribution of organic acids and bases of different pK$_a$ between the intestinal lumen pH 5.5 and plasma pH 7.4 separated by the gastrointestinal membrane under the assumption of passive diffusion. [ ] = concentrations, N = nonionized moiety, I = ionized moiety.

two compartments after steady state is reached, as seen in Figure 7-1.

At the steady state in unequal equilibrium distribution, the concentration of the nonionized form is the same in both compartments. But the concentrations of the ionized form are unequal due to the difference in pH. Therefore, the total concentration of the solute (nonionized and ionized forms) on both sides of the membrane is a function of the pH of the two aqueous compartments as well as of the pK$_a$ of the solute.

But we have to be aware of the fact that very few, if any, drugs actually obey the pH-partition hypothesis as just outlined. It is possible that even an ionized drug might be sufficiently lipid soluble to permeate the membrane (gastrointestinal barrier). On the other hand, the nonionized form of a drug might be insufficiently lipid soluble and therefore unable to cross the membrane. Furthermore, we must consider that this theory is not applicable when other transport mechanisms, such as active transport, are involved.

Regarding permeation of membranes, we have seen that the nonionized form of a drug is important. But we have not considered the drug-receptor interaction in the biophase. For this drug interaction with specific receptors a certain concentration of the ionized or unionized form of the drug is required. The degree of ionization in the biophase, in the plasma, having a pH of 7.4, can be calculated using Equations 7.10 and 7.11.

The question arises: what minimum percent of drug must be in nonionized form at the absorption site in order to be absorbed? The author calculated the degree of ionization at the absorption site for a number of drugs for which peroral or rectal absorption has been shown. It seems that drugs are absorbed by passive diffusion from the small intestine if at least 0.1 to 1 percent is in nonionized form, and from the rectum if at least 1–5 percent is in nonionized form. Since the degree of ionization is constant, immediately some of the ionized moiety becomes nonionized when the nonionized form has been absorbed. This process occurs so fast that even poorly nonionized drugs may be well absorbed from the gastrointestinal tract. Surface area definitely plays an important role in this process.

Selected References

1. Hogben, C. A. M., Tocco, D. J., Brodie, B. B. and Schanker, L. S.: On the Mechanism of Intestinal Absorption of Drugs, *J. Pharmacol. Exp. Ther. 125*:275 (1959).

2. Newton, D. W. and Kluza, R. B.: pK$_a$ Values of Medicinal Compounds in Pharmacy Practice, *Drug Intell. Clin. Pharm. 12*:546 (1978).

3. Ritschel, W. A.: pK$_a$ Values and Some Clinical Applications. In: *Perspectives in Clinical Pharmacy,* Francke, D. E. and Whitney, H. A. K., Editors. Drug Intelligence Publications, Hamilton, Ill., 1972, p. 325.

4. Schanker, L. S.: Physiological Transport of Drugs. In: Harper, N. J. and Simmonds, A. B., Editors. *Advances in Drug Research,* Academic Press, London-New York, 1964, p. 100.

8

Lipid/Water Partition Coefficient

The lipid/water partition coefficient denotes the ratio of the concentration of a drug in two immiscible or slightly miscible phases.

True Partition Coefficient (TPC)

The distribution law is exact only for ideal solutions under the following conditions:

1. When the two liquid phases are completely immiscible;
2. When the solute neither associates nor dissociates in either phase;
3. When the solute concentration is relatively low; and
4. When the solute is only slightly soluble in either phase.

Then:

$$TPC = \frac{C_1}{C_2} \tag{1}$$

TPC = true lipid/water partition coefficient
C_1 = drug concentration in the lipid phase
C_2 = drug concentration in the aqueous phase

In case a solute exists as undissociated single molecules in phase 2 (C_2) and as a bimolar species in phase 1 (C_1), a correction can be made:

$$PC' = \frac{\sqrt{C_1}}{C_2} \tag{2}$$

In case the solute dissociates in phase 2 (C_2) but not in phase 1 (C_1), a correction can be made following:

$$PC'' = \frac{C_1}{C_2(1-a)} \tag{3}$$

53

PC', PC" = partition coefficients for nonideal distribution
a   = degree of dissociation at a given pH

Apparent Partition Coefficient (APC)

In biopharmaceutics and for general purposes often nonideal systems are found and no correction is made. Any APC is valid only for a specified system, using a particular lipid phase (octanol, chloroform, cyclohexane, isopropyl myristate, etc.), a particular aqueous phase (buffer solution of particular pH), and at specified temperature (30°C, 37°C, etc.). The determination is done by dissolving the drug first in the aqueous or lipid phase, as illustrated below. Equilibration is done for a minimum of 3 hours:

$$APC = \frac{(C_2^o - C_2') \cdot a}{C_2' \cdot b} \tag{4}$$

APC = apparent lipid/water partition coefficient
C_2^o = drug concentration in aqueous phase before equilibration
C_2' = drug concentration in aqueous phase after equilibration
a   = volume of aqueous phase
b   = volume of lipid phase

    In Figure 8-1 the experimental set-up for determination of the lipid/water partition coefficient is shown.
    The partition coefficient can be considered as a measure of the relative affinity of a drug for two immiscible solvents, as well as an index of comparative solubilities in solvents, and as a parameter of the relative rate of partitioning from one phase into another. In general, with increasing polarity of the drug (ionization, introduction of hydroxyl, carboxyl, amino groups, etc.), water solubility increases at the expense of the solubility in the nonpolar solvent and, hence, the lipid/water partition coefficient decreases. Vice versa, decreasing the polarity of the drug (introduction of methyl or methylene groups, etc.) results in decreased water solubility and increased lipid/water partition coefficient.

    A change of pH in the aqueous phase alters the degree of dissociation of electrolytes. The nondissociated moiety is usually much more soluble in the nonpolar phase than the dissociated moiety. Therefore, with increasing pH, the partition coefficient of acidic drugs decreases and that of basic drugs increases. The pH will have a marked influence on penetration and absorption of weak electrolytes transported by passive diffusion since the pH of the physiological fluids at the

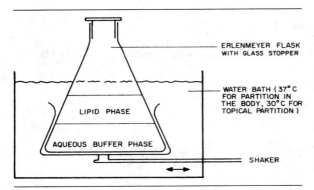

Figure 8-1. Experimental setup for determination of lipid/water partition coefficient.

site of absorption will determine the amount of nondissociated species present. A survey of body pH values is given in Table 8-1.

The lipid/water partition coefficient is a useful in vitro guide to the absorption potential of a drug. As the aqueous phase, a buffer solution is chosen having a pH of the physiologic fluid at the site of absorption. In vivo partitioning does not occur between two immiscible fluids, but does occur between physiological fluids separated by membranes. Since membranes which permit passive diffusion of lipid soluble, nonpolar drugs are lipoidal in nature, whereas lipid insoluble, polar drugs are restricted from passive diffusion, the lipid/water partition may be used to predict absorbability. However, it must be remembered that absorption of drugs can occur also by transport mechanisms other than that of passive diffusion.

As the lipid phase, octanol is usually employed. The use of the lipid/water partition coefficient to measure the absorption potential is reliable for absorption from the stomach, the buccal cavity, the colon, and the skin. In vitro data obtained for intestinal absorption are often erroneous because of the tremendous surface area of the small intestine, which compensates for poor solubility of the drug in the membrane.

Table 8-1. Body pH Values

LOCATION	MEAN	RANGE	REMARKS
Bile	6.9	5.6–8.0	Bile in liver: 7.7
			Bile in gallbladder: 6.8
Blood, arterial	7.40	7.35–7.45	
Blood, venous	7.37	7.32–7.42	
Cerebrospinal fluid	7.34	7.32–7.37	
Gastric fluid	2.0	Men: 1.92	
		Women: 2.59	Children: 0.9–7.7
Milk	6.6	6.6–7.01	
Pancreatic fluid	7.5	7.5–8.8	
Saliva	6.4	5.8–7.1	Children: 6.4–8.2
Sweat	4.5	4.0–6.8	
Urine	5.7	4.8–7.5	Children: 5.1–7.2
Feces	7.2	5.85–8.45	Children: 4.6–5.2
Stomach	1.5	1.0–3.5	
Duodenum	6.9	6.5–7.6	
Jejunum	6.9	6.3–7.3	
Ileum	7.6	6.9–7.9	
Colon	7.95	7.9–8.0	
Rectum	7.7	7.5–7.8	
Plasma	7.40		

The lipid/water partition coefficient is also an indicator for storage of drugs in fat. Since the minimum amount of fat is 10 percent of the body weight, and usually is in the range of 15–25 percent, in obesity even 50 percent or more, considerable quantities of drugs of high lipid solubility can be stored in fat. Drugs stored in fat are dissolved in it and are usually slowly released from the depot. (The slow release from the fat depot results, in the case of barbiturates, in the hangover phenomenon.)

It is commonly believed that an APC of log 4.2–5.5 represents the optimum range for drug absorption based on buccal and percutaneous studies. Recent in vitro investigations using cell culture systems revealed that when APC log was lower than 3.5, transepithelial permeability increased with the lipophilicity. In contrast, when APC log was between 3.5 and 5.2, the transepithelial permeability coefficient decreased with increasing lipophilicity. Consequently, it appears that in vitro APC data may only provide an indication of drug translocation which must be verified from studies performed in the intact organism.

It has been shown recently that the volume of distribution is related to the apparent partition coefficient and the extent of protein binding. It is possible to predict a drug's volume of distribution from the in vitro determination of the APC and the extent of protein binding (see also Chapter 16, Volume of Distribution and Distribution Coefficient).

Likewise, the APC may be estimated from knowledge of the apparent volume of distribution (V_d in L/kg) of a given drug, the body weight (BW in kg) of a patient, and the extent of drug binding to circulating plasma proteins (p = fraction of drug bound to protein). After determination of the V_d and p, which may represent patient-specific values or, for the purpose of estimation, age appropriate average values from the literature (see Appendix), the APC can be estimated according to Equation 8.5.

$$APC = \frac{[V_d/(BW \cdot (1-p))] - 0.9314}{0.1302} \tag{5}$$

Selected References

1. Cohnen, E., Flasch, H., Heinz, N. and Hempelmann, F. W.: Partition Coefficients and R_m-Values of Cardenolides, *Arzneim. Forsch.* 28:2179 (1978).

2. Doluisio, J. T. and Swintosky, J. V.: Drug Partitioning II, *J. Pharm. Sci.* 53:598 (1964).

3. Doluisio, J. T. and Swintosky, J. V.: Drug Partitioning III, *J. Pharm. Sci.* 54:1594 (1965).

4. Lien, E., Koda, R. T. and Tong, G. L.: Buccal and Percutaneous Absorption, *Drug Intell. Clin. Pharm.* 5:38–41 (1971).

5. Reese, D. R., Irwin, G. M., Dittert, L. W., Chong, C. W. and Swintosky, J. V.: Drug Partitioning I, *J. Pharm. Sci.* 53:591 (1964).

6. Ritschel, W. A. and Hammer, G. V.: Prediction of the Volume of Distribution from in vitro Data and Use for Estimating the Absolute Extent of Absorption, *Int. J. Clin. Pharmacol. Ther. Toxicol.* 18:298 (1980).

7. Wils, P., Warnery, A., Phung-Ba, V., Legrain, S. and Scherman, D.: High Lipophilicity Decreases Drug Transport Across Intestinal Epithelial Cells, *J. Pharmacol. Exp. Ther.* 269:654–658 (1994).

9

Physicochemical Factors Altering Biological Performance of Drugs

Particle Size

Particle size is of importance for drugs of low solubility in water or biological fluids such as stomach fluid, intestinal fluid, etc. The critical point seems to be if the solubility is less than 0.3 percent. (The U.S. FDA regulation on bioavailability lists 0.5 percent as the limit.) With decreasing particle size, surface area increases, thus increasing the area of solid matter being exposed to the dissolution media and, hence, dissolution rate increases (becomes more rapid). However, the actual solubility does not significantly change with particle-size reduction (micronization) in the range used in pharmaceutical manufacture:

$$\frac{dc}{dt} = k \cdot a \cdot (C_s - C_t) \tag{1}$$

$\dfrac{dc}{dt}$ = dissolution rate (amount per unit time) (Noyes-Whitney equation)

k = constant depending on intensity of agitation, temperature, structure of solid surface, and diffusion coefficient

a = surface area of undissolved solute

C_s = solubility of drug in solvent

C_t = concentration of dissolved drug at time t

Examples of drugs for which therapeutic differences have been found depending on particle size are: amphotericin, aspirin, bishydroxycoumarin (dicumarol), chloramphenicol, digoxin, fluocinolone acetonide, griseofulvin, p-hydroxypropiophenone, meprobamate, nitrofurantoin, phenobarbital, phenothiazine, phenylbutazone, prednisolone, procaine penicillin, reserpine, sodium para-aminosalicylate, spironolactone, sulfadiazine, sulfisoxazole, and tolbutamide.

The decrease in particle size is technically limited. The smallest particle sizes used are in the range of 1–10 μm. Particle size reduction is not a universal answer for all drugs of low solubility. For instance, if the dissolution rate is not the absorption rate-limiting step or, in cases where decomposition of the drug would be faster than the time needed for absorption (for example micronized penicillin G in gastric fluid), then micronization should be avoided.

Co-Solutes and Complex Formation

The question of co-solutes is of importance only for drugs of low solubility.

Salting-Out. If an electrolyte is added in solid form to a solution of an organic non-electrolyte, the ions of the added electrolyte require water for their hydration, and thereby reduce the amount of water available for the solution of the nonelectrolyte. The nonelectrolyte will be precipitated → salting out. See Figure 9-1.

Salting-In. Salting-in occurs when either the salts of various organic acids or organic-substituted ammonium salts are added to aqueous solutions of nonelectrolytes. In the first case, the solubilizing effect is associated with the anion, and in the second case with the cation. The added compound adds to the hydrophilicity of the solution. See Figure 9-2.

Clathrate Formation. Clathrates are formed if a substance is capable of forming channels, or cages which can take up another substance into the intraspace of the structure. Clathrate-forming substances are gallic acid, urea, thiourea, amylose, and zeolite. Clathrates are formed by crystallization of an organic solution of the clathrate-forming vehicle substance with the drug. See Figure 9-3.

The drug is in monomolecular dispersion in the clathrate complex. If exposed to water the clathrate-forming vehicle dissolves rapidly and exposes the single molecule of drug to the dissolution media.

Drugs used in clathrates are: vitamin A, sulfathiazole, chloramphenicol, and reserpine. Clathrates are stable in the dry form.

Solid-in-Solid Solution Complex. If a drug is dissolved in a *melt* of mannitol or a mixture of mannitol and other carbohydrates or of succinic acid, for example, and the mixture is solidified or crystallized, a solid-in-solid solution is obtained whereby the drug is in monomolecular dispersion. Other substances which yield solid-in-solid solution complexes are mixtures of creatinine and tartaric acid, and organic solutions containing either polyvinylpyrrolidone or polyethylene glycol. The liquid melt can be used for spray-congealing to obtain beads or the solidified melt may be milled.

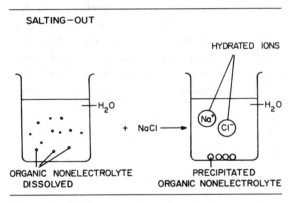

Figure 9-1. Schematic diagram of salting-out. Mechanism: reduction in free water.

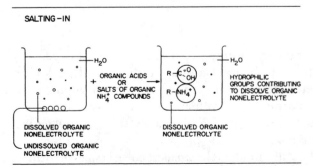

Figure 9-2. Schematic diagram of salting-in. Mechanism: increase in hydrophilic groups.

Upon exposure of the solid-in-solid material to water, the vehicle dissolves rapidly releasing the drug in monomolecular state. See Figures 9-4 and 9-5.

Examples of drugs used in solid-in-solid solutions are griseofulvin, chloramphenicol, acetaminophen, aminobenzoic acid, beta-cyclodextrin, and antihistamines in melts of urea, mannitol, succinic acid, etc., and of salicylic acid, sulfathiazole, prednisone, salicylamide, pentaerythritol tetranitrate, and griseofulvin in polyvinylpyrrolidone or polyethylene glycol solutions.

Chemical Variation

Chemical variations are made for two reasons: either to change the structure of the active compound in order to increase pharmacologic response, or to maintain the basic structure but change solubility by formation of either salts, esters, ethers, or complexes. The last group (salts, esters, ethers, complexes) is of biopharmaceutical importance. See Table 9-1.

Salts. In general, the salts of electrolytes have a higher solubility and a more rapid dissolution rate than the free acid or the free base. The dissolution rate of an acidic drug increases with increasing pH, but not to the same extent as the solubility increases with increasing pH (salt formation). The dissolution rate of a salt is relatively independent of the pH of the medium. See Figure 9-6. For example, the dissolution rate and the peak serum levels and area under blood level curves of penicillin V decrease from: K salt → Na salt → Ca salt → free acid → benzathine salt.

Esters. Chloramphenicol and erythromycin are absorbed from the gastrointestinal tract in form of free bases which, however, are unstable in acidic gastric fluid. For example, chloramphenicol esters dissolve at higher pH in the small intestine and are subsequently enzymatically hydrolyzed.

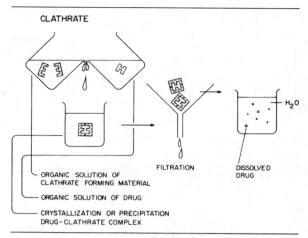

Figure 9-3. Schematic diagram of clathrate formation. Since the drug is entrapped in the clathrate in monomolecular state and the clathrate forming material dissolves readily in water, the drug is exposed to the water in molecular state and dissolves readily, too.

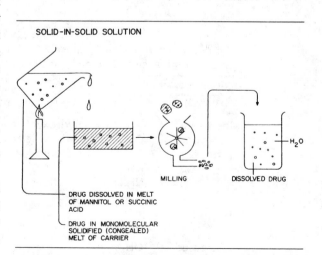

Figure 9-4. Schematic diagram of solid-in-solid solution. Since the carrier dissolves readily in water the drug is exposed to the water in monomolecular state and dissolves readily, too.

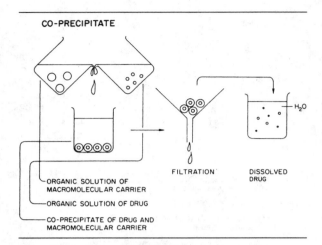

Figure 9-5. Schematic diagram of co-precipitate formation. Since the carrier goes rapidly into solution the drug is exposed in minute form to the water and dissolves readily, too.

Different esters have different rates of hydrolysis. Chloramphenicol palmitate is more readily hydrolyzed than chloramphenicol stearate.

Amorphous and Crystalline

Solid particles are either amorphous or crystalline. In general, the amorphous state is more soluble and has a higher dissolution rate than the crystalline form. Probably the crystalline form requires a higher amount of energy to free a molecule of drug from it than does the amorphous form. For example, amorphous novobiocin and amorphous chloramphenicol esters are biologically active while their crystalline forms are inactive.

Penicillin G should not be used in amorphous form PO because it is more rapidly dissolved and inactivated in stomach fluid than the crystalline form.

Anhydrous Form, Hydrates, and Solvates

Hydrates are addition-compounds of drug with water while solvates are addition-compounds of drug and organic solvent. Their physical properties differ greatly from the anhydrous form in respect to solubility and dissolution rate. For example, the anhydrous form of ampicillin,

Table 9-1. Examples of Chemical Modification of Drug Molecule to Either Increase or Decrease Solubility

CHEMICAL VARIATION TO OBTAIN		INTRODUCTION OF GROUPS		
Increased hydrophilic property	$-OH$	hydroxyl (alcoholic, phenolic)		
	$-COOH$	carboxylic acid		
	$-SO_3H$	sulfonic acid		
	$-NH_2$	primary		
	$-NHR$	secondary	amino	
	$-NR^1R^2$	tertiary	groups	$(R, R^1, R^2, R^3 =$ small alkyl groups)
	$+$			
	$-NR^1R^2R^3$	quaternary		
Decreased hydrophilic property	$-OH \rightarrow$	$-O-C-R$ $|| $ O		$(R =$ long chain alkyl group)
		e.g. fatty acid esters		

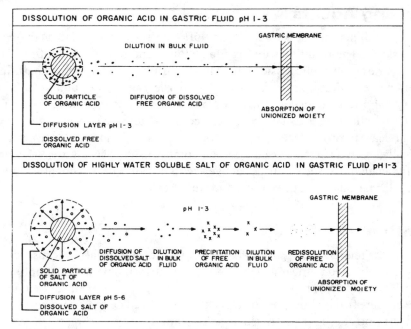

Figure 9-6. Schematic diagram of dissolution of an organic acid and a highly water soluble salt of an organic acid in gastric fluid.

caffeine, penicillins, glutethimide, para-aminosalicylic acid, and calcium phenobarbital dissolves more rapidly than the crystalline form and gives higher peak blood levels. Solvates of corticosteroids dissolve more readily than the nonsolvated form.

Polymorphism

Polymorphism is the phenomenon that a drug may exist in different crystalline forms, polymorphs. Polymorphism exists only in the solid state. The most stable form has highest stability but lowest dissolution rate. The least stable form usually has the most rapid dissolution rate. The unstable (metastable) forms convert more or less slowly into the more stable form. For example, cocoa butter when heated above 40°C forms a metastable polymorph which does not solidify above 26°C. Chloramphenicol palmitate appears in three different polymorphs, but only polymorph B is biologically active, since the other forms do not dissolve and are not hydrolyzed. Polymorphs may be stabilized by the addition of viscosity increasing agents in order to retard transition of one polymorph into another.

Viscosity

Increasing their viscosity prolongs the time of diffusion of solvent molecules to the surface of solids. It also prolongs the time of diffusion of dissolved drug molecules into the bulk of the solution. Disintegration and dissolution of tablets are decreased with increasing viscosity. Food increases the viscosity of gastrointestinal contents and, hence, often delays absorption of such drugs as ethanol, salicylic acid, and sulfonamides.

Solubilizing Agents

Drugs of low solubility may be brought into solution by the use of surface active agents (surfactants, tensides). The resulting solution is a colloidal and not a true solution. The drug is solubilized by the amphiphilic tenside which has hydrophilic and lipophilic parts in the molecule. The tenside molecules associate to form micelles, aggregates of 50 to 150 molecules until the critical micelle concentration is obtained (CMC). If the tenside concentration is below the CMC, the drug is usually well released. If the tenside concentration is above the CMC, drug release may be affected, especially if the product is not diluted upon administration (topically, rectally, intramuscularly, subcutaneously). See Figure 9-7. Drugs with increased bioavailability due to surface active agents are vitamin A, cephaloridine, heparin, riboflavin, salicylamide, spironolactone, and sulfisoxazole.

Adsorption

Adsorption is the tendency of a substance to accumulate at a surface, because molecules on any surface are subjected to the unbalanced forces of attraction perpendicular to the plane of the surface. Physical adsorption occurs when the valency requirements of each molecule on the surface are satisfied by bonding to adjacent molecules. The forces are known as van der Waal's. Adsorption and desorption usually occur rapidly.

Chemisorption occurs when the valency requirements of the surface molecules are not fully satisfied by nearby molecules. Usually strong bonds result by electron transfer which often requires activation energy (heating). Only monolayers are formed. For example, anticholinergics may be adsorbed to antacids (magnesium trisilicate, magnesium carbonate, aluminum compounds), lincomycin is adsorbed if an attapulgite-pectin preparation is administered simultaneously, promazine is adsorbed if given simultaneously with attapulgite or charcoal, anti-bacterials of cationic nature (quats) are adsorbed on bentonite. In all cases activity is reduced. Charcoal is used as an antidote because of its adsorptive properties.

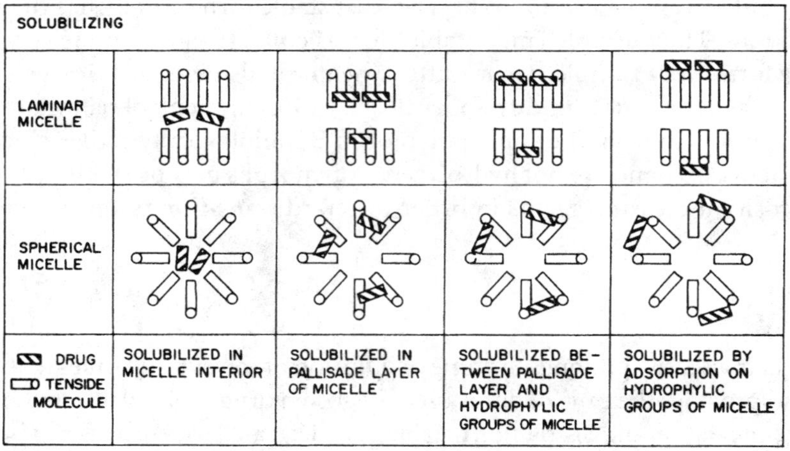

Figure 9-7. Schematic diagram of solubilization of drug in tenside micelles.

Manufacturing Factors

Many unit operations used in manufacture of drug products may decrease biological performance. In the case of tablets, increased compression force increases "hardness" (mechanical resistance) of tablets and prolongs disintegration and dissolution time. Increasing amounts of binders in granules and tablets increase "hardness" (mechanical resistance) of tablets and prolong disintegration and dissolution time. Increasing amounts of lubricants decrease hydrophilicity and wetting of tablets, thus prolonging disintegration and dissolution time.

"Hard" granules and high compression speed and high compression force may cause a rise in the temperature of tablets during the moment of compression to 75°C, at which temperature some drugs may sinter. A micronized drug may hence form larger aggregates. Heat used in manufacture of suppositories and ointments may cause some drugs to dissolve in the base. Upon cooling, the drug may crystallize and form large needles, thus prolonging the time of drug release.

Dissolution

When a drug substance dissolves in a dissolution medium, a cube root law most often is applicable, if sink conditions apply. An exponential decay of mass dissolved versus time is applicable, if nonsink conditions apply. In most cases, however, there will be a lag time due to interfacial effects. For the drug substance itself, the most important interfacial effect is that of the wetting of the planes of the solid. For hydrophilic solids, "wetting" is complete in the sense that the contact angle is zero. For less hydrophilic to hydrophobic substances, the contact angle increases, and if the contact angle is less than $\pi/4$, then the wetting is generally complete. However, this requires time.

For the dissolution under sink conditions, the cube root law with lag time takes the following form (M is mass not dissolved, t is time, t_i is the lag time, K is a cube root dissolution constant, and M_o is the original mass):

$$M^{1/3} = M_o^{1/3} - K \cdot (t - t_i) \tag{2}$$

Under nonsink dissolution into an adequate dissolution volume (V), it is exponential-asymptotic so that introducing a lag time for wetting would give:

$$C = (M_o/V) \cdot (1 - e^{-q \cdot (t - t_i)}) \tag{3}$$

It is noted, however, that the wetting is important in the beginning of the dissolution. If the area, A, wetted is linear in time, i.e., if:

$$A = f \cdot t \tag{4}$$

where f is a constant, then the lag time is given by:

$$t_i = A_o/f \tag{5}$$

It can be assumed that sink conditions apply prior to t_i, so that:

$$dm/dt = -k \cdot A \cdot S \qquad (6)$$

Substituting Equation 9.4 in Equation 9.6 gives:

$$dm/dt = -k \cdot (f \cdot t) \cdot S \qquad (7)$$

If the drug dissolves slowly and/or there is an excess present, then A may be assumed to be fairly constant, and equal to A_o, and in this case, Equation 9.7 integrates to:

$$M = M_o - (k \cdot f \cdot S/2) \cdot t^2 \qquad (8)$$

or:

$$C = (M_o - M)/V = (k \cdot f \cdot S/2V) \cdot t^2 \qquad (9)$$

where V is liquid volume and S is solubility. At $t = A_o/f$, the concentration is:

$$C' = (k \cdot S \cdot A_o^2/2V \cdot f) \qquad (10)$$

Since the dissolution occurs under sink conditions at the low time points, the profile is one of a parabola at first, which, at the point given in Equation 9.10 (where all the solid is wetted), becomes the straight line:

$$C' = k \cdot A_o \cdot S \cdot (t - t_i) \qquad (11)$$

If Equation 9.10 is inserted in Equation 9.11, it is found that:

$$t_i = (A_o - (1/2V)) \cdot (1/f) \qquad (12)$$

Conclusion

Pharmacotechnical factors, although of different kinds, may alter biological performance of drugs by changing the rate and extent of drug release (liberation) from the dosage form upon administration.

A prerequisite of drug absorption is that the drug be in aqueous (true) solution (except in the relatively rare case of pinocytosis). The process of bringing a drug into solution at the site of absorption is the liberation or drug release process. Drug release can be determined in vitro by means of a dissolution rate test for peroral and oral dosage forms, or by dialysis or diffusion methods for rectal and topical preparations.

Drug products having different release characteristics will result in different blood level curves in vivo. However, if the extent of drug release is identical, there will be identical areas under curves depicting blood level versus time. If the extent of drug release is identical but the release rates differ, the blood level versus time curves will show different absorption rate constants and different peak heights. The different absorption rate constants so obtained are artifacts because the actual absorption rates of a given drug should be the same for a given route of administration. The differences in absorption rates, however, are not caused by differences in the absorption pattern but by differences in the rate of drug release. Therefore, absorption rates obtained for one and the same drug, but in different dosage forms for the same route of administration, are "apparent" absorption rates. They are "apparent" because the true absorption rate is overlapped by release characteristics. An apparent change in absorption rate will be obtained if the dissolution rate or liberation rate of the drug is slower than the unrestricted absorption rate of the pure drug in solution. Absorption difficulties are encountered either with drugs of low solubility (solubility <0.3 percent) or with those which are released extremely slowly from the dosage form. In both cases, dissolution becomes the absorption rate-limiting step. A diagram of the influence of pharmacotechnical factors on the absorption rate is given in Figure 9-8.

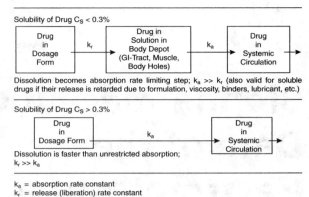

Figure 9-8. Influence of solubility and dissolution rate on the absorption rate constant.

Selected References

1. Barker, H.: The Role of Pharmaceutics in Drug Therapy, *Australas. J. Pharm. 49*:S33 (1968).

2. Carstensen, J. T.: *Theoretical Aspects of Interfacial and Surface Effects in the Dissolution of Drug Substances and Dosage Forms,* 132nd Annual APhA Meeting, San Antonio, February 16–21, 1985.

3. Garrett, E. R.: Physico-Chemical Factors: Drug Systems Affecting Availability and Reliability of Response, *J. Am. Pharm. Assoc. NS9*:110 (1969).

4. Mitchell, A. G.: Pharmaceutical Factors Affecting Drug Availability, *Australas. J. Pharm. 47*:559 (1966).

5. Münzel, K.: Der Einfluss der Formgebung auf die Wirkung eines Arzneimittels. In: *Progress in Drug Research,* Karger, S., Editor, Birkhäuser Verlag, Basel-Stuttgart, 1966, p. 204.

6. Plakogiannis, F. M. and Cutie, A. J.: *Basic Concepts in Biopharmaceutics,* Brooklyn Medical Press, Brooklyn, N.Y., 1977.

7. Polderman, J., Editor: *Formulation and Preparation of Dosage Forms,* Elsevier-North-Holland Biomedical Press, Amsterdam-New York-Oxford, 1977.

8. Ritschel, W. A.: *Angewandte Biopharmazie,* Wissenschaft-liche Verlagsgesellschaft, Stuttgart, 1973, pp. 52, 281.

9. Ritschel, W. A.: Physicochemical and Pharmaceutical Properties of Drugs and Dosage Forms Influencing the Results of Phase I Studies. In: *Advances in Clinical Pharmacology,* Kuemmerle, H. P., Shibuya, T. K. and Kimura, E., Editors, Urban and Schwarzenberg, Munich-Vienna-Baltimore, 1977, p. 116.

10. Swarbrick, J., Editor: *Current Concepts in the Pharmaceutical Sciences: Dosage Form Design and Bioavailability,* Lea and Febiger, Philadelphia, 1973.

10

Biopharmaceutical Data of the Gastrointestinal Tract

Anatomy and Function

The gastrointestinal (GI) tract comprises a tube system starting from the mouth to the anus. The **stomach** has a capacity of approximately 1.1 to 1.2 liters when filled; the empty stomach contains about 100 ml of stomach fluid. The esophagus has no true sphincter valve, but rather a type of sphincter (e.g., gastroesophageal junction) in its lower part. At the lower end of the stomach is the pylorus which has a powerful sphincter. The mechanism of the closed valve is to permit the transfer of liquid into the small intestine but to prevent the exit of solid food, except when the sphincter opens periodically for the transfer of food. The stomach wall is highly muscular and mixes the food with the gastric fluid. The mucous membrane of the stomach is divided by a system of furrows into areas of 1 to 6 mm in diameter. These furrows are again divided by tiny grooves. The invaginations formed by furrows are called gastric pits. The mucous membrane of the stomach contains many glands situated at the bottom of the gastric pits.

We distinguish between three types of glands: (1) **mucous glands,** which secrete mucus; (2) **chief cells (zymogenic cells),** which secrete pepsin and other enzymes; and (3) **parietal cells,** which secrete hydrochloric acid. The chief cells and the parietal cells, which are called gastric glands, are found throughout the body and the fundus of the stomach; they are not found in the pyloric region where only mucous glands are present. Most gastric glands are found in the body of the stomach; the fundus contains approximately one-third less.

The pyloric canal leads into the **small intestine** which is divided into three parts: the **duodenum,** the **jejunum,** and the **ileum.** There is no division between the three parts and one passes gradually into the other. The structures are generally the same and the differences are very small.

The outer part of the small intestine is a serous or fibrous coat called the serosa, followed by smooth muscle which is arranged in two layers. An outer longitudinal muscle and an inward circular muscle are responsible for peristalsis. The contraction of the longitudinal muscle shortens the gut while contraction of the circular muscle constricts it. The inner part of the intestinal lumen is the mucosa that contains glands which secrete the digestive juices.

The innermost lining of the mucosa is the epithelium which forms many villi which are finally responsible for most of the absorption.

The wall of the **duodenum** is deeply folded and contains the duodenal digestive glands. Also the secretory ducts of bile and pancreas open into the duodenum.

The **jejunum** and **ileum** have a high degree of motility and the lumen decreases gradually in diameter. The deep circular folds having the macrovilli and microvilli increase steadily through the jejunum and ileum.

The **microvilli** are microscopic small cellular processes directed to the center of the lumen of the small intestine. The enterocytes which comprise the microvilli also contain enzymes required for nutrient absorption (e.g., lactase) and drug metabolism (e.g., CYP3A4). The total surface area of the gastrointestinal tract is approximately 120 to 200 m^2. This is due to the enormous number of microvilli. (See Figure 6-1.)

The **ileocecal valve** is the border between the small intestine and the large intestine and prevents regurgitation of the cecal content into the ileum.

The structure of the **large intestine** is similar to that of the small intestine, but it does not have folds of the mucous membrane in the rectum, and there are no villi present. Therefore, the internal surface of the large intestine is smooth. The longitudinal muscular coat of the colon does not surround the wall completely, as is the case in the small intestine, but there are three muscular bands, called **taenia coli.**

The measurements of the different parts of the gastrointestinal tract are listed in Table 10-1.

The total time for certain types and certain quantities of food to pass through the entire gastrointestinal tract varies enormously in different individuals, and with changing conditions. The time required before the food is emptied from the stomach varies widely and may be up to five hours. Thus food (or a drug) may reach the colon where practically no absorption of drugs occurs; this may be only two and one-half hours in the most rapid passage, but it may also require eight hours or more. The food or drugs are stored in the colon for several hours, so that the total time spent between intake until rectal excretion is somewhere between sixteen and twenty-four hours or even longer.

Gastrointestinal Motility and Secretion

Secretions are produced by glands which are found throughout the entire gastrointestinal tract. The secretions mix with the food by means of peristalsis and digest it. We distinguish between two different types of secretions: (1) mucus, which is for the protection of the intestinal wall and (2) enzymes, which break the large chemical compounds in the food into simpler, smaller compounds. The gastrointestinal motility and secretions are summarized in Tables 10-2 and 10-3. In man, the greatest variation is in the gastric transit time (e.g., 0.3 to 9.2 h) whereas the small intestine transit time is within a more narrow range (e.g., 0.9 to 5.5 h). It should also be noted that the formulation of a drug product can often affect gastrointestinal transit time in individuals with a normally functioning GI tract (Table 10-4). Finally, in disease states where gastric and/or intestinal motility is altered (e.g., gastroesophageal reflux, diabetic gastroparesis, infectious diarrhea), the overall pattern of drug absorption may vary as both a consequence of drug formulation and disease.

Table 10-1. Biopharmaceutical Data of the Gastrointestinal Tract

ANATOMICAL UNIT	AVERAGE LENGTH [cm]	DIAMETER [cm]	VILLI PRESENT	ABSORPTION MECHANISM	pH	ENZYMES & OTHERS	AMOUNT OF SECRETION [ml/DAY]
Mouth cavity	15–20	10	—	Passive diffusion Convective transport	6.4	Ptyalin Maltase Mucin	Saliva: 500–1500
Esophagus	25	2.5	—	—	5–6	—	—
Stomach	20	15	—	Passive diffusion Convective transport Active transport(?)	1–3.5	Pepsin Lipase Rennin Hydrochloric acid	Gastric Fluid: 2000–3000
Duodenum	25	5	+	Passive diffusion Convective transport Active transport Facilitated transport Ion pair Pinocytosis	6.5–7.6	Bile Trypsin Chymotrypsin Amylase Maltase Lipase Nuclease CYP3A4/5 P-gp MRP OATP OCT	Bile: 250–1100 Pancreatic Juice: 300–1500

							Intestinal Fluid: 3000
Jejunum	300	5	++	Passive diffusion Convective transport Active transport Facilitated transport	6.3–7.3	Erepsin Amylase Maltase Lactase Sucrase CYP3A4/5 P-gp MRP OATP OCT	
Ileum	300	2.5–5	++	Passive diffusion Convective transport Active transport Facilitated transport Ion pair Pinocytosis	7.6	Lipase Nuclease Nucleotidase Enterokinase	—
Cecum	10–30	7	+	Passive diffusion Convective transport Active transport Pinocytosis	7.5–8.0	—	—
Colon	150	5	—	Passive diffusion Convective transport	7.9–8.0	—	—
Rectum	15–19	2.5	—	Passive diffusion Convective transport Pinocytosis	7.5–8.0	—	—

Table 10-2. Motility in the Gastrointestinal Tract

AREA	TYPE	SPEED	FREQUENCY	CONTROL MECHANISM	RESULT
Mouth	Chewing	Variable	Variable	Initiated voluntarily, proceeds reflexly	Reduction in size, mixing with saliva
Pharynx	Swallowing		Maximum 20/min	Initiated voluntarily, reflexly controlled by swallowing center	Clears mouth of food
Esophagus	Peristalsis	5 cm/sec	Depends on frequency of swallowing	Initiated by swallowing	Transport through esophagus
Stomach	Receptive relaxation		According to frequency of swallowing	Unknown	Filling of the stomach
	Tonic contractions		15–20/min	Inherent by plexuses	Mix and churn
	Peristalsis	Variable	1–2/min	Inherent	Mixing with gastric secretions, finally emptying of the stomach
	Hunger contractions			Low blood sugar level	"Feeding"

	Type of movement	Velocity	Frequency	Stimulus	Function
Small intestine	Peristalsis	1–2 cm/min	17–18/min	Inherent	Movement through tube
	Peristaltic rush	2–25 cm/sec			Transport
	Segmentation (regularly spaced, isolated, irregularly spaced, weak but regularly spaced)		13/min in jejunum, 8–10/min in ileum		Mixing
	Pendular		Variable	Inherent	Mixing
	Villus movements, shortening and waving		Variable	Villikinin	Facilitates absorption
Colon	Peristalsis		3–12/min	Inherent	Transport and absorption of water and electrolytes
	Mass movement		3–4/day	Stretch	Fills pelvic colon
	Haustrations		Lasting ca. 30 sec		Rolling over for water absorption
	Tonic		3–12/min	Inherent	Mixing
	Segmentation		3–12/min	Inherent	Mixing
	Defecation		Variable 1/day–3/week	Reflex triggered by rectal distention	Emptying of rectum

Table 10-3. Gastrointestinal Secretions and Principal Digestive Enzymes

LOCATION	SECRETION	ENZYME	SUBSTRATE	PRODUCT OR FUNCTION
Mouth	Saliva	Ptyalin	Starch	Dextrin and maltose
Stomach	Gastric juice (with HCl)	Pepsin	Proteins	Proteoses, peptones, polypeptides
		Rennin (esp. in infants)	Caseinogen	Casein
		Gastric lipase	Emulsified fats (cream, egg yolks)	Glycerol, fatty acids
Pancreas	Pancreatic fluid	Trypsin Chymotrypsin	Proteins and proteoses	Small polypeptides
		Peptidases	Peptides	Amino acids
		Nucleases	Nucleoproteins	Nucleosides, bases
		Amylase	Starch	Maltose
		Lipase	Fats	Glycerol, fatty acids
Liver	Bile	no enzymes		Emulsification of fats
Small intestine	Intestinal Juice	Peptidases	Polypeptides	Amino acids
		Lipase	Fat	Glycerol, fatty acids
		Sucrase	Sucrose	Glucose + fructose
		Maltase	Maltose	Glucose
		Lactase	Lactose	Glucose + galactose

Throughout the gastrointestinal tract mucus is secreted for lubrication and protection of the gastrointestinal wall.

Table 10-4. Transit (TT) and Arrival (AT) Times of Segments of the Normal Human GI Tract for Selected Pharmaceutical Dosage Forms

DOSAGE FORM	GASTRIC TT	SMALL INTESTINE TT	COLON AT	COLON TT
Tablets	2.7 ± 1.5	3.1 ± 0.4	4.4 ± 1.0	—
Pellets	1.2 ± 1.3	3.4 ± 1.0	4.5 ± 2.1	—
Capsules	0.8 ± 1.2	3.2 ± 0.8	3.9 ± 1.9	16.2
Oral Solution	0.3 ± 0.07	4.1 ± 0.5	4.4 ± 0.5	—

Data expressed as mean or mean $\pm$ SD hours for adult subjects with normal physiology

Gastrointestinal Absorption

Absorption is the process of transferring chemical substances from the gastrointestinal tract through its wall into the bloodstream and lymphatic stream. While there is no specific difference in absorption between drugs or food, there are different mechanisms of absorption and there are also differences in absorption at different parts of the GI tract.

Most of the absorption of food takes place in the small intestine. (See Table 10-5.) This very long and narrow tube has a tremendously large surface area due to the millions of macrovilli and microvilli. The macrovillus consists of loose connective tissue and a network of capillaries. It is covered by columnar epithelial cells. The capillaries come from an arteriole at the base of the macrovillus. The blood from the capillaries is then drained into the mesenteric veins. Each macrovillus also has a lacteal duct, which ends blindly at its top and joins a larger tube at its base, which is connected with the surrounding macrovilli. The tube system of lymph vessels of the intestine empties into larger vessels and finally into the thoracic duct.

Table 10-5. Absorption of Food

MATERIAL ABSORBED	AREA	ROUTE OF ABSORPTION
Water	Entire gastrointestinal tract	Blood and lymph capillaries into systemic circulation
Vitamins	Stomach and small intestine	Blood and lymph capillaries into systemic circulation
Inorganic salts	Small and large intestine	Blood and lymph capillaries into systemic circulation
Amino acids	Small intestine	Blood capillaries → portal vein → liver → synthesized into proteins or enzymes, systemic circulation
Sugars	Small intestine	Blood capillaries → portal vein— liver (energy) → systemic circulation (energy), excess stored as glycogen
Glycerides, glycerol fatty acids	Small intestine	Lacteals → thoracic duct → jugular vein → systemic circulation → fat depots or storage and synthesis into new products in the liver

Most drugs are absorbed by passive diffusion in the form of the nonionized moiety. Commonly the pH in the intestines is considered to be alkaline although this is not true. In the duodenum and the upper parts of the small intestine, the pH is slightly acidic to neutral. It is only in the terminal ileum and in the colon that we have a neutral to slightly alkaline pH.

Scarcely any absorption of food occurs from the large intestine, since it was not designed for such a function due to the absence of villi. However, large amounts of water are absorbed from the large intestine.

The passage of either food or drugs through the intestinal mucosa into the bloodstream and lymphatic stream is very complex and cannot be explained solely by the physical laws of diffusion, filtration, and osmosis. There are also active transport principles involved, based on energy utilization. Furthermore, there is a possibility of selective absorption, because some highly soluble inorganic salts such as sodium chloride are absorbed, whereas others, like sodium sulfate, are not. The same is true of many sugars which are readily absorbed, whereas other sugars, even with smaller molecular weight, are not absorbed. Apart from the specific mechanism of absorption for a particular drug which follows either passive diffusion, convective transport, active transport, facilitated transport, ion-pair absorption, or pinocytosis, we must consider many other factors, such as pK_a value of the drug, the pH of the drug product, whether it is buffered or unbuffered, the pH of the part of the GI tract involved, the solubility of the drug and its dissolution rate, the particle size, polymorphism, whether amorphous or crystalline, the viscosity of the drug environment, the influence of food taken concomitantly with the drug product, the stomach emptying rate, influence of diseases, etc. Additionally, the bioavailability of specific drugs may be influenced by the activity of drug-metabolizing enzymes (CYP3A4/5) and various efflux transporters (e.g., P-glycoprotein, MRP, OATP, OCT; see Chapter 6) that reside in enterocytes of the small intestine. Drugs that are substrates for CYP3A4/5 can be extensively metabolized by these enzymes (thereby increasing presystemic clearance) which have the same activity and affinity for the respective CYP3A isoforms that exist in the liver. Drugs that are substrates for these efflux transporters can be actively pumped back into the intestinal lumen, thereby increasing their excretion into stool and/or recycling them for availability of intestinal metabolism should they be substrates for enzymes present in the enterocytes that comprise the microvilli of the small bowel. Factors which influence gastrointestinal absorption are listed in Table 10-6.

As previously mentioned, most drugs are absorbed by passive diffusion. Only the nonionized moiety of the drug is absorbed. According to the pH partition hypothesis, the nonionized form has a higher lipid solubility. An acidic compound, if absorbed by passive diffusion, will therefore be absorbed primarily from the stomach. On the other hand, the solubility of the free acid may be much less than in the form of a salt, into which it is transformed in the intestines. But still, if an acidic drug is administered in the form of a salt and enters the stomach, it is precipitated as the free acid, which has such a fine particle size that dissolution occurs more rapidly than if it were administered in the large crystal form of its free acid. Even when a drug has a low pK_a value it still will be absorbed from the intestines. The reason is, according to the law of mass action, there is always a small proportion of nonionized drug which is available for absorption. Most of the acidic drug will be ionized in the intestines at pH values between 5 and 7 or even slightly more, but the very small amount of undissociated drug can be absorbed due to the large surface area of the small intestine. Then, according to the law of mass action, if the undissociated portion is withdrawn from the system by absorption, some of the ionized drug will become unionized and is then steadily absorbed.

Table 10-6. Factors Influencing Gastrointestinal Absorption

GROUP	FACTOR	EFFECT
Gastric emptying	Volume of meal	Increasing volume of ingested material results in initially increased gastric emptying, followed by decrease in emptying rate. Liquids are more rapidly emptied than solid material
	Type of meal	Fats decrease emptying rate
	Viscosity	Increasing viscosity reduces rate of emptying
	Osmotic pressure	Increasing osmotic pressure reduces rate of emptying
	Drugs	Anticholinergics, narcotics, analgesics, ethanol, bile salts, acidification decrease rate of emptying; glycerol and sodium bicarbonate increase rate of emptying
Intestinal motility, Transit time	Food Viscosity	Solid food delays transit time Increased viscosity delays transit time but decreases rate of dissolution and diffusion, too
	Drugs	Anticholinergics decrease motility and prolong transit time
Splanchnic blood flow	Food	Food uptake increases blood flow in splanchnic area
	Physical work	Hard physical work decreases blood flow in splanchnic area
Drug Interactions	Food	Drugs may interact with food components and form complexes of low solubility
	Enzyme activity	Enzymes in the GI tract may alter drugs through enzymatic reactions
	Mucus	Mucus of the GI tract may bind drugs and form complexes of low solubility
	Bile	Bile may form insoluble complexes with drugs; bile may increase wettability of drugs and accelerate dissolution rate

As soon as either food or drug has passed the epithelium of the gastrointestinal mucosa, there are two ways it can reach the systemic circulation. Most of the drugs, carbohydrates, amino acids, salts, and water enter through the villi, the small blood capillaries, and are conveyed by the superior and inferior mesenteric veins to the portal vein which then carries all of the venous blood from the small intestine, large intestine, stomach, and spleen to the liver. This pathway is the direct route of absorption. From the liver the drug and nutrients are taken by the hepatic veins to the inferior vena cava to the heart and thence to the entire circulation. Before the substances leave the liver and are further transported to the heart, they may undergo many changes by the liver, including their major metabolism. The second, or indirect route of gastrointestinal absorption is via the lacteals. Most of the fat is taken up by this route. The fat is in the lacteals in the form of an emulsion, which has a milky appearance. The contents of the lacteals and of the lymph vessels draining them are brought to the thoracic duct, which finally empties into the left subclavian vein near the heart.

Water is absorbed primarily from the small and large intestine. It is not only the water ingested; water is also absorbed from the gastrointestinal juices emptied into the tract. The total amount of water absorbed is approximately 5 liters/day or more.

Carbohydrates ingested are converted to monosaccharides, primarily to glucose. It is only in the form of monosaccharides that the body can utilize them. It is estimated that about 90 to 98 percent of the ingested carbohydrates are absorbed. The carbohydrates are absorbed by the direct channel via the blood capillaries.

Proteins ingested have to be converted to amino acids or to simple peptides before they can be absorbed, again through the direct channel via the blood capillaries. When proteins are introduced directly into the bloodstream without digestion, as in pathologic conditions, they are absorbed as such. Antibody formation within the bloodstream occurs and may cause allergic symptoms. The amount of proteins digested and absorbed depends on the type of food. Up to 99 percent of the proteins of milk, meat, and eggs are absorbed, but only 90 percent from whole wheat and roots, and only 25 percent from beans and potatoes.

Fats are hydrolized to fatty acids and glycerol. The fatty acids are emulsified by the bile salts and then pass, in the form of water-miscible compounds, into the intestinal epithelium where the complex between fatty acid and bile salts breaks up and the free fatty acids reunite with the absorbed glycerol to again form the fats. On leaving the epithelium, most of the fat enters the lacteals and the bloodstream via the lymphatic vessels through the thoracic duct at the left subclavian vein. Part of the fat also enters the circulation by the direct channel via the blood capillaries. The absorption of the fat-soluble vitamins A, D, E, and K is probably by the same route. After ingestion of fat-rich meals the concentration of fat in the blood rises, but soon falls off as the fat is utilized for the construction of phospholipids and similar compounds, or is deposited in depots, such as the subcutaneous fat depot or the intramuscular tissue.

Food and Bioavailability

Besides general information given in the preceding discussion and listed in Table 10-6 on factors influencing gastrointestinal absorption, one needs to also consider interactions between food and drugs other than binding, precipitation, adsorption, chelation, change in gastric and urinary pH, etc. Grapefruit juice may considerably increase peroral bioavailability of many CYP3A substrates by *inhibiting intestinal Phase I metabolism* by up to 300%, such as found for felodipine, nifedipine, nisoldipine, and nitrendipine. Many drugs are transported back from the enterocyte into the gastrointestinal lumen by the P-gp efflux transport system (see Chapter 6). If the grapefruit juice has higher affinity for P-gp than a drug, then the efflux may be inhibited and the bioavailability increases such as found for cyclosporine, vinca alkaloids, digoxin, fexofenadine, and others. Grapefruit juice has also affinity for the organic anion transport polypeptide, OATP, which would inhibit the influx of drugs transported by this system from the enterocyte to plasma, thus decreasing a drug's bioavailability.

Table 10-7. Methods Used To Assess the Absorption of Drugs and Drug Products (adapted from Hidalgo 2001 and Pelkonen et al. 2001)

METHODS	MODEL SYSTEM(S)	PURPOSE
In Vivo	Whole animal	Evaluate pharmacokinetics of absorption in an intact organism with comparable physiology to humans.
In Vitro	Excised tissue (perfused intestinal segments, everted sacs, intestinal mucosa, isolated enterocytes)	Determine absorption across different gastrointestinal segments by examining disappearance (uptake) of drug from lumen of gastrointestinal tissue containing absorptive cells and muscle, or cells alone (i.e., enterocytes maintained in culture).
	Membrane vesicles	Cell membrane preparations including brush-border and basolateral membrane vesicles suspended in buffer. Used to study drug uptake and/or metabolism.
	Cell cultures (Caco-2, canine kidney [MDCK], HT29)	Used to assess intestinal permeability as cells possess many of the transporters and enzymes present in normal human enterocytes.
	Artificial membranes (e.g., immobilized artificial membrane columns [IAM], parallel artificial membrane permeation assay [PAMPA])	Assesses drug permeation (absorption) based on lipophilicity using lipid surfaces that mimic cell membrane.
In silico	Computational (mathematical methods)	Prediction of absorption based upon molecular size, H-bonding capacity and consideration of the dynamic polar surface area.

Finally, one needs also to be aware of the fact that it has become common practice to "fortify" many processed foods, such as nonfat milk, orange juice, breakfast cereals, breads, noodles, and sugar, either with calcium, other minerals or vitamins, or both. Not informing patients about potential food-drug interactions with fortified foods may result in clinical failures with some drugs, such as the fluoroquinolones.

Assessment of Drug Absorption

Knowledge of the normal and abnormal physiology of the gastrointestinal tract and the physicochemical properties of a drug or drug product is key to comprehending the multifactorial determinants of drug absorption (e.g., influence of age, disease, pharmacogenetics of drug-metabolizing enzymes and/or transporters, interactions with concomitantly administered drugs or natural products). With regard to drug discovery, assessing the absorption of new pharmaceuticals before phase I clinical testing is increasingly possible and is attaining great importance in the drug development process. Approaches used for this purpose largely involve the application of in vitro, in vivo, and in silico model systems, examples of which are provided in Table 10-7.

Selected References

1. DeCoursey, R. M.: *The Human Organism*, 4th Ed., McGraw-Hill, Inc. New York 1974, p. 415.
2. Jacob, S. W. and Francone, C. A.: *Structure and Function in Man*, 3rd Ed., W. B. Saunders Co., Philadelphia 1974, p. 423.
3. Doherty, M. M. and Charman, W. N.: The Mucosa of the Small Intestine: Clinical Relevance as an Organ of Drug Metabolism. *Clin. Pharmacokinet.* 41:235–253 (2002).
4. Hidalgo, I. J.: Assessing the Absorption of New Pharmaceuticals. *Curr. Topics in Med. Chem.* 1:385–401 (2001).
5. McClintic, J. R.: *Basic Anatomy and Physiology of the Human Body*, J. Wiley & Sons, New York 1975, p. 444.
6. Pelkonen, O., Boobis, A. R., and Gundert-Remy, U.: In Vitro Prediction of Gastrointestinal Absorption and Bioavailability: An Experts' Meeting Report. *Eur. J. Clin. Pharmacol.* 57:621–629 (2001).
7. Shepro, D., Belamarich, F. and Levy, C.: *Human Anatomy and Physiology*, Holt, Rinehart and Winston, Inc., New York, 1974, p. 343.
8. Vander, A. J., Sherman, J. H. and Luciano, D. S.: *Human Physiology*, 2nd Ed., McGraw-Hill, Inc., New York, 1975, p. 355.
9. Wheeler, R., Neo., S.-Y., Chew, J., Hladky, S. B., Barrand, M. A.: Use of Membrane Vesicles to Investigate Drug Interactions with Transporter Proteins, P-glycoprotein and Multidrug Resistance-Associated Protein. *Int. J. Clin. Pharmacol. Ther.* 38:122–129 (2000).
10. Wallace, A. W. and Amsden, G. W.: Is it Really OK to Take this with Food? Old Interactions with a New Twist. *J. Clin. Pharmacol.* 42:437–443 (2002).
11. Lee, M., Min, D. I., Ku, Y. M. and Flanigan, M.: Effect of Grapefruit Juice on Pharmacokinetics of Microemulsion Cyclosporin in African American Subjects Compared with Caucasian Subjects: Does Ethnic Difference Matter? *J. Clin. Pharmacol.* 41:317–323 (2001).

11

Fluid Compartments and Circulatory System

Upon entering the systemic circulation, a drug is distributed within the body by the flow of blood and lymph within the arterial-venous system. Usually the biophase—the place of drug-receptor interaction—is not the bloodstream but in the tissue. To exert its pharmacological effect, a drug has to cross not one but many membranes. The vehicle bringing the drug molecule to the membrane and carrying it away is the biological fluid. Although the circulating bloodstream and lymph stream are confined to a tube system there is a constant exchange of fluid between the circulatory system and tissue.

Anatomy of Circulatory System

The center of the circulatory system is the heart. The venous blood is pumped through the right atrium and right ventricle of the heart via the pulmonary arteries into the lungs and, after oxygenation in the capillary network of the alveoli, returns via the pulmonary veins to the heart, entering it through the left atrium (pulmonary circulation). From the left ventricle the blood is pumped into the aorta which branches into smaller arteries supplying the upper part of the body (head, arms, chest) and lower part of the body (liver, kidney, GI tract, and legs) with oxygenated blood. The arteries branch into arterioles which finally branch into a fine network of capillaries (microcirculation) where the exchange of gases, nutrients, metabolic products, and drug distribution between circulatory system and tissue takes place. From the capillary bed the blood enters the venous system through venules which empty into veins and finally returns to the right atrium of the heart. A schematic diagram of the circulatory system is given in Figure 11-1.

Arteries, arterioles, capillaries, venules, and veins differ anatomically according to the function of the different segments of the circulatory tube system. They all have one common characteristic: the one cell layer thick endothelium which forms the capillaries is present in all other parts of the circulatory system, including the heart, as the inner lining of the tube system. Arteries consist of a single layer of endothelium (*tunica intima*), a middle coat (*tunica media*) of smooth muscle, elastic and fibrous tissue which permits constriction and dilatation, and an outer coat (*tunica externa* or *adventitia*) of fibrous tissue which gives firmness to

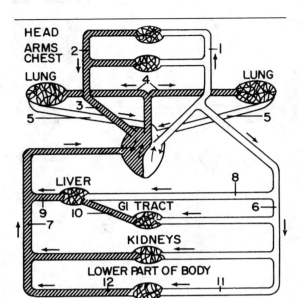

Figure 11-1. Schematic diagram of circulatory system.

 1 = Arteries to upper body
 2 = Veins from upper body
 3 = Superior vena cava
 4 = Pulmonary arteries
 5 = Pulmonary veins
 6 = Aorta
 7 = Inferior vena cava
 8 = Hepatic artery
 9 = Hepatic veins
10 = Portal vein
11 = Arteries to lower body
12 = Veins from lower body

the vessels. Arterioles consist of a single layer of smooth muscle cells. Venules consist of a single layer of endothelium covered with fibrous tissue. Veins, like arteries, have three layers; however, the middle and outer layers are thinner and fewer elastic fibers are present. Therefore veins collapse when cut. At intervals, semilunar valves are present.

The endothelial lining cells are supplied by blood flowing through the vessels. The cells of the middle and outer coats are supplied by tiny vessels known as "vessels of the vessels" (*vasa vasorum*). The smooth muscle cells of the middle coat are innervated by autonomic fibers controlled by the vasomotor center of the medulla (vasoconstriction, vasodilation).

The fibrous pericardium forms a loose-fitted inextensible sac around the heart, lined with the serous pericardium (parietal layer). The visceral layer of the serous pericardium (epicardium) covers the outer surface of the heart and adheres to it. Between the parietal and the visceral layers of the serous pericardium is the pericardial fluid (lubricating fluid). The pericardium protects the heart against friction. The heart wall is composed of the myocardium (cardiac muscle cells) and the endocardium (endothelial lining of the myocardium). The upper two chambers are the atria, and the lower two are the ventricles. The openings between the atria and ventricles are the atrioventricular orifices.

The blood is forced into the arteries at high pressure by the heart and is maintained at high pressure by the resistance offered by the arterioles, from which the capillary system supplies the tissue. At low pressure, the blood enters venules and finally veins, where valves keep the blood flowing towards the heart. Vasoconstriction and vasodilation of the larger blood vessels are controlled by the nervous system and by chemical "messengers" in the blood.

The volume of blood circulating each minute varies directly with the blood pressure gradient and inversely with the resistance opposing the blood flow. The mean arterial pressure varies directly with the cardiac minute output (cardiac minute output = heart rate · stroke volume). In Table 11-1 a schematic diagram of factors influencing the volume of circulating blood per minute is given.

In Figure 11-2 a comparison of anatomical structures with the different volumes of blood in the various anatomical parts of the arteriovenous system and the corresponding velocity and pressure of blood is given.

Table 11-1. Schematic Diagram of Control Mechanisms on Volume of Circulating Blood per Minute

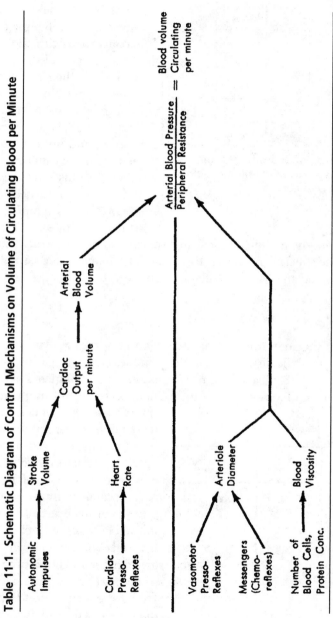

ANATOMICAL SEGMENT	ANATOMICAL STRUCTURE	VOLUME [cm³]	VELOCITY [cm·sec⁻¹]	PRESSURE [mm Hg]
AORTA	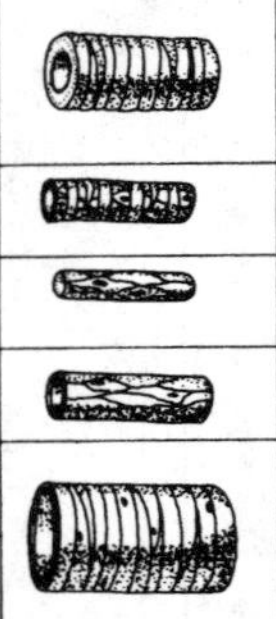	100	40	100
ARTERIES		325	40–10	100–80–40
ARTERIOLES		50	10–0.1	80–40–35
CAPILLARIES		250	<0.1	35–12
VENULES		300	<0.3	15–6
VEINS		2200	0.3–5	8–2
VENA CAVA		300	5–20	2–1

Figure 11-2. Comparison of anatomical segments of the arteriovenous system with volume, velocity of flow, and pressure of blood.

Homeostasis, the steady state which characterizes the internal environment of the healthy organism, is maintained by the circulation of blood and lymph. The lymphatic circulation is concerned with the recirculation of the interstitial fluid to the bloodstream and the maintenance of consistency of the blood itself. During the passage of the blood through the capillary network large molecules such as proteins and lipids (and also drugs) seep from the capillaries (along with water and salts) into the tissue spaces and are then returned to the bloodstream by the lymphatic capillaries which are collected by larger lymphatic vessels which empty into the thoracic duct (*ductus thoracicus*), which in turn empties near the heart into the subclavian vein. In Figure 11-3 a schematic diagram of exchange of substances between blood and lymph capillaries is given.

Microcirculation

An understanding of the anatomy and microcirculation of the capillary network is most important to comprehend the distribution of drugs in the body.

The major part of the capillary system arises as abrupt side branches of the thoroughfare channel where we find a muscle structure. The muscle cells form a ring around the entrance to the capillary. This ring is responsible for regulating the flow of the blood into the capillary network.

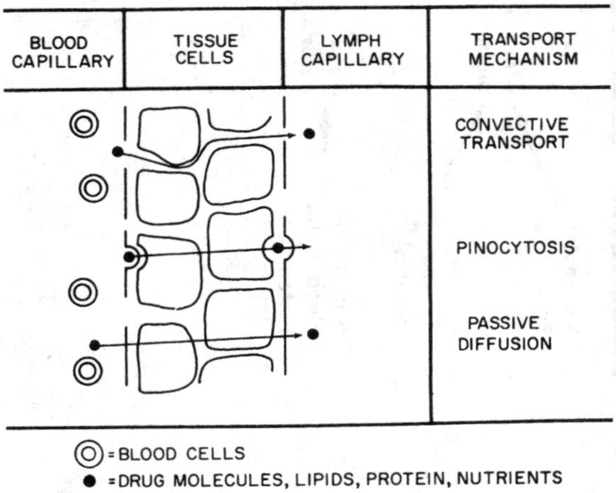

The microcirculatory system is present in every tissue of the body and the farthest capillary is within approximately 0.125 mm of any cell. The capillaries are formed by a single layer of flat endothelial cells, having a wall thickness of approximately 0.0025 mm. The diameter of capillaries is approximately 0.02 mm. Under the assumption that the average diameter of a human tissue cell is approximately 0.01 mm, and that the farthest capillary is within 0.125 mm of any cell, we can conclude that a drug molecule has to permeate through approximately up to 12 cells after it has been absorbed into systemic circulation in order to be

BLOOD CAPILLARY	TISSUE CELLS	LYMPH CAPILLARY	TRANSPORT MECHANISM
			CONVECTIVE TRANSPORT
			PINOCYTOSIS
			PASSIVE DIFFUSION

◎ = BLOOD CELLS
● = DRUG MOLECULES, LIPIDS, PROTEIN, NUTRIENTS

Figure 11-3. Schematic diagram of exchange of protein, lipids, nutrients, and drugs between blood and lymph capillaries.

distributed and reach the biophase. This explains the fast distribution of drugs, which is instant in the open one-compartment model and the central compartment of the open two-compartment model, and slower for those tissues comprising the peripheral compartment in the open two-compartment model.

The structures of the different organs and tissues in the body vary according to the characteristic needs of the tissues. Striated muscles, which contract rapidly and are under voluntary control, require more than 10 times as much blood for contraction than when at rest. To satisfy this requirement, each thoroughfare channel in striated muscle branches into 20 to 30 capillaries. On the other hand, glandular tissue requires only a minimum of blood supply and thus its thoroughfare channel may branch into only one or two capillaries. The skin protects the body from the outer environment. Here we find special shunts through which blood can pass directly from the arteries to the veins with a minimum loss of heat. Common for all types of tissue is a central thoroughfare channel whose muscle cells control the flow of blood into the capillaries.

The capillary network is the principal place of exchange and interchange of biological fluid, particularly between intravasal and interstitial fluid, but also with intracellular fluid. In oversimplification, we can compare living tissue as a collection of cells bathed in a fluid medium. The interstitial fluid brings nutrients and drugs to the cells and carries away waste products. The total length of capillaries in the adult is estimated to be 95,000 km. The microcirculation is controlled by messenger substances in the blood and specific chemical products of tissue metabolism.

In Figure 11-4 a schematic diagram is given of the anatomical boundaries between different fluids.

Body Fluids

The whole body fluid (WBF) in man comprises approximately 60 percent of the body weight. The WBF consists of intracellular fluid (ICF) and extracellular fluid (ECF). The ECF is further subdivided into plasma and interstitial fluid (ISF). The three fluid compartments for pharmacokinetic consideration are therefore: (1) intravasal fluid compartment, (2) interstitial fluid compartment, and (3) intracellular fluid compartment.

However, although these compartments are anatomical and morphological entities, exchange of fluid and of substances dissolved in them takes place between the compartments. The rate of exchange of drugs from one fluid compartment to another depends on many factors such as pK_a of drug, pH of fluid

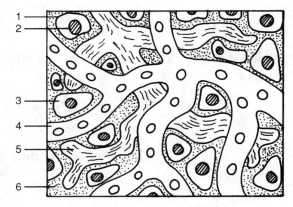

Figure 11-4. Anatomical boundaries between different body fluids.
1 = cell
2 = nucleus
3 = intracellular fluid
4 = blood capillary containing intravasal fluid (extracellular fluid)
5 = lymph capillary containing extracellular fluid
6 = interstitial fluid (extracellular fluid)

compartment, lipid/water partition coefficient, extent of protein binding, type of transport mechanism, and the rate of blood flow.

The whole body fluid (WBF) can be determined from the volume of distribution of any substance which is a nonelectrolyte and mixes or dissolves in water such as ethanol, antipyrine, D_2O, tritium oxide, etc.

The plasma volume, V_p, can be determined using indicators such as Evan's blue, trypan red, ^{131}I-albumin, tetraiodine, fluorescein, etc. It is 4.3 percent of the body weight in male adults. Since:

$$V_B = V_E + V_p \tag{1}$$

and:

$$H = \frac{V_E}{V_B} \cdot 100 \tag{2}$$

V_B = volume of blood
V_E = volume of erythrocytes
V_p = volume of plasma
H = hematocrit

then upon determination of V_p and H, one can calculate the total blood volume as expressed in Equation 11.3, which includes a correction factor for the plasma trapped in the erythrocyte volume:

$$V_B = V_p \cdot \frac{100}{100 - (0.87 \cdot H)} \tag{3}$$

The blood volume can also be calculated according to Equations 11.4 and 11.5 for males and females:

$$V_{B\ Men}[liter] = 0.3669 \cdot H^3[m] + 0.03219 \cdot BW[kg] + 0.6041 \tag{4}$$

$$V_{B\ Women}[liter] = 0.3651 \cdot H^3[m] + 0.03308 \cdot BW[kg] + 0.1833 \tag{5}$$

H = height
BW = body weight

The extracellular fluid (ECF) can be determined using indicators such as thiosulfate, mannitol, or inulin which equilibrate within the ECF only. The ECF comprises the plasma, easily diffusible and nondiffusible interstitial fluid, and the transcellular fluid as shown in Table 11-2. The ECF shows the largest variations among the fluid compartments between children and adults. In pharmacokinetic studies, it is important to realize that the volumes of the fluid compartments may change during the course of the day. During sleep the ISF is

Table 11-2. Fluid Compartments

COMPARTMENT	PERCENT OF BODY WEIGHT	REMARKS
Extracellular Fluid		
Plasma	4.3	4.1 percent in women $V_P = V_B - V_E$
Interstitium (easily diffusible fluid, including lymph)	9.0	$ISF = ECF - V_B$
Interstitium (non-diffusible fluid in connective tissue, cartilage and bones)	11.0	
Transcellular fluid (in GI tract, ureter, gall ducts, CNS, bulbi of eyes)	2.5	
Total in adults and aged	26.8	Thiosulfate method
Total in newborns	37.0	Thiosulfate method
Total in prematures	45.0	Thiosulfate method
Intracellular Fluid		
In adults	33.0	$ICF = WBF - ECF$
In aged	~20.0	$ICF = 0.67 \cdot CM$
In children	~37.0	(CM = cell mass)
Whole Body Fluid		
In adults	59.8	Percent of whole body fluid
In children 2–7 years	63.1	in women is 10–15 percent
In children up to 6 months	72.2	lower than in men.
In newborns up to 10 days	77.6	
In aged	M:45 F:37	
Blood Volume		
In adults	6.5–7.7	
In newborns	10.0	

increased. Intake of salt, edema, and drugs (amidopyrine, phenylbutazone, estrogens, testosterone, corticosteroids, anabolic hormones, ACTH) increase ECF, particularly the ISF. Any change in volume may change the drug concentration and, hence, result in fluctuations of blood level curves, within one subject and from subject to subject.

Water absorbed from the GI tract passes to the largest extent into the bloodstream, thus becoming part of the plasma compartment (water-loading). In order to maintain homeostasis, the plasma compartment has four routes for exit of fluid: kidneys, lungs, skin, and the interstitial compartment ISF. Fluid excreted via kidney, lung, and skin is irretrievably lost. The fluid passing into the interstitial fluid may further pass into cells or may move back into the bloodstream or pass into the lymph stream. From the latter route it is returned into the bloodstream. In order to maintain homeostasis, the input of fluid into the body has to be equal to the output from the body. The input in the adult comprises approximately 2500 ml/day out of which 2300 ml/day are ingested (food and drink) and 200 ml/day are metabolic water. The output comprises approximately 2500 ml/day (lungs 300, skin 500, urine 1500, feces and mouth 200 ml/day).

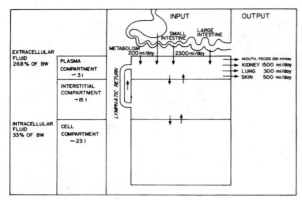

Figure 11-5. Relationship between fluid compart-ments and fluid input and output.

The interrelationship between the fluid compartments and input and output is shown in the schematic diagram of Figure 11-5.

The blood flow rates (Table 11-3) are of paramount importance for various pharmacokinetic processes, such as: the mesenteric blood flow rate for absorption in order to maintain a large concentration gradient across the intestinal epithelium, the liver blood flow rate in case of first-pass effect and rate of metabolism, blood flow rates in tissues for drug distribution to peripheral compartments, and renal blood flow rate for urinary excretion.

The blood flow rates may vary widely between rest and exercise (Table 11-3). As well, blood flow rates decrease with age beyond age of 25 years. The decrease may range from 0.35 percent per year in the brain to 1.9 percent per year in the kidney.

Table 11-3. Blood Flow Rates in Healthy Adult Humans

ORGAN	PERCENT OF CARDIAC OUTPUT	PERCENT OF BODY WEIGHT	FLOW RATE [ml · min⁻¹ · 100 g tissue⁻¹]	AVERAGE FLOW RATE IN ORGAN [ml · min⁻¹]	RANGE BETWEEN REST AND MAXIMUM EXERCISE [ml · min⁻¹]
Lungs	100	1.5	400	4200	4000–6100
Kidneys	20	0.5	350	1225	1100–1400
Liver	24	2.8	85	1666	500–3000
Heart	4	0.5	84	294	200–1000
Brain	12	2.0	55	770	750–2100
G.I. Tract	24	2.8	72	1400	700–5500
Skeletal Muscle	23	40.0	5	1400	750–18000
Muscle, Deltoid			11.6		
Muscle, Vastus			10.8		
Muscle, Gluteus			9.6		
Forearm			1.9		
Skin	6	10.0	5	350	200–3800
Adipose Tissue	10	19.0	3	399	

Selected References

1. Dost, F. H.: *Grundlagen der Pharmakokinetik,* 2nd Ed., Georg Thieme Verlag, Stuttgart, 1968, p. 5.
2. Langley, L. L., Telford, I. R. and Christensen, J. B.: *Dynamic Anatomy and Physiology,* 4th Ed., McGraw-Hill, New York, 1974, p. 466.
3. Mapleson, W. W.: An Electric Analogue for Uptake and Exchange of Inert Gases and Other Agents, *J. Appl. Physiol. 18:*197 (1963).
4. Shepro, D., Behamarich, F. and Levy, C.: *Human Anatomy and Physiology: A Cellular Approach,* Holt, Reinhart and Winston, Inc., New York, 1974, p. 312.

12

Binding of Drugs to Biological Material

Blood plasma contains 93 percent water. The balance of 7 percent consists of different dissolved compounds, primarily proteins. The main protein fraction is albumin which constitutes approximately 5 percent of the total plasma. Proteins are found not only in plasma but also in tissue. Many drugs are bound to plasma and tissue proteins. The extent of protein binding of a drug is influenced by many factors but within a certain dosage level it remains within a relatively small, more or less constant range. Usually drug binding occurs on albumin, although drugs may be bound to different types of protein. Albumin has the ability to reversibly bind drug molecules to its surface. The chemical structure of a drug influences the extent of its binding to proteins. Many substances of low molecular weight are almost completely bound to plasma proteins. Only the free drug, unbound by protein, can exert a pharmacological action by interaction with receptors. A schematic diagram of drug-protein binding, distribution, and drug-receptor interaction is given in Figure 12-1.

Human serum albumin has a molecular weight of approximately 67,500 and is composed of 20 different amino acids. The different kinds of amino acids and their relative position in the protein molecule determine the binding of drugs. The basic groups of the amino acids arginine, histidine, and lysine are responsible for binding acidic drugs and the acidic groups of the amino acids aspartic acid, glutamic acid, and tyrosine are responsible for binding basic drugs. At blood pH of 7.4, the acidic carboxyl groups are protonized to positive ions. These groups form positively and negatively charged sites on the protein molecule attracting ions of opposite charge by electrostatic forces. Drugs can be bound to albumin by van der Waal's forces, by hydrophobic bonds, by hydrogen bonds, and by ionic bonds. Acidic drugs are strongly bound to albumin, usually one or two molecules per molecule albumin. Basic, positively charged drugs are weakly bound to a larger number of sites on the albumin molecule. Often interactions between basic drugs and protein are without clinical importance.

Although albumin constitutes the largest proportion of plasma proteins and is predominantly responsible for binding of drugs, there is another protein fraction, α_1-acid glycoprotein (AAG), which has received considerable attention during the past years. AAG, also known as orosomucoid, is an α_1-globulin, having a molecular weight of 41,000 to 45,000, and consists of a linear polymer of amino acids with branching chains of carbohydrate. The plasma concentration of AAG is normally only 0.6 to 0.8 g/l. AAG has only one high affinity binding site and binds only basic, highly lipophilic drugs. Drugs for which significant binding to AAG in plasma has been found are listed in Table 12-1.

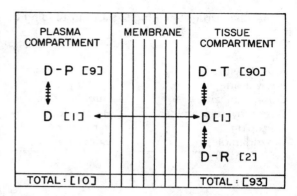

Figure 12-1. Distribution and binding of a hypothetical drug to plasma and tissue proteins.
D   = free unbound drug
D-P = drug bound to plasma protein
D-T = drug bound to tissue protein
D-R = drug bound to receptors in the biophase
[]   = concentrations
↔   = true equilibrium at steady state
⇎   = constant ratio of distribution at steady state

Drug binding to protein is usually rather nonspecific, i.e., many drugs bind to the same binding sites (receptors) on the protein molecule. The drug with the higher affinity will, therefore, displace a drug of lower affinity from its binding site by competition. Since only the non-protein-bound fraction is free for pharmacological action, intensity of pharmacological response, side effects, and toxicity increase upon displacement from protein binding sites. This is of importance only in drugs highly bound to protein. If, for instance, a drug is normally 98 percent bound to protein and another drug given simultaneously competes for the same binding sites and displaces some of the first drug so that it becomes only 94 percent bound, the level of free, non-protein-bound drug increases from 2 to 6 percent, or 200 percent more free drug.

The extent of protein binding is determined in vitro by dialysis, ultracentrifugation, ultrafiltration, Sephadexgel filtration, molecular filtration, electrophoresis, or by agar plate test. The extent of protein binding is usually given in percentage. However, one must be aware that percent bound is a function of the capacity of the protein and the concentration of the drug bound in the environment.

Calculation of Protein Binding

Drug binding to protein can be considered as a reversible process as given in Equation 12.1:

$$[D]+[P] \underset{K_d}{\overset{K_a}{\rightleftarrows}} [D-P] \tag{1}$$

[D]   = concentration of free drug [M/l]
[P]   = concentration of free protein [M/l]
[D−P]= drug-protein complex concentration
K_a = association constant
K_d = dissociation constant = $1/K_a$

The association constant is expressed by Equation 12.2:

Table 12-1. Drugs Showing Significant Binding to α_1-Acid Glycoprotein

Alfentanil	Disopyramide	Lofentanil	Pindolol
Alprenolol	Erythromycin	Meperidine	Prazosin
Amitriptyline	Etidocaine	Methadone	Propranolol
Bupivacaine	Fentanyl	Nortriptyline	Quinidine
Chlorpromazine	Fluphenazine	Oxprenolol	Sufentanil
Desmethylimipramine	Haloperidol	Perazine	Thioridazine
Diazepam	Imipramine	Perphenazine	Timolol
Dipyridamole	Lidocaine	Phencyclidine	Trihexyphenidyl

$$K_a = \frac{[D-P]}{[D] \cdot [P]} \tag{2}$$

The drug-protein complex can be expressed by Equation 12.3:

$$[D-P] = K_a \cdot [D] \cdot [P] \tag{3}$$

The quantity of binding r is defined as moles of drug bound divided by total moles of protein present:

$$r = \frac{[D-P]}{[D-P]+[P]} \tag{4}$$

Upon substitution $[D-P]$ in Equation 12.4 by Equation 12.3 and dividing by $[P]$ one obtains Equation 12.5:

$$r = \frac{K_a \cdot [D]}{1 + K_a \cdot [D]} \tag{5}$$

If there are more independent binding sites a series of equations results which can be summated to Equation 12.6 for the total quantity of binding r_{total}:

$$r_{total} = \frac{N \cdot K_a \cdot [D]}{1 + K_a \cdot [D]} \tag{6}$$

N = number of binding sites.

Since [D] can be measured and r can be calculated from total and free drug concentrations and the protein concentration, one can determine N and K_a upon plotting. Figure 12-2 shows three different methods for drug-protein binding plots.

Pharmacokinetic Importance of Protein Binding

Drug-protein binding is of influence on the distribution equilibrium of drugs. Plasma proteins may exert a "buffer and transport function" in the distribution process. Only the free, non-protein-bound fraction of drug can leave the circulatory system and diffuse into tissue. The equilibrium between free and bound drug acts as a "buffer" system, since a relatively constant concentration of free drug can be maintained over a relatively long period of time due to the dissociation of the drug-protein complex. The "transport" function of plasma proteins is of importance for drugs of low solubility in water. Often hydrophobic drugs are found to be considerably bound to plasma proteins, and also to erythrocytes.

In Figure 12-3 a schematic diagram is given for drug distribution in the organism. Once equilibrium is established, it is assumed that the free, unbound concentration of drug is identical in all compartments.

If the free drug fraction, f_u, the free drug concentration, $f_u \cdot C$, and the bound drug concentration, $(1 - f_u) \cdot C$, are substituted into Equation 12.2 and rearranged, the fraction of free drug is:

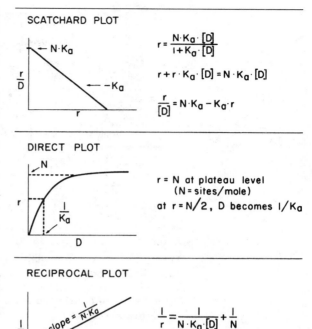

SCATCHARD PLOT

$$r = \frac{N \cdot K_a \cdot [D]}{1 + K_a \cdot [D]}$$

$$r + r \cdot K_a \cdot [D] = N \cdot K_a \cdot [D]$$

$$\frac{r}{[D]} = N \cdot K_a - K_a \cdot r$$

DIRECT PLOT

r = N at plateau level
(N = sites/mole)
at r = N/2, D becomes $1/K_a$

RECIPROCAL PLOT

$$\frac{1}{r} = \frac{1}{N \cdot K_a \cdot [D]} + \frac{1}{N}$$

Figure 12-2. Methods for plotting drug-protein binding data in order to obtain information on the number of binding sites per mole and the association rate constant.

$$f_u = \frac{1}{1 + K_a \cdot [P]} \qquad (7)$$

Hence, f_u depends only on the unbound protein concentration [P], and the association constant K_a. Considering the apparent volume of distribution of a drug and its relationship to plasma and tissue distribution, the V_d can be characterized as follows:

$$V_d = V_p + V_T \cdot \frac{f_u}{f_T} \qquad (8)$$

V_p = volume of plasma
V_T = volume of tissue
f_u = free fraction of drug in plasma
f_T = free fraction of drug in tissue

Since most drugs have a $V_d \gg V_p$, Equation 12.8 can be simplified to:

$$V_d = V_T \cdot \frac{f_u}{f_T} \qquad (9)$$

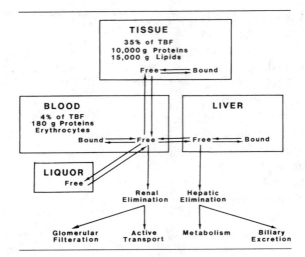

Figure 12-3. Schematic diagram of drug distribution in the body based on the concept of binding to biologic material. Only the free fraction is available for distribution and elimination. TBF = total body fluid.

which, upon multiplication of both sides by the concentration, gives the amount of drug in the body:

$$V_d \cdot C = \frac{V_T \cdot f_u \cdot C}{f_T} \tag{10}$$

Upon rearrangement the free drug concentration, $f_u \cdot C$, is obtained:

$$f_u \cdot C = V_d \cdot C \cdot \frac{f_T}{V_T} \tag{11}$$

This indicates that the free drug concentration is independent of plasma binding, but is dependent on tissue binding. The total drug concentration, C, is the ratio of free drug concentration divided by the free drug fraction.

The distribution equilibrium of drugs is significantly influenced by the affinity of low molecular weight substances to macromolecular structures in blood and tissue. The adult man has approximately 0.18 kg plasma proteins, 10 kg macromolecular structures in tissue (proteins, nucleic acids, etc.), and 15 kg fat. Lipophilic substances can pass easily through membranes and interact with macromolecules and fat in tissue. The quantitative relation of plasma to tissue macromolecules indicates that plasma protein binding should not be of significant influence on the distribution equilibrium of drugs of extremely high lipid solubility unless they have an extremely high affinity for plasma proteins, such as some hormones and vitamins. Plasma protein binding is of significant influence on the distribution equilibrium if the drug is polar and, therefore, diffuses slowly into tissue. If additionally, such a substance has a high affinity for plasma proteins, displacement from its protein binding sites may result in a change of distribution equilibrium and an altered pharmacological response. Lipophilic drugs can be bound more extensively to erythrocytes than to plasma proteins.

Disease and Protein Binding

Diseases may cause hypoalbuminemia as found in patients with burns, cancer, cardiac failure, cystic fibrosis, enteropathy, inflammations, liver impairment, malabsorption, nephrotic syndrome, renal failure, sepsis, and trauma. Also hypoalbuminemia is found in geriatric patients, after prolonged immobilization, during pregnancy, after prolonged stress, and in smokers.

Not only may the albumin concentration in plasma be reduced, but, additionally, the exchange of protein between plasma and the interstitial compartment, which normally proceeds at a rate of 5 percent plasma protein per hour (plasma to interstitial fluid by capillary filtration; return via the thoracic duct), may be hampered. The diffusion from plasma to the interstitial fluid is increased by inflammatory processes, during pregnancy, with use of oral contraceptives, in diabetes, and in septic shock and traumatic pulmonary edema. A decreased return of albumin from the interstitial fluid to plasma is found in neoplastic diseases, prolonged immobilization, cardiogenic shock, artificial respiration, and hemodynamic pulmonary edema. In some conditions hyperalbuminemia is found such as in patients with benign tumors, myalgia, neuroses, psychoses, schizophrenia, and paranoia.

In contrast to other proteins capable of binding drugs (e.g., AAG) and hormones (e.g., thyroid binding globulin, retinol binding protein, growth hormone binding protein), albumin has a relatively slow "turn-over" rate with a half-life of approximately 20 hours in man. As well, certain disease states can reduce the binding affinity of weak acids by producing conformational changes in the three dimensional structure of the protein. Examples include glycosylation of albumin in patients with poorly controlled diabetes mellitus and carbamylation of albumin in patients with uremia. Finally, the presence of acidosis and endogenous competing ligands (e.g., free fatty acids) can also reduce the capacity of drug binding to albumin.

Diseases may decrease the extent of plasma protein binding. Drugs for which such a decrease has been documented in liver diseases (chronic hepatitis, viral hepatitis, toxic hepatitis, cirrhosis, steatosis, hepatic tumors) and in renal diseases (acute and chronic renal failure, nephrosis) are listed in Table 12-2.

The free steady state drug concentration may not change in nephrotic patients; however, the time course of free drug may change during the dosing interval resulting in higher peak and lower trough concentrations.

In acute renal failure the concentration of total plasma proteins, particularly of albumin, is significantly reduced (up to approximately 25 percent) which may result in reduced protein binding (found

Table 12-2. Drugs Showing Decreased Extent of Protein Binding in Liver and/or Renal Diseases

LIVER DISEASES	RENAL DISEASES
Dapsone	Barbiturates
Diazepam	Cardiac glycosides
Morphine	Chlordiazepoxide
Phenytoin	Clofibrate
Prednisolone	Diazepam
Quinidine	Diazoxide
Tolbutamide	Furosemide
Triamterene	Morphine
	Phenylbutazone
	Phenytoin
	Salicylates
	Sulfonamides (some)
	Triamterene

Table 12-3. Pathological Conditions in which Plasma Concentration of α_1-Acid Glycoprotein is Increased

Cancer	Carcinoma, leukemia, lymphoma, malignant melanoma, myeloma
Inflammation	Crohn's disease, inflammatory polyarthritis, pneumonia, rheumatoid arthritis, ulcerative colitis, systemic erythematosus
Myocardial Infarction Trauma	Burns, extensive tissue damage, surgery, transplantation

to be approximately 20 to 50 percent of the amount of drug in μg bound per mg albumin, for 6 drugs studied). Under pathological conditions, the concentration of plasma AAG may increase considerably (up to 10-fold) as listed in Table 12-3.

Displacement from Protein Binding

The quantitative and clinical importance of displacement from protein binding depends on the total amount of drug in the body that is bound to plasma protein before displacement, the extent of displacement, the extent of binding to tissue structures, and the apparent volume of distribution. The actual increase in free drug concentration in plasma upon displacement of a drug highly bound to plasma proteins (> 80 to 90 %) depends on the apparent volume of distribution. If the V_d is large, the increase may be minimal; if it is small, the free plasma concentration and the concentration in the biophase may significantly rise and elicit a significant increase in intensity of drug action or toxicity. Displacement will be clinically important only if the V_d is less than 0.15 L/kg.

If the process of elimination is by glomerular filtration and metabolism in the hepatocyte, most displaced drugs will have a shortened elimination half-life. If the process of elimination is by active tubular secretion or metabolism after the drug has been actively transported into the hepatocyte, displacement will usually result in a prolonged elimination half-life.

Examples of clinical importance for displacement of drug from its plasma protein binding are listed in Table 12-4, and some facts on binding of drugs to biological material and its consequences are listed in Table 12-5.

Table 12-4. Displacement of Drugs from Their Plasma Protein Binding Sites by Other Drugs Given Concomitantly

DRUG DISPLACED	BY CONCOMITANT DRUG
Warfarin and other highly bound coumarin-type anticoagulants	Clofibrate Ethacrynic acid Mefenamic acid Nalidixic acid Oxyphenbutazone Phenylbutazone Chloral hydrate
Tolbutamide	Phenylbutazone Salicylates Sulfisoxazole

Table 12-5. Summary of Binding of Drugs to Biological Material and Storage

BINDING OF DRUGS:
— In plasma and tissue
— Primarily to protein, especially albumin and α_1-acid glycoprotein
— Is reversible (exception N-mustards, P-containing anticholinesterases)
— By weak bonds (van der Waal's and ionic bonds)
— Has mostly unspecific binding capacity for many drugs
— May be specific to tracer proteins (Cu $\rightarrow$ ceruloplasmin; Fe $\rightarrow$ siderophillin; hemin $\rightarrow$ haptaglobin, hemoglobin and hemopexin; insulin, thyroxine and cortisone $\rightarrow$ specific proteins)
— To one or two binding sites on the albumin molecule for acidic drugs; to one binding site on α_1-acid glycoprotein for basic drugs
— Can be displaced by other drugs with higher affinity (competition)
— Delays urinary excretion of drugs (protein bound drugs are not filtered through glomeruli)
— Increases elimination half-life (bound drugs cannot be metabolized and are not excreted)
— Is limited (limited binding capacity of the protein for the drug; saturation)

CONSEQUENCES:
— If two substances compete for the same binding sites the one with less affinity will be displaced, resulting in higher concentration of free drug. Only the free (not protein bound drug) is available for drug receptor interaction, hence pharmacologically active. The increased amount of free drug may result in toxicity (displacement of tolbutamide by sulfonamides $\rightarrow$ hypoglycemic coma; displacement of bilirubin by sulfonamides, salicylates etc. $\rightarrow$ kernicterus; displacement of warfarin by phenylbutazone $\rightarrow$ hemorrhage).
— The higher the protein binding of a drug the more severe toxic reaction is expected upon displacement, or if protein concentration is reduced (hypoalbuminemia, acute renal failure).
— Protein binding is the reason that certain drugs require higher loading doses and why lower maintenance doses have to be given.

STORAGE IN DEPOTS:
Some drugs are specifically stored in pools, such as vitamin B_{12} and antimalarials in the liver, chloroquine in the retina, iodine in the thyroid gland and drugs with extremely high lipid solubility (short acting barbiturates) in fat.

CONSEQUENCES:
The dose sizes of repeated doses should be equal to the amount which can be adequately metabolized by the body or eliminated from the body.

Uptake of Drugs by Red Blood Cells

Erythrocytes, red blood cells (RBC), have a lipid membrane perforated by positively charged aqueous channels of various diameters. Drug molecules may enter the cell by passing through the aqueous channels or by dissolving in the lipid membrane. The rate of drug entry is controlled primarily by the drug's lipid solubility, which is affected by the drug's ionization at physiologic pH (7.4) or altered pH in acidosis or alkalosis. Drugs bound to or taken up by erythrocytes are listed in Table 12-6.

The mechanisms and consequences of binding of drugs to erythrocytes can be summarized as follows:

Table 12-6. Binding or Uptake of Drugs to Erythrocytes

Acetazolamide	Chlorpromazine	Haloperidol	Pentazocine
Alfentanil	Clonazepam	Hydromorphone	Pentobarbital
Amantadine	Coumarin	Imipramine	Perphenazine
Amiodarone	Cyclosporine	Lidocaine	Phenytoin
Amitriptyline	Dapsone	Lithium	Prochlorperazine
Amobarbital	Desipramine	Lofentanil	Promazine
Artemisinin	Desmethylchlorpromazine	Lorazepam	Propranolol
Aspirin	Desmethyldiazepam	Mefloquine	Quinidine
Auranofin	Diazepam	Meperidine	Quinine
Bepridil	Digoxin	Methazolamide	Sufentanil
Bupivacaine	Doxepin	Methotrexate	Theophylline
Butaperazine	Doxycycline	Methotrimeprazine	Trifluoperazine
Chlorambucil	Fentanyl	Myocrisin	Triflupromazine
Chloroguanide	Flurazepam	Nortriptyline	
Chloroquine	Folate	Oxazepam	

- Lipophilic molecules may dissolve in the lipid material of the erythrocyte membrane and may cross it.
- Anions can be attracted to and enter the positively charged pores of erythrocytes.
- Lipophilic drugs may be adsorbed to the erythrocyte membrane (membrane stabilization) [chlorpromazine] due to a change of shape of membrane proteins, a change of shape of membrane, and membrane extension, sometimes leading to change of the shape of RBC [lidocaine, bupivacaine]. Drugs adsorbed to the erythrocyte membrane may inhibit the deformability of RBC, thus becoming lodged in capillaries. In turn, macrophages may recognize and remove such RBC. This could result in an increase in free drug concentration.
- Often the distribution in RBC [fentanyl, sufentanil, alfentanil, lofentanil, bepridil] follows: Hematocrit × fraction distributed to RBC = % distributed to RBC.
- Binding within erythrocytes to carbonic anhydrase [acetazolamide], oxyhemoglobin A and S [phenothiazines], or nucleoside transport system [benzodiazepines].
- Binding to erythrocytes may be age-dependent [meperidine], and concentration dependent [diazepam].
- The erythrocyte binding sites for drugs are: intracellular proteins, hemoglobin, carbonic anhydrase, cell membrane, and ATPase.
- Extended stay at high altitude results in increase (often doubling) of number of erythrocytes. Hence, drugs highly bound to RBC (such as meperidine) may become ineffective due to lack of free, unbound drug.
- Beneficial effects of RBC binding include a lower tissue uptake and lesser retention in critical organs like the kidney in the case of auranofin.

Binding (uptake) to erythrocytes, C_E, is determined from binding of drug in whole blood, C_B, and in plasma, C_P, and the hematocrit:

$$C_E = \frac{[C_B - C_P \cdot (1-H)] \cdot 100}{C_B} \tag{12}$$

where C_E is % of drug bound to RBC, C_B is the drug concentration in whole blood in µg/ml, C_P is the drug concentration in plasma in µg/ml, and H is the hematocrit as a fraction.

Selected References

1. Craig, W. A. and Welling, P. G.: Protein Binding of Antimicrobials: Clinical Pharmacokinetics and Therapeutic Implications, *Clin. Pharmacokinet. 2*:252 (1977).

2. Gugler, R. and Azarnoff, D. L.: Drug Protein Binding and the Nephrotic Syndrome, *Clin. Pharmacokinet. 1*:25 (1976).

3. Iberb, N. and Fluckiger, R.: Nonenzymatic Glycosylation of Albumin in vivo. Identification of Multiple Glycosylated Sites. *J. Biol. Chem. 261*(29):13542-3 (1986).

4. Jusko, W. J. and Gretch, M.: Plasma and Tissue Binding of Drugs in Pharmacokinetics, *Drug Metab. Rev. 5*:43 (1976).

5. Kearns, G. L., Kemp, S. F., Turley, C. P. and Nelson, D. L.: Protein Binding of Phenytoin and Lidocaine in Pediatric Patients with Type I Diabetes Mellitus, *Dev. Pharmacol. Ther. 11*:14–23 (1988).

6. Levy, R. H. and Moreland, T. A.: Free Drug Levels: Why, When, and How?, *Ther. Drug Monit. 5*:1 (1983).

7. Meuldermans, W. E. G., Hurkmans, R. M. A. and Heykants, J. J. P.: Plasma Protein Binding and Distribution of Fentanyl, Sufentanil, Alfentanil, and Lofentanil in Blood, *Arch. Int. Pharmacodyn. 257*:4–19 (1982).

8. Paxton, J. W.: Alpha$_1$-Acid Glycoprotein and Binding of Basic Drugs, *Methods Find. Exp. Clin. Pharmacol. 5*:635 (1983).

9. Rao, M. N. A. and Kumar, A.: Quantitative Activity Studies on Erythrocyte Binding of Salicylates. *Indian J. Exp. Biol. 23*:574–575 (1985).

10. Reidenberg, M. M. and Affrime, M.: Influence of Disease on Binding of Drugs to Plasma Proteins, *Ann. N.Y. Acad. Sci. 226*:115 (1973).

11. Ritschel, W. A., Paulos, C., Arancibia, A., et al.: Pharmacokinetics of Acetazolamide in Healthy Volunteers after Short- and Long-term Exposure to High Altitude, *J. Clin. Pharmacol. 38*:533 (1998).

12. Shanker, L. S., Johnson, J. M. and Jeffrey, J. J.: Rapid Passage of Organic Ions Into Human Red Cells, *Am. J. Physiol. 207*:503–508 (1964).

13. Shanker, L. S., Nafpliotis, P. A. and Johnson, J. M.: Passage of Organic Bases Into Human Red Cells, *J. Pharmacol. Exp. Ther. 133*:325–331 (1961).

14. Sjogvist, F., Borga, O. and Orme, M. L. E.: Fundamentals of Clinical Pharmacology. In: *Drug Treatment,* Avery, S., Editor. Adis Press, Sydney; Lea and Febiger, Philadelphia, Churchill Livingstone, Edinburg, 1976, p. 1.

15. Tillement, J. P., Lhoste, F. and Giudicelli, J. F.: Diseases and Drug Protein Binding, *Clin. Pharmacokinet. 3*:144 (1978).

16. Worner, W., Preissner, A. and Rietbrock, N.: Drug-protein Binding Kinetics in Patients with Type I Diabetes, *Eur. J. Clin. Pharmacol. 43*:97–100 (1992).

13

Drug Biotransformation

Most drugs that are administered to patients must possess some degree of lipophilicity to be absorbed from the gastrointestinal tract. Once absorbed, they circulate in blood bound to plasma proteins, such as albumin, and distribute into fat with relative tissue:blood ratios determined to a great extent by their degree of lipophilicity. As a result, lipophilic compounds are not readily excreted by the kidney into urine. Rather, conversion to more water-soluble or hydrophilic products is required to facilitate drug removal (i.e., clearance) from the body. This "conversion" takes place through a process known as *biotransformation*.

Most tissues and organs possess the ability to biotransform lipophilic drugs into more water-soluble metabolites. Because of its strategic location and specialized architecture, the liver is quantitatively the most important organ involved in drug biotransformation. However, other organs such as the small intestine, lung, and skin that interface with the external environment are also capable of drug/xenobiotic biotransformation and thus play important roles in protecting the organism from the potential harmful effects of some compounds.

Chemical modification of drugs generally results in termination of biological activity through decreased affinity for receptors or other cellular targets as well as more rapid elimination from the body. Thus, detoxification is an important function of drug biotransformation. However, detoxification is not the only biological consequence of drug biotransformation processes. In some cases, such as the conversion of prodrugs to a pharmacologically active form, bioactivation results in increased pharmacologic activity. Furthermore, the production of chemically reactive metabolites capable of binding irreversibly to cellular macromolecules such as proteins and nucleic acids may lead to toxicologic consequences (e.g., acetaminophen hepatotoxicity, carcinogenicity from heterocyclic hydrocarbons, teratogenicity from phenytoin).

Drug biotransformation can be a very complex process since there are several ways in which lipophilic compounds may be converted to more hydrophilic products. In general, there are several important characteristics that distinguish enzymes involved in drug biotransformation from other enzymes. First is the concept of *broad substrate specificity* whereby a single enzyme (isozyme) may metabolize a large variety of chemically diverse compounds. Secondly, many different enzymes may be involved in the biotransformation of a single drug;

this is a characteristic known as *enzyme multiplicity.* One example of product multiplicity is racemic warfarin where at least seven hydroxylated metabolites have been identified and are produced by different isoforms of cytochromes P450. Finally, a given drug may undergo several different reaction types; this is a substrate property often referred to as *polyfunctionality.* In man, the specificity and/or multiplicity of drug metabolizing enzymes, as well as the kinetic properties of the interaction between a substrate and enzyme, is generally determined directly from in vitro experiments using microsomes prepared from human tissue (e.g., liver) or cell lines which express a particular enzyme. Alternatively, indirect expressions of substrate characteristics can be inferred from pharmacokinetic studies where the clearance of a test compound is compared to the clearance or metabolite profile of another drug whose biotransformation has been previously characterized as being dependent upon a particular enzyme.

The numerous biotransformation reactions are conventionally classified into two main types, *phase I* and *phase II,* that generally occur sequentially. *Phase I reactions* introduce or reveal (e.g., by oxidation, reduction, or hydrolysis) a functional group within the substrate that can serve as a site for subsequent conjugation (i.e., phase II type) reactions. Phase I enzymes are found in several subcellular compartments including the cytoplasm (e.g., alcohol and aldehyde dehydrogenases, aldehyde oxidase, sulfoxide reductase) and mitochondria (e.g., monoamine oxidase, ketone reductases). Reductases which metabolize quinone, nitro, and ketone functional groups can be found associated with the cytoplasm and endoplasmic reticulum. Microsomal monooxygenases such as flavin-containing monooxygenases and, more importantly, the cytochromes P450 are quantitatively the most important oxidative enzymes responsible for drug biotransformation. *Phase II reactions* (e.g., conjugation by endogenous substrates such as sulfate, acetate, glucuronic acid, glutathione, and glycine) further increase water solubility and thereby facilitate elimination. Phase II enzymes include the glucuronosyl transferases (UGTs), sulfotransferases (STs), arylamine *N*-acetyl transferases (NAT1 and NAT2), glutathione *S*-transferases (GSTs), and methyl transferases (catechol *O*-methyl transferase, thiopurine *S*-methyl transferases, and several *N*-methyl transferases), all of which play an important role in the biotransformation of xenobiotics.

Cytochromes P450

The cytochromes P450 (or more properly, the hemethiolate P450s) represent a superfamily of heme-containing proteins that catalyze the metabolism of many lipophilic endogenous substances (e.g., steroids, fatty acids, fat-soluble vitamins, prostaglandins, leukotrienes, and thromboxanes) and exogenous compounds. In humans, 36 genes and 5 putative pseudogenes which code for the P450 enzymes have been described to date. These enzymes can be functionally divided into two distinct classes: (1) the steroidogenic enzymes expressed in specialized tissues such as the adrenal glands, gonads, and placenta, and (2) the P450s involved in the metabolism of drugs, pesticides, and environmental contaminants. The complement of known human cytochromes P450 is illustrated in Figure 13-1.

P450 nomenclature is based on evolutionary considerations and uses the root symbol "CYP" for *cy*tochrome *P*450. As reflected by Figure 13-1, P450s that share at least 40% homology are grouped into families denoted by an Arabic number following the CYP root. Subfamilies, designated by a letter, appear to represent clusters of highly related genes. Members of the human CYP2 family, for example, have greater than 67% amino acid

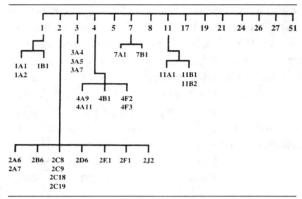

Figure 13-1. The human cytochromes P450 superfamily. Subfamilies are designated by letter and individual P450s in a subfamily are numbered sequentially.

sequence homology. Individual P450s in a subfamily are numbered sequentially (e.g., CYP3A4, CYP3A5). Cytochromes P450 that have been identified as being important in human drug biotransformation are predominantly found in the CYP1, CYP2, and CYP3 gene families.

Figure 13-2A indicates the relative content of cytochrome P450 isoforms in adult human liver. It is important to note that the relative contribution of a P450 isoform to the biotransformation of compounds used therapeutically may be disproportionate to its level of expression in liver (Figure 13-2B).

CYP3A4, CYP2D6, and members of the CYP2C subfamily (CYP2C8, CYP2C9, CYP2C19) are involved in the oxidative biotransformation of the majority of drugs used therapeutically in humans. Substrates for CYP3A4 (Table 13-1) are structurally diverse ranging from relatively small drugs like dapsone (molecular weight 248) to relatively large compounds such as cyclosporin A (molecular weight 1208). CYP2D6 substrates (Table 13-2) also represent many different chemical classes but share some common structural features. Specifically, prototypical CYP2D6 substrates possess a nitrogen atom that is positively charged at physiological pH located 5 or 7 Å from a lipophilic group. Conversely, CYP2C9 substrates (Table 13-3) contain a negatively charged group at physiological pH as well as a hydrophobic region between the anionic site and the site of oxidation. With the general exception of methylxanthines, CYP1A2 is only a relatively minor contributor to the biotransformation of therapeutic drugs (Table 13-4) that preferentially are metabolized by other CYP isoforms (e.g., CYP2D6 and CYP3A4). CYP2E1 substrates tend to be small organic compounds such as ethanol, chlorzoxazone, and isoflurane. It should be noted that CYP2E1 does play a significant role in the bioactivation of acetaminophen where the reactive

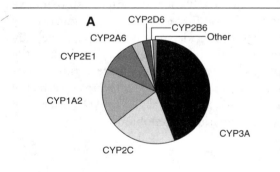

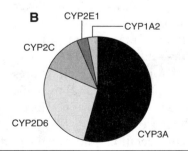

Figure 13-2. A. Relative content of cytochrome P450 isoforms in adult human liver microsomes. B. Relative contribution of cytochrome P450 isoforms to drug biotransformation.

Table 13-1. Example Substrates of CYP3A4

SUBSTRATES	REACTION(S)	ALTERNATE PATHWAYS
acetaminophen	NAPQI formation	
amiodarone astemizole	N-deethylation	
carbamazepine cisapride	10, 11-epoxidation	
cortisol	6-beta hydroxylation	
cyclosporine	N-demethylation	
dapsone	N-hydroxylation	
diazepam diltiazem	3-hydroxylation	[2C19: N-demethylation]
erythromycin estrogens felodipine	N-demethylation	
imipramine ketoconazole lidocaine lovastatin methylprednisolone midazolam	N-demethylation	[2D6: 2-hydroxylation]
nifedipine	pyridine formation	
progesterone	6-beta hydroxylation	
propafenone quinidine	N-dealkylation	
rapamycin ritonavir	O-demethylation	
tacrolimus	O-demethylation	
taxol	3'-hydroxylation	[2C8: 6α-hydroxylation]*
terfenadine	N-dealkylation	
testosterone	6-beta hydroxylation	
theophylline	8-hydroxylation	
troleandomycin triazolam	N-dealkylation	
verapamil	N-dealkylation, N-demethylation	[1A2]
warfarin	(S)-4'-hydroxylation	[2C9: (S)-7-hydroxylation]

Previously characterized representative reactions for specific substrates are denoted
[:] denotes alternate CYP enzyme and representative alternate pathway
*denotes primary pathway for biotransformation of taxol

Table 13-2. Example Substrates of CYP2D6

SUBSTRATES	PRIMARY REACTION(S)	ALTERNATE PATHWAYS
alprenolol	aromatic hydroxylation	
amiodarone	aromatic hydroxylation	
amitriptyline	benzylic hydroxylation	
bufurolol captopril	1'-hydroxylation (benzylic); (4-hydroxylation)	
clomipramine clozapine	aromatic hydroxylation	
codeine	O-demethylation	
debrisoquine	4-hydroxylation	
desipramine	aromatic hydroxylation	
dextromethorphan	O-demethylation	[3A4: N-demethylation]
encainide	O-demethylation; N-demethylation	
flecainide flunarizine fluoxetine haloperidol	O-dealkylation	
imipramine	2-hydroxylation	[3A4: N-demethylation]
metoprolol mexiletine	aliphatic hydroxylation; O-dealkylation	
nortriptyline paroxetine perphenazine	benzylic hydroxylation	
phenformin	aromatic (ρ)-hydroxylation	
propafenone	5-hydroxylation	
propranolol	4-hydroxylation	
sparteine	N-hydroxylation	
thioridazine	S-oxidation	
timolol	?O-dealkylation	

Previously characterized representative reactions for specific substrates are denoted
[:] denotes alternate CYP enzyme and representative alternate pathway

(i.e., electrophilic) metabolic product (i.e., N-acetylbenzoquinoneimine or NAPQI) can produce hepatic and renal damage. Tables 13-1 through 13-4 are intended to provide representative examples of therapeutic substrates for the cytochromes P450.

Sources of Variability in Drug Biotransformation Activity

There is considerable interindividual variability in the hepatic expression of the cytochromes P450. For any individual, the pathway and rate of a given compound's metabolic clearance

Table 13-3. Example Substrates of CYP2C9

SUBSTRATES	PRIMARY REACTION(S)	ALTERNATE PATHWAYS
diclofenac	hydroxylation	
ibuprofen	hydroxylation	(UGT2B7: glucuronidation)
naproxen	hydroxylation	
phenytoin	4-hydroxylation	
piroxicam	hydroxylation	
tenoxicam	hydroxylation	
tolbutamide	hydroxylation	
S-warfarin	(S)-7-hydroxylation	

Previously characterized representative reactions for specific substrates are denoted
[:] denotes alternate enzyme and representative alternate pathway

is a function of that individual's unique phenotype with respect to the forms and amounts of P450 species expressed. Interindividual variability in drug biotransformation activity is a consequence of the complex interplay among genetic (e.g., genotype, phenotype, gender, race/ethnic background), environmental (e.g., diet, disease, concurrent medication, xenobiotic exposure), and developmental factors (e.g., somatic growth in infants, children, and adolescents; senescence in the elderly).

The term *pharmacogenetics* was proposed to describe the study of genetically determined variations in drug response. Over the past several years, the importance of genetic *polymorphisms* (i.e., more than one form) in drug metabolizing enzyme activities has become more apparent as clinicians have become increasingly aware of the numbers of clinically useful drugs that are metabolized by polymorphically expressed enzymes and the proportion of treated patients who are affected. By definition, a *pharmacogenetic polymorphism* is a monogenic trait that is caused by the presence in the same population of more than one allele at

Table 13-4. Example Substrates of CYP1A2

SUBSTRATES	REACTION(S)	ALTERNATE PATHWAYS
caffeine	3-demethylation	
phenacetin	O-deethylation	
theophylline	3-demethylation; 8-hydroxylation	[3A4: 8-hydroxylation]
acetaminophen*	NAPQI formation	[2E1, 3A4]
imipramine*	N-dealkylation	[2D6, 3A4]
propafenone*	N-dealkylation	[2D6, 3A4]
verapamil*	N-dealkylation	[3A4]
warfarin*	(R)-6-hydroxylation	[2C9/10]

Previously characterized representative reactions for specific substrates are denoted
[:] denotes alternate CYP enzyme and representative alternate pathway
*denotes reaction not primary/predominant in biotransformation of substrate

the same gene locus and more than one phenotype in regard to drug interaction (i.e., metabolism) with the organism. For a drug metabolizing enzyme to be polymorphic in its expression, the frequency of the least common allele which controls its production must be more than 1%.

Of the CYP enzymes involved in drug biotransformation, CYP2C19 and CYP2D6 are polymorphically expressed. The CYP2D6 poor-metabolizer (PM) phenotype is found in approximately 5 to 10% of Caucasians and North Americans of African descent, and about 1 to 2% of Asian subjects. The PM phenotype for CYP2D6 results in inefficient metabolism of more than 30 therapeutic entities including several β-receptor antagonists, antiarrhythmics, antidepressants, antipsychotics, and morphine derivatives (Table 13-2). The molecular basis for the lack of CYP2D6 activity is now well understood. Specifically, many different mutations in the CYP2D6 gene have been identified including point mutations, one-base pair deletions, and deletion of the entire gene. With current genotyping technologies, CYP2D6 poor metabolizers can be identified by screening of genomic DNA for 17 of the most common alleles.

CYP2C19 or "mephenytoin hydroxylase" deficiency is present in 3–5% of the Caucasian population and in approximately 20% of the Asian population. It is inherited as an autosomal recessive trait, and four defective alleles have been identified to date. Although several allelic variants of CYP2C9 have been identified, current information suggests that phenotypic expression of the various isoforms may be substrate dependent (e.g., warfarin, tolbutamide). Polymorphic expression of CYP1A2 and CYP3A4 have been reported in the literature but have not been definitively established. Nevertheless, the activities of these enzymes between normal individuals can vary widely, up to 50- to 60-fold, depending on the method used (e.g., administration of pharmacologic substrates with assessment of "turnover" by quantitation of parent drug and metabolite(s)) for phenotyping.

The activities of several phase II drug metabolizing enzymes in humans are also polymorphically expressed. Inheritance of two nonfunctional N-acetyltransferase-2 (NAT2) alleles is associated with the slow acetylator phenotype although allelic variants of the NAT1 gene also occur. The relative proportion of rapid and slow acetylators (NAT2) varies considerably with ethnic or geographic origin. For example, the percentage of slow acetylators is 5% among Canadian Eskimos, approximately 55% in Caucasians and African Americans residing on the North American continent, and approaches 90% in some Mediterranean populations. Several mutations in glucuronosyl transferase-1 (UGT1) genes have been reported with reductions in bilirubin conjugation activity (e.g., Crigler-Najjar syndrome, Gilbert's syndrome) being the major consequence of inheriting two defective alleles. Polymorphic activity of UGTs involved in drug biotransformation (e.g., UGT2B subfamily) has been suggested, but conclusive data are not yet available. Several methyl transferases are polymorphically expressed including catechol O-methyl transferase (COMT) and thiopurine S-methyl transferase (TPMT). Approximately 1 in 300 individuals possesses two nonfunctional TPMT alleles and is at increased risk for profound suppression of the bone marrow if treated with compounds (i.e., TPMT substrates) such as azathioprine, 6-mercaptopurine, or 6-thioguanine. Consequently, an 8–15-fold reduction in dose is required to minimize the risk of toxicity in an affected patient.

The activity of drug metabolizing enzymes can be modulated by many nongenetic factors including (but not limited to) age, diet, concurrent drug administration, infection, environmental factors, and developmental processes. For example, the activities of several cytochromes P450 are reduced during viral infections with the accompanying risk of concentration-dependent adverse events for drugs which have a narrow therapeutic index. Grapefruit juice, a common dietary constituent which contains the bioflavinoid naringenin, is capable of dramatically reducing CYP3A4 activity in the enterocytes. Likewise, several drugs are associated with decreased clearance of concomitantly administered agents through inter-actions (e.g., competitive or noncompetitive inhibition of enzyme activity) at the drug bio-transformation level, frequently involving the cytochromes P450. Finally, the ontogeny of drug metabolizing enzyme activity can produce dynamic and dramatic changes ranging from a virtual absence at birth to activity exceeding adult levels in infants as young as three to six months of age. It is important to note that, in most instances, functional alterations in drug biotransformation capacity are enzyme- and isoform-specific. Accordingly, broad gener-alizations regarding the many possible interactions of drug metabolizing enzymes are not necessarily appropriate and cannot be based solely on the ability of a given enzyme to bio-transform a given substrate.

Drug Interactions

Drug interactions involving the cytochromes P450 have gained considerable attention over the last 20 years since the initial reports of the ability of cimetidine to alter the clear-ance of many commonly used drugs (e.g., benzodiazepines, phenytoin, phenobarbital, theophylline) and, most recently, the well publicized interaction between terfenadine and concurrently administered inhibitors of CYP3A4 (e.g., erythromycin and ketoconazole). In view of all the potential drug-drug interactions that may occur on a metabolic basis, the clinician can use substrate-specific information concerning drug metabolizing enzymes to predict individuals potentially at increased risk for drug-drug interactions. There are, however, important considerations/caveats that must be recognized before cat-alogued information (e.g., that contained in Tables 13-1, 13-2, 13-3, and 13-4) concern-ing drug metabolism is transformed into data which are interpreted to be of potential clinical significance and hence may be of therapeutic utility. Several of these considera-tions are listed as follows:

- The amount and activity of constitutively expressed enzyme(s);
- The therapeutic index of the compound in question and the degree to which the drug is dependent upon a particular biotransformation pathway for the majority of its elimination from the body versus the availability of alternate pathways;
- The potential impact of inducers or inhibitors relative to constitutive enzyme expres-sion (e.g., the magnitude of induction/inhibition relative to subject phenotype);
- The impact of age/development/gender on enzyme activity;
- For competing substrates, the kinetic characteristics which describe the interaction between the substrate and its respective enzyme(s);
- The impact of concomitant disease state, pharmacotherapy, and other extrinsic fac-tors (e.g., nutrition, environmental chemicals) on enzyme activity; and
- The contribution of extrahepatic enzymes (and their ontogeny) to the total bio-transformation process.

A list of clinically relevant inducers and inhibitors of specific CYP isoforms and selected Phase II enzymes is presented in Table 13-5.

Table 13-5. Major Drug Metabolizing Enzymes in Man: Examples of Inhibitors and Inducers of Potential Clinical Importance

ENZYME	INHIBITOR(S)	INDUCER(S)
CYP1A2	α-naphthoflavone, quinolones (enoxacin > ciprofloxacin >ofloxacin), furafylline, cimetidine, ritonavir	cigarette smoke, omeprazole, cruciferous vegetables, charcoal broiled meat
CYP2C9	sulfaphenazole, sulfinpyrazone, chloramphenicol, fluconazole	rifampin
CYP2C19	tranylcypromine, fluoxetine, fluvoxamine, omeprazole	rifampin
CYP2D6	fluoxetine, quinidine, cimetidine, haloperidol, paroxetine, ritonavir	none known
CYP2E1	disulfiram, 4-methylpyrazole	ethanol, isoniazid
CYP3A4	azole antifungals, macrolide antibiotics (erythromycin, troleandomycin, clarithromycin), naringenin (from grapefruit), cimetidine, ethinyl estradiol, fluoxetine, fluvoxamine, indinavir, ritonavir, danazol, omeprazole, quinine, sertraline	carbamazepine, rifampin, dexamethasone, phenytoin, phenobarbital, isoniazid, griseofulvin, phenylbutazone
NAT2	none known	none known
UGT*	none known	phenobarbital, cigarette smoke, cruciferous vegetables
ST*	salicylic acid, benzoic acid, naproxen	phenobarbital, 3-methylcholanthrene
TPMT*	none known	none known

*denotes presence of multiple isoforms which may differ with respect to inhibitor and/or inducer specificity
Adapted from Leeder and Kearns (1997) and Singer et al. (1997)

Ontogeny of Drug Metabolizing Enzymes

Pharmacokinetic data reported over the past two decades clearly demonstrate that development markedly influences the absorption, distribution, excretion, and metabolism of many xenobiotics. With respect to many of the processes which govern drug biotransformation, genetically determined events which control this process appear to vary as a consequence of development. For most enzymes involved in drug biotransformation, fetuses and newborns may be considered to be phenotypically "slow" or "poor" metabolizers. In most instances, infants will acquire a phenotype consistent with their genotype at some point later in the developmental process, usually during the first year of life. Although research targeted specifically to characterizing the maturation of drug biotransformation pathways is in its infancy, some information can be obtained from pediatric pharmacokinetic and phenotyping studies.

Phenotyping studies with dextromethorphan in children suggest that catalytic activity of CYP2D6 comparable to adults is present at least by 10 years of age, and probably much earlier. CYP2C proteins and characteristic catalytic activities are not expressed to an appreciable extent in fetal liver, but clinical data for phenytoin suggest that CYP2C9 activity is attained by one to six months of age, significantly exceeds adult activity by three to ten years of age, and reestablishes adult activity following the completion of puberty. Functional CYP1A2 does not appear to be present to any appreciable extent in human fetal liver, and activity is very low in neonates maturing to adult levels by postnatal age 120 days. Toddlers and young children appear to have CYP1A2 activity that exceeds adult values and down-regulates to adult values at the conclusion of puberty. In contrast to CYP1A2 and CYP2D6, relatively high levels of a functional CYP3A isoform are present during embryogenesis (days 50–60 of gestation), primarily as catalytically active CYP3A7. In vitro studies with fetal and neonatal liver microsomes indicate that CYP3A7 activity is maximal during the first week and progressively declines thereafter whereas CYP3A4 expression is essentially nonexistent in the fetus but increases after birth to reach levels that are 30–40% of adult activity after one month. Pediatric clinical pharmacokinetic data for CYP3A4 substrates are consistent with higher activity in children relative to adults. While the decline to adult levels presumably is a function of hormonal changes during puberty, this has not been rigorously studied to date.

With respect to phase II enzymes, the ontogeny of NAT2 has been examined in vitro and in vivo. During the first 50 days of postnatal life, virtually all infants are phenotypically slow acetylators. Concordance between NAT2 genotype and phenotype is reached by approximately 10 months, with adult activity fully expressed by three years of age. TPMT appears to be present in human fetal liver at levels that are approximately one-third that observed in adult liver. In newborn infants, peripheral blood TPMT activity is reported to be 50% greater than in race-matched adults and demonstrates a distribution of activity that is consistent with the polymorphism characterized in adults. Finally, the ontogeny of UGT activity during the first six months is dynamic and isoform specific as reflected by acquisition of competence for the conjugation of bilirubin by one month of age as compared to reduced glucuronidation of chloramphenicol and acetaminophen (both UGT substrates) through six months of age. Additional examples and discussion of the ontogeny of important drug metabolizing enzymes are also presented in Chapter 24 (Pediatric Pharmacokinetics).

As described earlier, the developmental pattern of drug metabolizing enzyme activity is traditionally viewed as being limited in newborns, rapidly increasing in the first year of life to levels in toddlers and older children that may exceed adult capacity and declining to adult levels by the conclusion of puberty. From the aforementioned discussion it is apparent that this "pattern" is overly simplistic and not representative of the true ontogeny for drug metabolizing enzymes in humans. At present, the factors which are responsible for both the up- and down-regulation of the activity for drug metabolizing enzymes during development are not known. Given the fact that this activity appears to be temporally associated with somatic growth, it is likely that the neuroendocrine factors (e.g., growth hormone, IGF-1) which modulate protein formation during development likewise regulate the formation and/or activity of certain drug metabolizing enzymes (e.g., cytochromes P450). When one considers that each organ has a unique complement of P450s and phase II enzymes, organ-specific developmental patterns (e.g., acquisition of CYP3A4 activity in the liver and small intestine) add an additional element of complexity to the whole process of ontogeny for drug metabolizing enzymes. Nonetheless, this process remains responsible for age-dependent differences in the pharmacokinetics (e.g., clearance, half life) of drugs which are substrates for one or more drug metabolizing enzymes and have significant nonrenal clearance.

Specific Factors which Can Influence Drug Metabolism

Stereoselectivity in Drug Metabolism

In view of the fact that the majority of chiral synthetic or semisynthetic drugs are marketed as racemates, consideration must be given to the potential stereoselective metabolism of chiral xenobiotics. Both phase I and phase II metabolic reactions are potentially capable of discriminating between enantiomers. For drug enantiomers with low hepatic extraction, a difference in the intrinsic clearance will be directly reflected in the hepatic clearance. This, in turn, results in stereoselectivity in the resultant plasma concentrations after both oral and IV drug administration. In contrast, for highly extracted enantiomers (i.e., those with a high hepatic extraction ratio) a difference in intrinsic clearance may not result in significant alterations in stereoselectivity of plasma drug concentrations. Stereoselective drug metabolism may involve the substrate (including chiral inversion and first-pass metabolism) and/or metabolite(s). In man, stereoselectivity in metabolism has been demonstrated for several common drugs. Selected examples include albuterol (sulfation), amphetamine (deamination), fenfluramine (deethylation), ibuprofen (inversion-*R*), mephobarbital (hydroxylation-*R*), mephenytoin (demethylation-*R* and 4-hydroxylation-*S*), mexiletine (glucuronidation-*R*), normephenytoin (demethylation-*R* and aromatic hydroxylation-*S*), phenytoin (parahydroxylation), oxazepam (glucuronidation-*S*), propranolol (4-hydroxylation-*R*), and tocainide (conjugation-*R*). Warfarin provides perhaps the best examples of some of the clinical implications of stereoselective drug metabolism. Specifically, the *S*-enantiomer of warfarin (which is 5–10 times more potent than the *R*-enantiomer) is 7-hydroxylated by CYP2C9 while the *R*-enantiomer is hydroxylated (10-hydroxylation and 4′-hydroxylation) by CYP3A4. As a consequence pharmacogenetic, developmental, and environmental factors which could alter the activity of either CYP2C9 or CYP3A4 have the ability to change the disposition characteristics of the respective enantiomers and thus impact the pharmacodynamics of warfarin in a significant fashion.

Chronopharmacokinetics and Drug Metabolism

Diurnal variation (i.e., circadian rhythm) has also been shown to impact the activity of selected phase I and phase II enzymes capable of metabolizing xenobiotics in man. In the case of acetaminophen conjugation, diurnal variation in the activity of glucuronosyltransferase and sulfotransferase isoforms appears to explain the chronopharmacokinetics of this compound and perhaps other drugs as well. The basic mechanisms by which diurnal variation alters the activity of drug metabolizing enzymes are not completely understood but may involve neuroendocrine regulation. As well, other physiologic alterations known to have a circadian pattern (e.g., drug protein binding, hepatic blood flow) could potentially impact drug metabolism by altering the free fraction of drug available for hepatic clearance and/or the efficiency of presentation of xenobiotics to the liver.

First-Pass Effect

Drug absorbed from the stomach, duodenum, jejunum, ileum, or following deep rectal administration is carried by the portal circulation to the liver where it is subject to biotransformation before reaching the systemic circulation. Substantial drug biotransformation may also occur in the gastrointestinal epithelium during the course of absorption. The process of drug biotransformation prior to becoming systemically available is referred to as the *first-pass effect* or *presystemic clearance* and represents one means by which the systemic availability of the drug is reduced. Incomplete release from the dosage form, chemical degradation, physical complexation, microbial biotransformation, and accelerated gastrointestinal transit may also contribute to presystemic clearance of drugs and hence be responsible in part for poor oral bioavailability.

The quantitative importance of the first-pass effect depends upon the rate of drug absorption, the rate of biotransformation, and the biotransformation capacity for a particular drug. For example, if the amount of drug administered is small but capacity and rate of drug biotransformation is high, a large fraction of the drug may undergo biotransformation, thereby reducing the extent of bioavailability. As the administered dose increases, first-pass metabolism may become saturated and in this way increase the extent of bioavailability as reflected in Figure 13-3.

Since the intestinal mucosa is second only to the liver in terms of CYP3A4 expression, it is therefore not surprising that drugs exclusively or highly metabolized by CYP3A4 are subject to considerable first-pass metabolism. Calcium channel blockers such as nifedipine are prime examples. For other drugs that are dependent on other P450 isoforms in addition to CYP3A4 for their biotransformation, the extent of the first-pass effect will be determined by the relative abundance of CYP3A4 relative to the other P450s and transport proteins (e.g., P-glycoprotein) in the liver and intestinal mucosa. By extension, P450 inhibitors such as grapefruit juice (a CYP3A4 inhibitor; Table 13-5) that exert their inhibitory activity primarily at the level of small bowel enterocytes can be expected to most profoundly influence those drugs subject to extensive first-pass metabolism (e.g., CYP3A4 substrates such as nifedipine, felodipine, midazolam, terfenadine, and saquinavir).

In its simplest form, the extent of the first-pass effect can be estimated by comparing the areas under the plasma concentration-time curve (AUC) following intravenous (AUC_{iv}) and oral (AUC_{po}) administration, after correcting for the doses administered and assuming complete absorption. By determining the area under the concentration-time curve for the parent drug and its metabolite(s), it is possible to differentiate between first-pass effect and incomplete absorption. For example, if absorption is complete but there is a first-pass effect, then the ratio of AUC_{po}/AUC_{iv} for the parent drug will be less than unity while the AUC_{po}/AUC_{iv} ratio for the metabolite(s) will be approximately 1. Conversely, if there is incomplete absorption and *no* first-pass effect, the

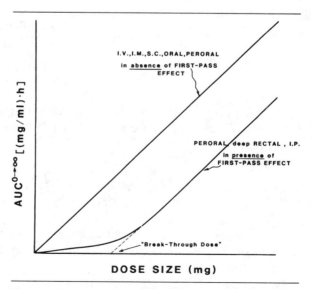

Figure 13-3. Schematic diagram showing determination of "break-through dose" to saturate first-pass metabolism.

AUC_{po}/AUC_{iv} ratios for parent compound and metabolite(s) will be approximately the same, and both will be less than 1.

The fraction of drug reaching systemic circulation in the presence of first-pass effect, f_{FPE}, may be estimated from IV blood concentration-time data under the assumption of complete absorption.

$$f_{FPE} = 1 - \frac{D_{I.V.}}{LBF \cdot AUC_{I.V.}^{0 \to \infty}} \tag{1}$$

f_{FPE} = fraction of drug reaching systemic circulation in presence of first-pass effect
D_{IV} = dose given IV [μg]
LBF = average liver blood flow rate = 90,000 [ml/h]
$AUC_{IV}^{0 \to \infty}$ = total area under the IV blood concentration-time-curve [(μg/ml) · h]

Since the total clearance is the ratio of the dose to the total area under the curve:

$$Cl_{tot} = \frac{D}{AUC^{0 \to \infty}} \tag{2}$$

Equation 13.1 can also be expressed as follows:

$$f_{FPE} = 1 - \frac{Cl_{tot}[ml/h]}{LBF[ml/h]} \tag{3}$$

In the case of practically complete metabolism, the fraction of drug perorally absorbed in the presence of first-pass effect can be calculated from PO data according to Equation 13.4, if one knows the fraction of drug absorbed, f:

$$f_{FPE} = \frac{LBF[ml/h] \cdot f}{LBF[ml/h] + \dfrac{D[\mu g] \cdot f}{AUC_{P.O.}^{0 \to \infty}[(\mu g/ml) \cdot h]}} \tag{4}$$

In the case of complete absorption and complete metabolism the actual liver blood flow, which may vary between 500 and 3,000 ml/min, can be calculated according to Equation 13.5:

$$LBF = \frac{D_{I.V.} \cdot D_{P.O.}}{D_{P.O.} \cdot AUC_{I.V.}^{0 \to \infty} - D_{I.V.} \cdot AUC_{P.O.}^{0 \to \infty}} \tag{5}$$

In the case in which the drug is partly metabolized and partly eliminated in unchanged form via the kidney, the actual LBF can be calculated according to Equation 13.6:

$$LBF = \frac{D}{AUC_{I.V.}^{0 \to \infty} - AUC_{P.O.}^{0 \to \infty}} - \frac{Cl_{ren}}{1 - \dfrac{AUC_{P.O.}^{0 \to \infty}}{AUC_{I.V.}^{0 \to \infty}}} \tag{6}$$

In order to differentiate between first-pass effect, f_{FPE}, and incomplete absorption, f, the method by Harris and Riegelman can be used. The drug must be administered IV and PO, and the area under the concentration-time curve must be determined for both the parent drug, p, and the metabolite(s), m. Then the ratios of AUC upon PO and IV administration, corrected for differences in dose sizes, are compared between parent drug and metabolite. The evaluation is done according to Table 13-6.

Michaelis-Menten or Saturation Kinetics

Enzyme reactions are usually best described by the Michaelis-Menten equation:

$$\frac{dC}{dt} = -\frac{V_{max} \cdot C}{K_m + C} \tag{7}$$

where dC/dt is the rate of decreasing drug concentration at time t, V_{max} is the theoretical maximum rate of the process, and K_m is the Michaelis-Menten constant. If $C \gg K_m$, then K_m can be removed from the denominator of Equation 13.7, and C cancels out. Hence, the equation is simplified to:

$$\frac{dC}{dt} = -V_{max} \tag{8}$$

indicating that the rate of change of concentration equals a constant, i.e., it follows zero-order kinetics.

Whenever a biotransformation process catalyzed by specific enzymes is limited by the availability or capacity of the system, saturation occurs. This is true not only for metabo-

Table 13-6. Differentiation between Incomplete Absorption and First-Pass Effect

Complete Absorption and *no* First-Pass Effect	
$R_p \cong 1$	$R_m \simeq 1$
Complete Absorption *and* First-Pass Effect	
$R_p < 1$	$R_m \simeq 1$
Incomplete Absorption and *no* First-Pass Effect	
$R_p \qquad = \qquad R_m < 1$	
Incomplete Absorption *and* First-Pass Effect	
$R_p \qquad < \qquad R_m < 1$	
Unchanged Drug: p	Metabolite (s): m

$$R_p = \frac{AUC_{P.O.p.}^{0 \to \infty} \cdot D_{I.V.p.}}{AUC_{I.V.p.}^{0 \to \infty} \cdot D_{P.O.p.}} \qquad R_m = \frac{AUC_{P.O.m.}^{0 \to \infty} \cdot D_{I.V.p.}}{AUC_{I.V.m.}^{0 \to \infty} \cdot D_{P.O.p.}}$$

lism but for all other capacity-limited processes such as in absorption, distribution, and elimination.

For most drugs the therapeutic concentration is in a range where $C << K_m$. Hence, in simplification, dC/dt approaches first-order kinetics. Therefore, first-order kinetics is usually applicable for describing disposition of drugs and to calculate dosage regimens.

If, however, the dose size is increased beyond a threshold level, such as in case of poisoning, overdosing, and hepatic and renal impairment, saturation kinetics may be observed with any drug. In this case, elimination half-life and clearance are prolonged and change with dose.

There are a few drugs which obey Michaelis-Menten kinetics even within their normal dose range in patients without metabolic, hepatic, or renal disorders. Such drugs are:

5′-Bromo-2-deoxyuridine
Bromouracil
Carbamazepine
Cinromide
5′-Deoxy-5-fluorouridine
Diltiazem
Ethanol
5-Fluorouracil
Hydralazine
4-Hydroxybutyrate
Nicardipine

Nitroglycerin
Penicillamine
Phenytoin
Prednisolone
Propoxyphene
Propranolol
Salicylamide
Salicylate
Theophylline
Verapamil

Prediction of In Vivo Pharmacokinetics from In Vitro Data

For many years, researchers have used in vitro liver systems (e.g., microsomes prepared from human liver or from insect cells transfected to express specific human drug-metabolizing enzymes, hepatocyte cultures, liver slices, perfused organ preparations) to study and extrapolate the in vivo clearance of drugs. For many drugs, hepatic clearance is a major determinant for the overall pharmacokinetic properties (e.g., plasma clearance, first-pass effect, elimination half-life). The utility of in vitro approaches to predict in vivo hepatic metabolic clearance is predicated upon the assumption that nonhepatic clearance mechanisms (e.g., biliary secretion, renal clearance, pulmonary clearance) do not appreciably contribute to the total plasma clearance of the drug under study.

In vivo extrapolation of in vitro data is primarily based upon the determination of in vitro clearance (calculated from K_m and V_{max} values based upon in vitro biotransformation of a drug using one or more of the aforementioned liver systems) and secondarily upon in vivo parameters such as hepatic mass, hepatic blood flow, and unbound fraction of the drug in blood. Important factors to consider in determining in vitro clearance include:

- availability and orientation of the specific drug-metabolizing enzyme being evaluated,
- specificity of the drug-metabolizing enzyme (i.e., isoform specificity) for the model substrate being evaluated,
- assessment of biotransformation at clinically relevant (e.g., therapeutic) substrate concentrations,
- genotype and phenotype of the drug-metabolizing enzyme(s) being evaluated,

- incubation conditions as they compare to the in vivo environment,
- in vitro enzyme stability, and
- protein binding and/or uptake of drug (e.g., presence of active drug transporters in intact cells versus their absence in microsomes) by cells.

Difficulties in the extrapolation of in vitro data to the in vivo condition reside with:

- accurate assessment of hepatic mass relative to the amount of drug-metabolizing enzyme present;
- differences in the amount and/or activity of drug-metabolizing enzymes that occur consequent to development, disease, concomitant drug treatment (e.g., other drugs capable of inhibiting or inducing a given enzyme), and/or normal pharmacogenetic variability (e.g., different phenotypes for a given drug-metabolizing enzyme);
- accurate prediction of hepatic blood flow during disease conditions and their treatment; and
- knowledge of the extent of protein binding throughout the normal range of "therapeutic" drug concentrations.

The availability of microsomes that selectively express recombinant human drug-metabolizing enzymes has engendered renewed interest in using in vitro drug metabolism data (also known as reaction phenotyping) to predict metabolic drug-drug interactions in vivo. As would be anticipated, predictive accuracy is best for enzymes that are not polymorphically expressed or where a polymorphism does not have apparent functional consequences (e.g., CYP3A4) and when the majority of metabolism occurs via a single enzyme. Also, the use of specific pharmacologic probes for in vivo phenotyping (see Chapter 39) permits the use of a "bridging strategy" to assess whether in vitro results can be successfully translated to predict pharmacokinetic characteristics of specific drugs. Approaches such as these are now being considered by regulatory agencies (e.g., the United States Food and Drug Administration) to predict potentially significant drug-drug interactions in humans without the need for conducting confirmatory clinical investigations (e.g., extrapolation of CYP3A4 induction by St. John's Wort to many drug substrates metabolized by this specific isoform).

Finally, in silico methods are being developed to enable translation of in vitro drug metabolism data to in vivo pharmacokinetics via computer simulation. Programs such as SIMCYP® incorporate variability into such predictions through step-by-step integration of patient demographics, disease states, anatomical, physiological (e.g., liver mass, amount of drug-metabolizing enzyme), biochemical (e.g., enzyme activity), and genetic (e.g., genotype, phenotype) information. Also whole body pharmacokinetic models can used that apply principles of physiologically based pharmacokinetic modeling and integrate information on drug-metabolizing enzyme activity to predict drug disposition in theoretical patients based on their age and disease states.

Selected References

1. Bjornsson, T. D., Callaghan, J. T., Einolf, H. J., Fischer, V. Gan, L., Grimm S., et al.: The Conduct of In Vitro and In Vivo Drug-Drug Interactions Studies: a PhRMA Perspective. *J. Clin. Pharmacol.* 43:443–469 (2003).
2. Boobis, A. R., Edwards, R. J., Adams, D. A., et al.: Dissecting the Function of Cytochrome P450, *Br. J. Clin. Pharmacol.* 42:81–89 (1996).

3. Davit, B., Reynolds, K., Yuan, R., Ajayi F., Conner, D., Fadiran, E., Gillespie, B., et al.: FDA Evaluations Using In Vitro Metabolism to Predict and Interpret In Vivo Metabolic Drug-Drug Interactions: Impact on Labeling. *J. Clin. Pharmacol. 39*:899–910 (1999).

4. Donato, M. T. and Castell, J. V.: Strategies and Molecular Probes to Investigate the Role of Cytochrome P450 in Drug Metabolism. *Clin. Pharmacokinet. 42*:153–178 (2003).

5. Gibaldi, M. and Perrier, D.: Route of Administration and Drug Disposition, *Drug Metab. Rev. 3*:185 (1974).

6. Harris, P.A. and Riegelman, S.: Influence of the Route of Administration on the Area Under the Plasma Concentration-Time Curve. *J. Pharm Sci. 58*:71–75 (1969).

7. Jamali, F., Mehvar, R. and Pasutto, F. M.: Enantioselective Aspects of Drug Action and Disposition: Therapeutic Pitfalls, *J. Pharm. Sci. 78*:695–715 (1989).

8. Labrecque, G. and Belanger, P. M.: Biological Rhythms in the Absorption, Distribution, Metabolism and Excretion of Drugs, *Pharmacol. Ther. 52*:95–107 (1991).

9. Leeder, J. S. and Kearns, G. L.: Pharmacogenetics in Pediatrics: Implications for Practice, *Pediatr. Clin. North Am. 44*:55–77 (1997).

10. Masimirembwa, C. M., Bredberg, U., and Andersson, T. B.: Metabolic Stability for Drug Discovery and Development: Pharmacokinetics and Biochemical Challenges. *Clin. Pharmacokinet. 42*:515–528 (2003).

11. May, G.: Genetic Differences in Drug Disposition, *J. Clin. Pharmacol. 34*:881 (1994).

12. Nestorov, I.: Whole Body Pharmacokinetic Models. *Clin. Pharmacokinet. 42*:883–908 (2003).

13. Pirmohamed, M., Madden, S. and Park, B. K.: Idiosyncratic Drug Reactions: Metabolic Bioactivation as a Pathogenic Mechanism, *Clin. Pharmacokinet. 31*:215–230 (1996).

14. Rettie, A. E., Wienkers, L. C., Gonzalez, F. J., et al.: Impaired (S)-Warfarin Metabolism Catalyzed by the R144C Allelic Variant of CYP2C9, *Pharmacogenetics 4*:39–43 (1994).

15. Riegelman, S. and Rowland, M.: Effect of Route of Administration on Drug Disposition, *J. Pharmacokinet. Biopharm. 1*:419 (1973).

16. Singer, M. I., Shapiro, L. E. and Shear, N. H.: Cytochrome P-450 3A: Interactions with Dermatologic Therapies, *J. Am. Acad. Dermatol. 37*:765–771 (1997).

17. Slaughter, R. L. and Edwards, D. J.: Recent Advances: The Cytochrome P450 Enzymes, *Ann. Pharmacother. 29*:619–624 (1995).

14

Compartment Models

Models are used to describe and interpret a set of data obtained by experimentation. A model in pharmacokinetics is a hypothetical structure which can be used to characterize with reproducibility the behavior and the "fate" of a drug in biological systems when given by a certain route of administration and in a particular dosage form.

A compartment is an entity which can be described by a definite volume and a concentration (of drug contained in the volume). Usually the behavior of a drug in biological systems can be described by a one-compartment model or a two-compartment model. Sometimes it is necessary to employ multicompartment models. One should begin by determining whether experimental data can be fitted to a one-compartment model. And only if no fitting is obtained, one continues trying more sophisticated models.

Actually, the human body is a multimillion compartment model considering drug concentration in different organelles, cells, or tissues. However, in the living body we have access to only two types of body fluid—blood (or plasma or serum) and urine. Compartment models in pharmacokinetics are, therefore, used to fit experimental data from blood level versus time curves or urinary cumulative excretion versus time curves to models. A certain type of model is not necessarily specific for a particular drug. Often a blood level versus time curve upon extravascular administration can be fitted to a simple one-compartment model, whereas the blood level versus time curve upon intravascular administration is best fitted to a two-compartment model.

Two or more compartments can be linked together because a drug may move back from one compartment into another and back. The movement occurs at different rates (speeds) and is described by distribution rate constants.

Open One-Compartment Model

We are talking about an open one-compartment model if the drug entering the body (input) distributes (equilibrates) instantly between the blood and other body fluids or tissues. In an open one-compartment model the drug is not necessarily (and indeed is rarely) confined

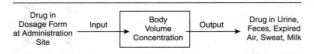

Figure 14-1. Concept of open one-compartment model.

to the circulatory system. The drug may occupy the entire extracellular fluid, "soft" tissue, or the entire body; however, distribution occurs instantly and is not "pooled" in a specific area (Figure 14-1).

Open Two-Compartment Model

We are talking about an open two-compartment model if the drug entering the body (input) does not instantly distribute (equilibrate) between the blood and those other body fluids or tissues which it eventually reaches. The distribution of the drug in blood and other "soft" tissues, on the one hand, and into other "deep" tissues, on the other hand, occurs at different rates (speeds). Eventually a steady state will be reached which terminates the "distribution" phase. From such data we cannot necessarily say to which specific tissues or organs a drug was slowly distributed. We may postulate from the pK_a value and lipid/water partition coefficient, but a definite answer may be obtained only by biopsy, animal experiments, the use of radioactive materials, and whole body scintillation. The body fluids or tissues which are in equilibrium with the circulatory system comprise the central compartment which is accessible through blood sampling. Those body fluids or tissues into which the drug distributes slowly comprise the peripheral compartment which is not accessible by blood sampling (Figure 14-2).

The term "open" in conjunction with a compartment model refers to the fact that we do not have a closed system but have a unidirectional input and output into and out of the system.

Figures 14-3 and 14-4 give the characteristics, models, and schematic blood level curves for the open one-compartment model and the open two-compartment model upon intravascular and extravascular administration. A summary and the general blood level equations for the open one-compartment and the open two-compartment models are given in Figure 14-5.

Decision on Compartment Model

Visual Inspection of Semilog Plot

Plot concentration-time data on a semilog plot. To make the decision whether the one- or two-compartment model applies, one first finds the terminal slope. A straight line is drawn through the terminal points of the plot by inspection. The terminal line is then back-extrapolated to the ordinate. If no concentration-time data points lie above the line, the one-compartment model is applicable. But if the peak concentration is markedly above this line, it must be assumed that the plot represents a two- or higher-compartment model as shown in the schematic diagram of Figure 14-6.

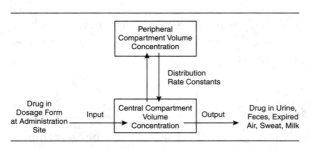

Figure 14-2. Concept of open two-compartment model.

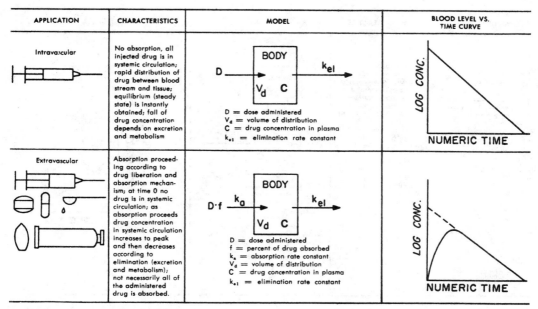

APPLICATION	CHARACTERISTICS	MODEL	BLOOD LEVEL VS. TIME CURVE

Figure 14-3. Characteristics of the open one-compartment model.

Modified Method of Saunders and Natunen

If upon IV and extravascular administration the first portion of the curve or the peak is above the back-extrapolated monoexponential line of the tail end of the curve, an open two- or higher-compartment model is applicable.

Sometimes the data points are somewhat scattered and it is not easy to determine the model under question. We have adopted a modification of the method by Saunders and Natunen for testing the applicability of the open one- or the open two-compartment model. If the points are scattered in a way in which it seems questionable which type of model shall be used, first a least squares is performed on all data points (NOTE: "All data points" means all points of the decaying portion of a curve, i.e., after the peak), and the antilogarithm of the intercept V_4 is determined. Then a least squares is done with the last half of data points and the antilogarithm of this intercept V_3 is determined (Figure 14-7). In the case of an uneven number of data points, the middle point is omitted. The following inequality expression is used:

$$(V_4 - V_3)/V_3 < 0.1 \tag{1}$$

If the inequality expressed in Equation 14.1 is satisfied, the open one-compartment model is used; if it is not satisfied, the open two-compartment model is employed. If there are enough data points at hand, one could even go further and inspect the data for eventual applicability of an open three-compartment model, as seen in Figure 14-7, again applying Equation 14.1, whereby V_4 and V_3 are substituted by V_6 and V_5. In any case, there must be at least three data points for each regression analysis.

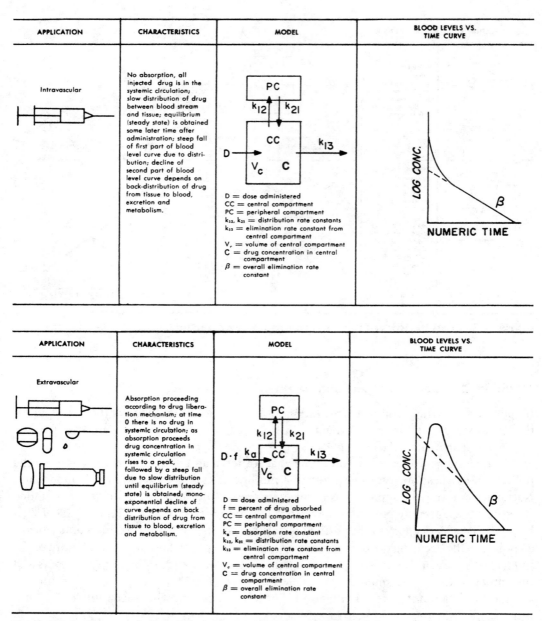

Figure 14-4. Characteristics of the open two-compartment model.

BLOOD LEVEL (on semi-log paper)	ROUTE OF ADMINISTRATION	COMPARTMENT MODEL	BLOOD LEVEL EQUATION (µg/ml)
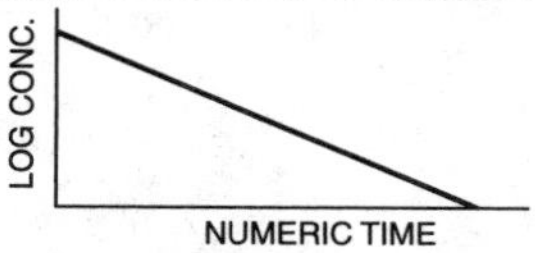 LOG CONC. / NUMERIC TIME	Intravascular (intravenous; intracardiac; intra-arterial)	open one	$C(t) = C(0) \cdot e^{-k_{el} \cdot t}$
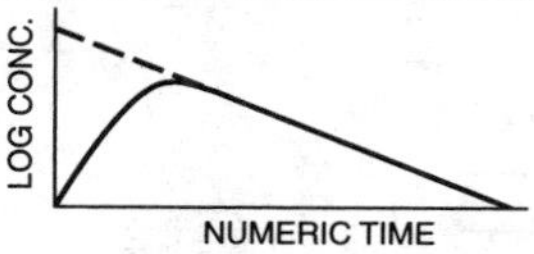 LOG CONC. / NUMERIC TIME	Extravascular (oral; peroral; rectal; intramuscular; subcutaneous; intracutaneous)	open one	$C(t) = B \cdot e^{-k_{el} \cdot t} - A \cdot e^{-k_a \cdot t}$
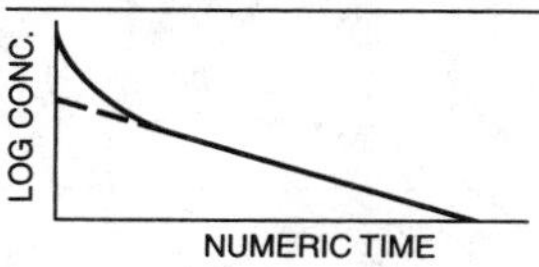 LOG CONC. / NUMERIC TIME	Intravascular (intravenous; intracardiac; intra-arterial)	open two	$C(t) = B \cdot e^{-\beta \cdot t} + A \cdot e^{-\alpha \cdot t}$
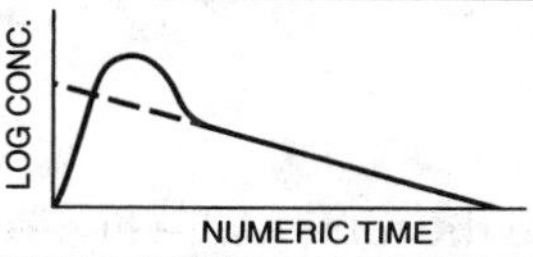 LOG CONC. / NUMERIC TIME	Extravascular (oral; peroral; rectal; intramuscular; subcutaneous; intracutaneous)	open two	$C(t) = B \cdot e^{-\beta \cdot t} + A \cdot e^{-\alpha \cdot t} - C(0) \cdot e^{-k_a \cdot t}$

Figure 14-5. Summary of compartment models, route of administration, and blood, serum, or plasma concentration equations.

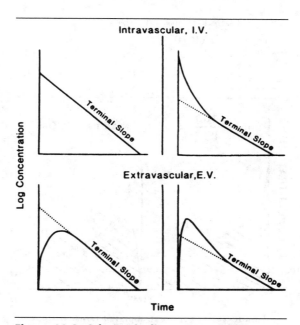

Figure 14-6. Schematic diagram to visually decide on applicable compartment model, based on back-extrapolated terminal slope.

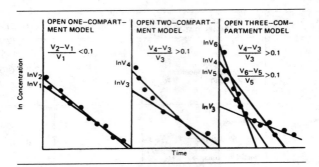

Figure 14-7. Schematic diagram on decision of applicable compartment model based on the method by Saunders and Natunen.

AUC Method

Determine the AUC above the back-extrapolated terminal slope and the total AUC (Figure 14-8). If Equation 14.2 results in less than 5 percent then the open one-compartment model is justified:

$$\frac{\text{AUC}_{\text{above back–extrapolated terminal slope}}}{\text{AUC}(0^{\to\infty})} \cdot 100 < 5\% \tag{2}$$

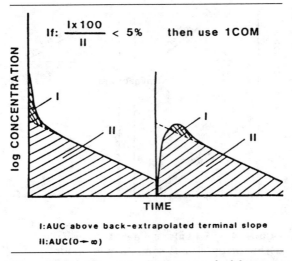

Figure 14-8. Schematic diagram on decision on applicable compartment model based on the area under the curve above the back-extrapolated terminal slope.

Selected References

1. Berlin, N. I., Berman, M., Berk, P. D., Phang, J. M. and Waldmann, T. A.: The Application of Multi-Compartmental Analysis to Problems of Clinical Medicine, *Ann. Intern. Med.* 68:423 (1968).

2. Berman, M. and Schoenfeld, R.: Invariants in Experimental Data on Linear Kinetics and the Formulation of Models, *J. Appl. Physics* 27:1361 (1956).

3. Dost, F. H.: *Grundlagen der Pharmakokinetik,* Georg Thieme Verlag, Stuttgart, 1968, p. 33.

4. Krüger-Thiemer, E.: Continuous Intravenous Infusion and Multicompartment Accumulation, *Eur. J. Pharmacol.* 4:317 (1968).

5. Levy, G., Gibaldi, M. and Jusko, W. J.: Multicompartment Pharmacokinetic Models and Pharmacologic Effects, *J. Pharm. Sci.* 58:422 (1969).

6. Riggs, D. S.: *A Critical Primer—The Mathematical Approach to Physiological Problems,* M.I.T. Press, Cambridge, Mass. 1967, p. 193.

7. Ritschel, W. A.: Graphic Approach to Clinical Pharmacokinetics, 2nd Ed., J. R. Prous, Barcelona, 1984, p. 20.

8. Ritschel, W. A.: Fundamentals of Pharmacokinetics. In: *Methods of Clinical Pharmacology,* Kuemmerle, H. P., Ed. Urban and Schwarzenberg, Munich-Vienna-Baltimore, 1978, pp. 133–166.

9. Ritschel, W. A.: Planning, Executing and Evaluating the Pharmacokinetics in Phase I Studies. In: *Advances in Clinical Pharmacology,* Vol. 13, "Problems of Clinical Pharmacology in Therapeutic Research: Phase I," H. P. Kuemmerle, T. K. Shibuya and E. Kimura, Editors, Urban and Schwarzenberg, Munich, 1977, pp. 212–247.

10. Saunders, L. and Natunen, T.: A Statistical Approach to Pharmacokinetic Calculations, *J. Pharm. Pharmacol.* 24:94P–99P (1972).

11. Teorell, T.: Kinetics of Distribution of Substances Administered to the Body I. The Extravascular Modes of Administration, *Arch. Int. Pharmacodyn.* 57:205 (1937).

12. Teorell, T.: Kinetics of Distribution of Substances Administered to the Body II. The Intravascular Modes of Administration, *Arch. Int. Pharmacodyn.* 57:226 (1937).

13. Wagner, J. G.: Drug Accumulation, *J. Clin. Pharmacol.* 7:84 (1967).

14. Wagner, J. G.: Pharmacokinetics 1. Definitions, Modeling and Reasons for Measuring Blood Levels and Urinary Excretion, *Drug Intell.* 2:38 (1968).

15. Wagner, J. G.: Pharmacokinetics 8. Construction of Percent Absorbed-Time Plots Based on the Two-Compartment Open Model, *Drug Intell.* 3:82 (1969).

16. Wagner, J. G.: *Fundamentals of Clinical Pharmacokinetics,* Drug Intelligence Publications, Hamilton, Ill., 1975, p. 63.

15

Determination of Rate Constants

Rate constants in pharmacokinetics characterize the change of drug concentration in a particular reference region. They give the "speed" at which a drug enters a compartment (absorption rate constant), distributes between a central and peripheral compartment(s) (distribution rate constants), and is eliminated from the systemic circulation (elimination rate constant). Additionally, many more rate constants can be described, such as those for each metabolic pathway and for each pathway of excretion.

Rate constants in pharmacokinetics are usually of first-order. An exception is alcohol which is eliminated by zero-order kinetics. However, even though first-order kinetics usually applies, there are instances when first-order kinetics changes to zero-order kinetics. This is known as dose-dependent kinetics. Examples are the following: (1) overloading of metabolic processes when large doses are given (more drug is present than there are metabolic systems to handle it), (2) competition for one type of metabolic process by two different drugs, and (3) when active transport mechanisms are overloaded (there is more drug present than there are carriers to handle it).

The elimination rate constant k_{el} in the open one-compartment model and the rate constant β in the open two-compartment model have different meanings. In the open one-compartment model k_{el} is the rate constant describing the loss of unchanged drug from the systemic circulation by either elimination (if the drug is not metabolized), regardless of pathway of excretion, or due to metabolism. In the latter case we refer to it as the overall elimination rate constant, often termed K. In the open two-compartment model, β is a hybrid constant for which everything discussed above applies in analogy. Additionally, we have an overlapping due to variations in the distribution process. The relation of the hybrid constants α and β with the specific micro rate constants can be described as follows:

$$\alpha + \beta = k_{12} + k_{21} + k_{13} \qquad (1)$$

$$\alpha \cdot \beta = k_{21} \cdot k_{13} \qquad (2)$$

The hybrid rate constants α and β are given by Equations 15.3 and 15.4.

$$\alpha = 0.5 \cdot \left[(k_{12} + k_{21} + k_{13}) + \sqrt{(k_{12} + k_{21} + k_{13})^2 - 4 \cdot k_{21} \cdot k_{13}} \right] \tag{3}$$

$$\beta = 0.5 \cdot \left[(k_{12} + k_{21} + k_{13}) - \sqrt{(k_{12} + k_{21} + k_{13})^2 - 4 \cdot k_{21} \cdot k_{13}} \right] \tag{4}$$

If a drug product is given extravascularly, the rate constant for the input or entry of drug into systemic circulation is described by the absorption rate constant k_a. Different drug products (from different manufacturers) containing the identical drug and administered by the same route of administration usually result in different blood levels due to different rates of absorption (see Chapter 36). However, the true absorption rate should be a constant for a particular drug and a particular route of administration, subject to biological variation only. Hence, the differences in rate of absorption of a particular drug from different dosage forms are explained by the fact that we measure "apparent" absorption rates. The true absorption rate would be obtained if the drug were in aqueous true solution at the site of absorption. Apparent absorption rates are observed upon administration of a drug product from which the drug must first be liberated (released) before it can be absorbed. In any case, where the liberation rate constant of a drug from a dosage form is slower than the unrestricted (true) rate of absorption, an apparent absorption rate is obtained.

However, one has to be aware of the complications due to the anatomical and physiological factors involved, too, particularly in gastrointestinal absorption. An example is griseofulvin. With this drug, a solution results in a smaller total amount of drug absorbed than when it is given in the form of capsules or tablets. This is due to the faster transit time of the solution through the duodenum where the drug is absorbed, in comparison to the slower transit time of the solid dosage forms.

ELIMINATION RATE CONSTANT, OPEN ONE-COMPARTMENT MODEL, INTRAVASCULAR (See Figure 15-1)

$$k_{el} = \frac{\ln C_1 - \ln C_2}{t_2 - t_1} [h^{-1}] \tag{5}$$

$C(0)$ = drug concentration at time 0, obtained by back-extrapolation of monoexponential declining line

C_1, C_2 = drug concentrations at corresponding times t_1 and t_2

k_{el} = overall elimination rate constant

ELIMINATION RATE CONSTANT AND ABSORPTION RATE CONSTANT, OPEN ONE-COMPARTMENT MODEL, EXTRAVASCULAR (See Figure 15-2)

$$k_{el} = \frac{\ln C_1 - \ln C_2}{t_2 - t_1} [h^{-1}] \tag{6}$$

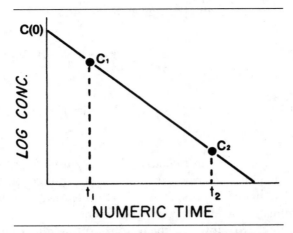

Figure 15-1. Determination of overall elimination rate constant in the open one-compartment model upon intravascular route of administration using blood level data.

$$k_a = \frac{\ln C_{1\,\text{diff}} - \ln C_{2\,\text{diff}}}{t_2' - t_1'} [\text{h}^{-1}] \qquad (7)$$

$$C(0) = B = A[\mu g/ml] \qquad (8)$$

C(0) = hypothetical drug concentration at time 0, obtained by back-extrapolation of monoexponential declining line

k_{el} = overall elimination rate constant

k_a = absorption rate constant

B = intercept of back-extrapolated monoexponential elimination slope with ordinate

A = intercept of monoexponential absorption slope with ordinate

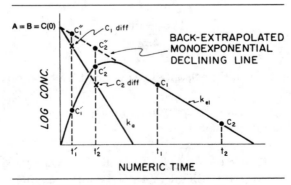

Figure 15-2. Determination of overall elimination rate constant and absorption rate constant in the open one-compartment model upon extravascular route of administration using blood level data.

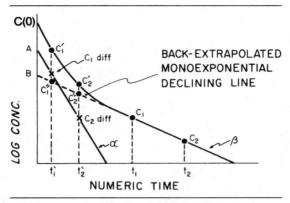

Figure 15-3. Determination of terminal β-phase rate constant, α-phase rate constant, distribution rate constants between central and peripheral compartment, and elimination rate constant from the central compartment in the open two-compartment model upon intravascular route of administration using blood level data.

C_1, C_2 = drug concentrations at corresponding times t_1 and t_2 of the elimination phase

C_1', C_2' = actual drug concentrations at corresponding times t_1' and t_2' during the absorptive phase

C_1'', C_2'' = graphically found hypothetical drug concentrations on back-extrapolated monoexponential declining slope at times t_1' and t_2'

$C_{1\,diff}$ = difference between actual plasma point of absorptive phase C_1' and the concentration on back-extrapolated monoexponential line C_1'' at same time t_1'

$C_{2\,diff}$ = difference between actual plasma point of absorptive phase C_2' and the concentration on back-extrapolated monoexponential line C_2'' at same time t_2'

ELIMINATION RATE CONSTANT AND DISTRIBUTION RATE CONSTANT, OPEN TWO-COMPARTMENT MODEL, INTRAVASCULAR (See Figure 15-3)

$$\beta = \frac{\ln C_1 - \ln C_2}{t_2 - t_1} [h^{-1}] \tag{9}$$

$$\alpha = \frac{\ln C_{1\,diff} - \ln C_{2\,diff}}{t_2' - t_1'} [h^{-1}] \tag{10}$$

$$C(0) = A + B \, [\mu g/ml] \tag{11}$$

$$k_{12} = \frac{A \cdot B \cdot (\beta - \alpha)^2}{C(0) \cdot (A \cdot \beta + B \cdot \alpha)} [h^{-1}] \tag{12}$$

$$k_{21} = \frac{A \cdot \beta + B \cdot \alpha}{C(0)} [h^{-1}] \tag{13}$$

$$A = \frac{\alpha - k_{21}}{\alpha - \beta} \cdot \frac{D}{V_c} [\mu g/ml] \tag{14}$$

$$B = \frac{k_{21} - \beta}{\alpha - \beta} \cdot \frac{D}{V_c} [\mu g/ml] \tag{15}$$

$$k_{13} = \frac{C(0)}{A/\alpha + B/\beta} [h^{-1}] \tag{16}$$

$C(0)$ = drug concentration at time 0 [obtained from $A + B = C(0)$]
β = overall elimination (slow disposition) slope (rate constant)
α = distribution (fast disposition) slope
B = intercept of back-extrapolated monoexponential elimination slope β with ordinate
A = intercept of distribution slope α with ordinate
C_1, C_2 = drug concentrations at corresponding times t_1 and t_2 of the elimination phase
C_1', C_2' = actual drug concentrations at corresponding times t_1' and t_2' during the distributive phase
C_1'', C_2'' = graphically found hypothetical drug concentrations on back-extrapolated monoexponential declining slope β at times t_1' and t_2'
$C_{1\,diff}$ = difference between actual plasma point of distributive phase C_1' and the concentration on back-extrapolated monoexponential line C_1'' at same time t_1'
$C_{2\,diff}$ = difference between actual plasma point of distributive phase C_2' and the concentration on back-extrapolated monoexponential line C_2'' at same time t_2'
k_{12} = distribution rate constant for transfer from central to peripheral compartment
k_{21} = distribution rate constant for transfer from peripheral to central compartment
k_{13} = elimination rate constant from central compartment

ELIMINATION RATE CONSTANT, ABSORPTION RATE CONSTANT, AND DISTRIBUTION RATE CONSTANTS, OPEN TWO-COMPARTMENT MODEL, EXTRAVASCULAR (See Figure 15-4)

$$\beta = \frac{\ln C_1 - \ln C_2}{t_2 - t_1} [h^{-1}] \tag{17}$$

$$\alpha = \frac{\ln C_{1\,diff} - \ln C_{2\,diff}}{t_2' - t_1'} [h^{-1}] \tag{18}$$

$$k_a = \frac{\ln C_{a^1} - \ln C_{a^2}}{t_2^* - t_1^*} [h^{-1}] \tag{19}$$

$$C(0) = A + B[\mu g/ml] \tag{20}$$

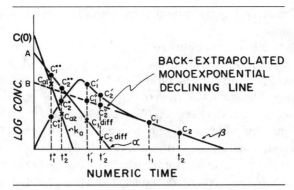

Figure 15-4. Determination of terminal β-phase rate constant, α-phase rate constant, distribution rate constants between central and peripheral compartment, elimination rate constant from the central compartment, and absorption rate constant in the two-compartment model upon extravascular route of administration using blood level data.

$$k_{12} = \frac{A \cdot B \cdot (\beta - \alpha)^2}{C(0) \cdot (A \cdot \beta + B \cdot \alpha)} [h^{-1}] \tag{21}$$

$$k_{21} = \frac{A \cdot \beta + B \cdot \alpha}{C(0)} [h^{-1}] \tag{22}$$

$$k_{13} = \frac{C(0)}{A / \alpha + B / \beta - C(0) / k_a} = \frac{C(0)}{AUC^{0 \to \infty}} [h^{-1}] \tag{23}$$

$$A = \frac{(\alpha - k_{21}) \cdot k_a}{(\alpha - \beta) \cdot (k_a - \alpha)} \cdot \frac{D \cdot f}{V_c} \tag{24}$$

$$B = \frac{(k_{21} - \beta) \cdot k_a}{(\alpha - \beta) \cdot (k_a - \beta)} \cdot \frac{D \cdot f}{V_c} \tag{25}$$

C(0) = hypothetical drug concentration at time 0 [obtained from A + B = C(0)]
β   = overall elimination (slow disposition) slope (rate constant)
α   = distribution (fast disposition) slope
k_a = absorption slope (rate constant)
B   = intercept of back-extrapolated monoexponential elimination slope β with ordinate
A   = intercept of distribution slope α with ordinate
C_1, C_2 = drug concentrations at corresponding times t_1 and t_2 of the elimination phase
C_1', C_2' = actual drug concentrations at corresponding times t_1' and t_2' during distributive phase
C_1'', C_2'' = graphically found hypothetical drug concentrations on back-extrapolated monoexponential slope β at times t_1' and t_2'
Read for all blood level data until terminal slope is reached.

C_1^*, C_2^* = actual drug concentrations at corresponding times t_1^* and t_2^* during absorptive phase

$C_{1\,diff}, C_{2\,diff}$ = calculate differences between C'_{index} and C''_{index}. Force straight line through last few concentration points of $C_{index\,diff}$ at t'_{index}, and calculate α.

C_1^{**}, C_2^{**} = graphically found concentrations on α-slope at t for all drug concentrations until blood level curve enters α-slope

C_{a1}, C_{a2} = calculate differences between C_{index}^{**} and $C_{index\,diff}$ at t for all drug concentrations until blood level curve enters α-slope. Plot these data, force straight line through all $C_{a\,index}$ points, and calculate k_a

k_{12} = distribution rate constant for transfer from central to peripheral compartment

k_{21} = distribution rate constant for transfer from peripheral to central compartment

k_{13} = elimination rate constant from central compartment

$AUC^{0\to\infty}$ = total area under the curve

Other Methods to Estimate k_a

Many different methods have been described in the literature for estimating k_a. Only a few simple ones will be mentioned here.

C_{max}-Truncated AUC Method (One-Compartment Model)

The C_{max}-truncated AUC method is described by:

$$k_a = \frac{C_{max}}{AUC^{t_{max}\to\infty} - C_{max}/k_e}[h^{-1}] \tag{26}$$

C_{max} = peak concentration

$AUC^{t_{max}\to\infty}$ = area under the curve from peak concentration to infinity

Nomogram Method (One- and Two-Compartment Model)

A nomogram is available (see Franke and Ritschel reference) to estimate k_a from t_{max} and k_{el} in the one-compartment model, or from t_{max} and α (instead of k_{el}) for the two-compartment model.

Absorption Time Method (One- and Two-Compartment Model)

From a log drug concentration-time plot, the time is read when the actual blood level curve is still just distinguishable before entering the terminal, monoexponential line in the one-compartment model, or when the actual blood level curve is still distinguishable before entering the descending distribution phase in the two-compartment model. Under the assumption that at time zero 100 percent of the drug is unabsorbed and at the end of the absorption time is 1 percent unabsorbed, k_a can be estimated (see also Chapter 23):

$$k_a = \frac{4.61}{\text{time of absorption in h}}[h^{-1}] \tag{27}$$

Estimation of k_{el} from Accumulation Studies

When a drug accumulates from the first dose until steady state is reached upon multiple dosing, a ratio, R, can be calculated from the trough concentration after the first dose, $C_{min\ 1}$, and that at steady state, C_{min}^{ss}:

$$R = \frac{C_{min}^{ss}}{C_{min\ 1}} \tag{28}$$

$$t_{1/2} = \frac{\tau \cdot (\ln 0.5)}{\ln(1 - 1/R)}[h] \tag{29}$$

$$k_{el} = 0.693 / t_{1/2}[h^{-1}] \tag{30}$$

Influence of k_a and k_{el} on t_{max}, C_{max}, and $AUC^{0 \to \infty}$

It is important to realize that a change in either k_a and/or k_{el} may profoundly influence the course of a drug blood concentration-time curve and pharmacokinetic parameters. k_a may be different due to different drug release rates from the dosage forms (i.e., solution, capsule, tablet, sustained release tablet, etc.), due to disease (i.e., malabsorption, intestinal atrophy, Crohn's disease), or due to stomach content (i.e., fasting; application before, during, or after meals; viscosity of gastric content; etc.), k_{el} may change due to renal or hepatic impairment, myocardial infarction, etc.

The peak time, t_{max}, and the peak concentration, C_{max}, are functions of the input (k_a) and output (k_{el}) rate constants. In the one-compartment open model t_{max} can be calculated by Equation 15.31, and in the two-compartment model t_{max} can be estimated by Equation 15.32.

$$t_{max} = \frac{\ln(k_a/k_{el})}{k_a - k_{el}}[h] \tag{31}$$

$$t_{max} \approx \frac{\ln(k_a/\alpha)}{k_a - \alpha}[h] \tag{32}$$

The influence of changes in k_a at constant (unchanged) k_{el} and in k_{el} at constant (unchanged) k_a on t_{max}, C_{max}, and AUC is shown in Table 15-1.

Table 15-1. Influence of Changes in Absorption or Elimination Rate Constants on Peak Time, Peak Concentration, and Total Area under the Curve

Change in	k_{el} unchanged: $k_a \downarrow$ (slower)	$k_a \uparrow$ (faster)	k_a unchanged: $k_{el} \downarrow$ (slower)	$k_{el} \uparrow$ (faster)
t_{max}	→	←	→	←
C_{max}	↓	↑	↑	↓
$AUC^{0 \to \infty}$	same	same	↑	↓

Selected References

1. Bjornsson, T. D. and Shand, D. G.: Estimation of Kinetic Parameters from a Two-Point Determination of Drug Accumulation Factor, *Clin. Pharmacol. Ther.* 26:540 (1979).

2. Carpenter, O. S., Northam, J. I. and Wagner, J. G.: Use of Kinetic Models in the Study of Antibiotic Absorption, Metabolism and Excretion. In *Antibiotics—Advances in Research, Production and Clinical Use,* Herold, M. and Gabriel, W., editors, Butterworth, London, 1965, p. 165.

3. Dominguez, R. and Pomerene, E.: Calculation of the Rate of Absorption of Exogenous Creatinine, *Proc. Soc. Exp. Biol. N.Y.* 60:173 (1945).

4. Franke, E. K. and Ritschel, W. A.: A New Method for Quick Estimation of the Absorption Rate Constant for Clinical Purposes Using a Nomograph, *Drug Intell. Clin. Pharm.* 10:77 (1976).

5. Loo, J. C. K. and Riegelman, S.: New Method for Calculating the Intrinsic Absorption Rate of Drugs, *J. Pharm. Sci.* 57:918 (1968).

6. Wagner, J. G. and Nelson, E.: Per Cent Absorbed Time Plots Derived from Blood Level and/or Urinary Excretion Data, *J. Pharm. Sci.* 52:610 (1963).

16

Volume of Distribution and Distribution Coefficient

The volume of distribution is not a "real" volume but an artifact. It is a parameter of a particular model used to fit experimental data. The volume of distribution depends on many factors such as blood flow rate in different tissues (between <2 to >500 ml blood/100 g tissue/min.), lipid solubility of the drug, partition coefficient of drug and different types of tissue, pH, and binding to biological material. The volume of distribution is often proportional to the body weight. However, obesity and edema produce abnormal deviations. In obesity, the volume of distribution of hydrophilic drugs is lower than expected from the body weight. In edematic patients, the volume of distribution of hydrophilic drugs is larger than expected from the body weight.

Since blood is the only accessible body fluid in which we can determine the drug concentration, and since we know in the case of intravascular administration the amount of drug injected directly into the bloodstream, we are able to determine the volume of distribution as soon as the drug has equilibrated (steady state) by dividing the dose administered IV by the initial drug concentration in blood C(0). However, this is valid only in the open one-compartment model. In the case of extravascular administration, this procedure is permissible only if the dose administered is multiplied by the percentage or fraction of dose actually absorbed.

Upon intravascular administration the drug is immediately in the bloodstream. Upon extravascular administration, the drug is absorbed into the bloodstream. If a drug is in the bloodstream it does not necessarily mean that it can immediately produce a pharmacologic response. To become effective, the drug must combine with receptors which usually are not in the bloodstream but in tissue. In order to enter the biophase, the drug must leave the bloodstream and enter other biological fluids. Usually the drug first enters intercellular spaces and then the cells. But even if the drug is in the cell, it may still not reach the biophase because the cell plasma is not a homogeneous fluid but contains organelles which are again surrounded by membranes. If the receptors are in organelles, the drug must permeate (diffuse) into these corpuscular bodies. The drug does not leave the bloodstream completely but equilibrates with the other fluid and tissue compartments according to type of mechanism of transport, pK_a of drug, pH, lipid/water partition coefficient, and binding to biological material (Figure 16-1).

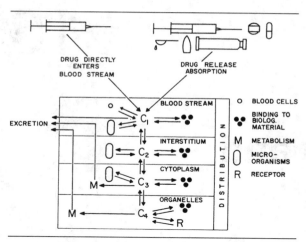

Figure 16-1. Schematic diagram of the distribution of a hypothetical drug in the body.

To exert its pharmacological effect, a drug must cross not one but many membranes. This process may occur extremely rapidly (open one-compartment model) or slowly (open two-compartment model). Let us consider a well vascularized tissue such as muscle, where capillaries have diameters of approximately 0.02 mm and where the farthest capillary is within approximately 0.125 mm of any cell. Since the cells can be assumed to have diameters of approximately 0.01 mm, a drug molecule must only permeate through approximately 10–12 cells to be distributed throughout this tissue.

The volume of distribution is that hypothetical volume one would obtain if all of the drug would be in the bloodstream based on the actual drug concentration found in blood. If the volume of distribution in an adult is approximately 5 liters, it means that the drug is confined to the circulatory system solely. The minimum volume of distribution must be at least equal to the plasma volume (approximately 4.3 percent of body weight). If the volume of distribution in an adult is between 10 and 20 liters, or between 15 and 27 percent of the body weight, we assume that the drug is distributed in the extracellular fluid. If the volume of distribution in an adult is 25–30 liters, or 35–42 percent of body weight, we may assume that the drug is distributed in intracellular fluid. If the volume of distribution in an adult is approximately 40 liters, or 60 percent of the body weight, we assume that the drug is distributed in the whole body fluid.

However, the volume of distribution may even exceed the actual total body weight and may reach 100 or 200 or even more liters for an adult of 70 kg body weight. This indicates that the drug either goes specifically to "deep" tissue in peripheral compartments or is stored or pooled somewhere in the peripheral compartment, such as fat or is bound to specific biological material.

The volume of distribution is a characteristic drug parameter for an individual patient having a particular volume of distribution. If the volume of distribution is divided by the patient's body weight, the distribution coefficient Δ' is obtained which is a general drug parameter valid for all adult patients of normal body weight and normal body stature and frame. Multiplying the distribution coefficient by the body weight of a particular patient yields the volume of distribution of the drug in this particular patient. However, this procedure is not applicable in obese and edematous patients.

The distribution coefficient Δ' is the key for the possibility to translate a given blood level vs time curve, obtained with one patient, to a blood level curve applicable to another patient of different body weight. It is, further, the key in calculating individual dose sizes and dosing intervals. In the case of first-pass effect, f must be multiplied by f_{FPE}.

The equations for the different volumes of distribution are listed in Table 16-1.

Table 16-1. Volume of Distribution

OPEN ONE-COMPARTMENT MODEL, INTRAVASCULAR

$$V_d = \frac{D}{C(0)} [ml] \tag{1}$$

$$V_{d\,area} = \frac{D}{k_{el} \cdot AUC} [ml] \tag{2}$$

$$V_d = \frac{Cl_{tot}}{k_{el}} \tag{3}$$

$$\Delta' = \frac{V_d}{BW} [ml/g] \tag{4}$$

OPEN ONE-COMPARTMENT MODEL, EXTRAVASCULAR

$$V_d = \frac{D \cdot f}{B} \cdot \left(\frac{k_a}{k_a - k_{el}} \right) [ml] \tag{5}$$

$$V_d = \frac{Cl_{tot}}{k_{el}} \tag{6}$$

$$V_{d\,area} = \frac{D \cdot f}{k_{el} \cdot AUC} [ml] \tag{7}$$

$$\Delta' = \frac{V_d}{BW} [ml/g] \tag{8}$$

OPEN TWO-COMPARTMENT MODEL, INTRAVASCULAR

$$V_c = \frac{D}{C(0)} [ml] \tag{9}$$

$$V_{d\,ss} = \frac{k_{12} + k_{21}}{k_{21}} \cdot V_c [ml] \tag{10}$$

$$V_{d\,ss} = Cl * (AUMC^{0 \to \infty} / AUC^{0 \to \infty}) \tag{11}$$

$$t_{1/2} = \ln 2 * (AUMC^{0 \to \infty} / AUC^{0 \to \infty}) \tag{12}$$

$$B = \frac{D \cdot (k_{21} - \beta)}{V_c \cdot (\alpha - \beta)} [\mu g/ml] \tag{13}$$

$$V_{d\,extrap} = \frac{D}{B} = \frac{V_c \cdot (\alpha - \beta)}{(k_{21} - \beta)} [ml] \tag{14}$$

$$V_{d\,area} = V_{d\,ss} + \frac{k_{13} - \beta}{k_{21}} \cdot V_c [ml] \tag{15}$$

$$V_{d\,area} = V_{d\,ss} + D \cdot \frac{A \cdot \beta \cdot (\alpha - \beta)}{(A \cdot \beta + \alpha \cdot B)^2} [ml] \tag{16}$$

(Continued)

Table 16-1. Volume of Distribution, *Continued*

$$V_{d\,area} = \frac{D}{AUC^{0\to\infty} \cdot \beta}[ml] \tag{17}$$

$$V_{d\beta} = \frac{D \cdot \alpha}{B \cdot \alpha + A \cdot \beta}[ml] \tag{18}$$

$$V_{d\beta} = \frac{k_{13} \cdot V_c}{\beta}[ml] \tag{19}$$

$$V_{d\beta} = \frac{Cl_{tot}}{\beta}[ml] \tag{20}$$

$$\Delta'_c = \frac{V_c}{BW}[ml/g] \tag{21}$$

$$\Delta'_\beta = \frac{V_{d\beta}}{BW} \tag{22}$$

$$\Delta'_{ss} = \frac{V_{d\,ss}}{BW}[ml/g] \tag{23}$$

OPEN TWO-COMPARTMENT MODEL, EXTRAVASCULAR

$$V_c = \frac{k_a \cdot f \cdot D \cdot (k_{21} - k_a)}{-C(0) \cdot (\beta - k_a) \cdot (\alpha - k_a)}[ml] \tag{24}$$

$$V_{d\,ss} = \frac{k_{12} + k_{21}}{k_{21}} \cdot V_c[ml] \tag{25}$$

$$V_{d\,ss} / f = Cl^* (AUMC^{0\to\infty} / AUC^{0\to\infty}) \tag{26}$$

$$B = \frac{D \cdot f \cdot (k_{21} - \beta)}{V_c \cdot (\alpha - \beta)}[\mu g/ml] \tag{27}$$

$$V_{d\,extrap} = \frac{D \cdot f}{B} = \frac{V_c(\alpha - \beta) \cdot (k_a - \beta)}{k_a \cdot (k_{21} - \beta)} \tag{28}$$

$$V_{d\,area} = V_{d\,ss} + \frac{k_{13} - \beta}{k_{21}} \cdot V_c[ml] \tag{29}$$

$$V_{d\,area} = V_{d\,ss} + D \cdot f \frac{A \cdot \beta \cdot (\alpha - \beta)}{(A \cdot \beta + \alpha \cdot \beta)^2}[ml] \tag{30}$$

$$V_{d\,area} = \frac{D \cdot f}{AUC^{0\to\infty} \cdot \beta}[ml] \tag{31}$$

$$V_{d\beta} = \frac{D \cdot f \cdot \alpha \cdot k_a}{(\alpha \cdot k_a \cdot B)(\beta \cdot k_a \cdot A)(\alpha \cdot \beta \cdot C(0))}[ml] \tag{32}$$

(Continued)

Table 16-1. Volume of Distribution, *Continued*

$$V_{d\beta} = \frac{k_{13} \cdot V_c}{\beta} \, [ml] \tag{33}$$

$$V_{d\beta} = \frac{Cl_{tot}}{\beta} \, [ml] \tag{34}$$

$$\Delta'_c = \frac{V_c}{BW} \, [ml/g] \tag{35}$$

$$\Delta'_\beta = \frac{V_{d\beta}}{BW} \tag{36}$$

$$\Delta'_{ss} = \frac{V_{d\,ss}}{BW} \, [ml/g] \tag{37}$$

V_d	=	volume of distribution [ml]
V_c	=	volume of central or plasma compartment [ml]
$V_{d\,extrap}$	=	volume of distribution by the extrapolation method [ml]
$V_{d\,area}$	=	volume of distribution by the area method [ml]
$V_{d\beta}$	=	volume of distribution during β-phase [ml]
$V_{d\,ss}$	=	volume of distribution at steady state [ml]
Δ'_{index}	=	distribution coefficient [ml/g]
D	=	dose size administered [µg]
f	=	fraction of drug absorbed [fraction of 1]
BW	=	body weight [g]
k_2	=	absorption rate constant [h^{-1}]
k_{el}	=	elimination rate constant in the open one-compartment model [h^{-1}]
k_{12}	=	distribution rate constant for transfer of drug from central to peripheral compartment [h^{-1}]
k_{21}	=	distribution rate constant for transfer of drug from peripheral to central compartment [h^{-1}]
k_{13}	=	elimination rate constant from central compartment [h^{-1}]
α	=	fast disposition rate constant [h^{-1}]
β	=	slow disposition rate constant [h^{-1}]
C(0)	=	intercept of back-extrapolated monoexponential line with ordinate upon intravascular administration in the open one-compartment model [µg/ml] or— intercept of back-extrapolated monoexponential line with ordinate upon extravascular administration resulting in hypothetical drug concentrations at time 0 in the open one-compartment model = B in [µg/ml] or—drug concentration upon intravascular administration in the open two-compartment model = A + B, in [µg/ml] or—hypothetical drug concentration at time 0 in the open two-compartment model upon extravascular administration = A + B, in [µg/ml]
A	=	intercept of monoexponential declining line of a slope with ordinate in the open two-compartment model [µg/ml]
B	=	intercept of monoexponential declining line of b slope with the ordinate in the open two-compartment model [µg/ml]
$AUC^{0\rightarrow\infty}$	=	total area under the curve [(µg/ml) $\cdot$ h]
$AUMC^{0\rightarrow\infty}$	=	area under the first moment curve [(µg/ml) $\cdot$ h^2]

The primary purpose of a volume of distribution is to be able to relate the concentration of a drug in plasma, blood, or serum to the total amount of drug present in the body at any time. However, none of the different expressions for the volume of distribution holds true over all time periods of the blood level curve. Since $V_{d\,ss}$ is independent of the rate constant for elimination, it is the definition of choice for use in correlating data from one patient to another by the distribution coefficient Δ'. In case it is important to know the total amount of drug present in the body at any time after the β-phase has been reached, then $V_{d\beta}$ or $V_{d\,area}$ (which is equivalent to $V_{d\beta}$) is the definition of choice.

For calculating dose sizes and dosing intervals $V_{d\,ss}$ or $V_{d\beta}$ should be used except for calculating the loading dose for IV infusion. In the latter case the V_c (volume of central compartment) should be used. Even $V_{d\,extrap}$ which is always an overestimate of the "real" situation can be of value because it allows one to make a rapid estimate of the volume of distribution.

In the one-compartment model there is only one volume of distribution, V_d. In multi-compartment models we find four volumes, the order of magnitude is $V_{d\,extrap} > V_{d\beta} > V_{d\,ss} > V_c$. $V_{d\beta}$ and $V_{d\,area}$ are identical in magnitude but determined by different approaches.

The ratio $V_c/V_{d\,extrap}$ is indicative of the degree of multicompartmental character of the concentration-time profile. The smaller the numerical value of $V_c/V_{d\,extrap}$ and the larger the value of the quantity $1 - (V_c/V_{d\,extrap})$, the greater the multicompartmental character. A large value of $1 - (V_c/V_{d\,extrap})$ indicates a pronounced distribution phase.

The quantity $(V_{d\,extrap}/V_{d\beta}) - 1$ is the fractional error in the total clearance when one assumes an open one-compartment model instead of a two- or higher-compartment model. Multiplying the quantity $(V_{d\,extrap}/V_{d\beta}) - 1$ by 100 gives the percent error in Cl_{tot}.

The ratio $V_{d\,ss}/V_{d\beta}$ indicates how well the one-compartment model predicts average amounts of drug in the body when actually a multiple-compartment is applicable. The closer $V_{d\,ss}/V_{d\beta}$ is to unity the better will be the prediction of average amounts in the body at steady state.

The quantity $(V_{d\,ss}/V_c) - 1$ is a direct measure for k_{12}/k_{21} in the two-compartment model or $k_{12}/k_{21} + k_{12}/k_{31}$ in the three-compartment model. The larger the quantity $(V_{d\,ss}/V_c) - 1$ (i.e., > 10), the larger is the proportion of the total amount of drug in the peripheral compartment(s). The smaller the quantity $(V_{d\,ss}/V_c) - 1$ (i.e., < 1), the larger is the proportion of the total amount of drug in the central compartment.

Estimate of the Volume of Distribution from In Vitro Data

It has been demonstrated that there is a relationship between the volume of distribution expressed as distribution coefficient, Δ', and the fraction of protein binding, p, and the apparent lipid/water partition coefficient, APC. The various volumes of distribution can be estimated from the in vitro data of APC (n-octanol/buffer pH 7.4) and from the extent of protein binding (4% human albumin pH 7.4 solution).

For the one-compartment open model:

$$V_d = (0.0955 \cdot APC + 1.2232) \cdot (1-p) \cdot BW[ml] \qquad (38)$$

For the two-compartment open model:

$$V_c = (0.0397 \cdot APC + 0.0273) \cdot (1-p) \cdot BW[ml] \qquad (39)$$

$$V_{d\,ss} = (0.1141 \cdot APC + 0.6611) \cdot (1-p) \cdot BW[ml] \tag{40}$$

$$V_{d\beta} = (0.1302 \cdot APC + 0.9314) \cdot (1-p) \cdot BW[ml] \tag{41}$$

Apparent Volume of Distribution in Renal Failure

Severe renal impairment (i.e., reduction in renal function by $\geq 50\%$) produces alterations in the apparent volume of distribution for specific drugs. Reductions in the concentrations of circulating proteins capable of drug binding (e.g., albumin, alpha-1-acid glycoprotein) occur consequent to filtration of these proteins by a damaged glomerular basement membrane. Accumulation of urea and other "middle-molecules" in the plasma of patients with severe renal failure produces conformational changes (e.g., carbamylation) of albumin, thereby reducing its affinity for binding acidic drugs. Accordingly, for drugs extensively bound to albumin, the increase in free fraction which occurs in renal failure commonly increases the apparent volume of distribution. Specific examples (i.e., V_d "normal" versus "renal failure") include the following: cefazolin (0.13 versus 0.17 L/kg), furosemide (0.11 versus 0.18 L/kg), naproxen (8.3 versus 11.9 L/kg), moxalactam (9.1 versus 21.4 L/kg), and phenytoin (0.64 versus 1.4 L/kg). Also, consequent to disturbances in fluid and electrolyte homeostasis and plasma oncotic pressure, patients with severe renal impairment have expansion of the extracellular, intracellular, and/or total body water spaces ranging in severity from mild edema to ascites (e.g., as seen with severe nephrotic syndrome). In this instance, the apparent volume of distribution of drugs which can partition to these body water spaces (e.g., aminoglycoside antibiotics, methylxanthines, beta-lactam antibiotics, vancomycin) may be increased significantly over "normal" values.

Finally, increases in the apparent volume of distribution (V_d) for drugs produced by severe renal impairment may likewise increase the apparent elimination half-life. As reflected by Equation 16.42, half-life ($t_{1/2}$) increases in association with increases in V_d in situations where total body clearance (Cl) remains stable:

$$t_{1/2} = (0.693 \cdot V_d) / Cl \tag{42}$$

Selected References

1. Benet, L. Z. and Ronfeld, R. A.: Volume Terms in Pharmacokinetics, *J. Pharm. Sci.* 58:639 (1969).

2. Cucinell, S. A. and Perl, W.: Application of Clearance and Volume of Distribution to the Plateau Principle of Drugs, *J. Pharm. Sci.* 59:1423 (1970).

3. Dost, F. H.: *Grundlagen der Pharmakokinetik*, Georg Thieme Verlag, Stuttgart, 1968, p. 31.

4. Fillastre, J.-P. and Singlas, E.: Pharmacokinetics of Newer Drugs in Patients with Renal Impairment (Part I), *Clin. Pharmacokinet.* 20:293–310 (1991).

5. Fillastre, J.-P. and Singlas, E.: Pharmacokinetics of Newer Drugs in Patients with Renal Impairment (Part II), *Clin. Pharmacokinet.* 20:389–410 (1991).

6. Gibaldi, M. and Perrier, D.: Drug Elimination and Apparent Volume of Distribution in Multicompartment Systems, *J. Pharm. Sci.* 61:952 (1972).

7. Lam, Y. W. F., Banerji, S., Hatfield, C. and Talbert, R. L.: Principles of Drug Administration in Renal Insufficiency, *Clin. Pharmacokinet.* 32:30–57 (1997).

8. Perrier, D. and Gibaldi, M.: Relationship Between Plasma and Serum Drug Concentration and Amount of Drug in the Body at Steady State Upon Multiple Dosing, *J. Pharmacokinet. Biopharm.* **1**:17 (1973).

9. Riggs, D. S.: *A Critical Primer—The Mathematical Approach to Physiological Problems,* M.I.T. Press, Cambridge, Mass. 1967, p. 168.

10. Riegelman, S., Loo, J. and Rowland, M.: Concept of a Volume of Distribution and Possible Errors in Evaluation of this Parameter, *J. Pharm. Sci.* **57**:128 (1968).

11. Ritschel, W. A. and Hammer, G. V.: Prediction of the Volume of Distribution from in vitro Data and Use for Estimating the Absolute Extent of Absorption, *Int. J. Clin. Pharmacol. Ther. Toxicol.* **18**:298 (1980).

12. Wagner, J. G. and Northam, J. I.: Estimation of Volume of Distribution and Half-Life of a Compound After Rapid Intravenous Injection, *J. Pharm. Sci.* **56**:529 (1967).

13. Wagner, J. G.: Significance of Ratios of Different Volumes of Distribution in Pharmacokinetics, *Biopharm. Drug Dispos.* **4**:263 (1983).

17

Excretion and Clearance of Drugs

Excretion of drugs is the final elimination (or loss of drug) from the body. Drugs may be eliminated from systemic circulation by different pathways, i.e., into urine, bile, intestines, saliva, alveolar air, sweat, and milk. Only if the drug is not reabsorbed—for example, from urine, bile, intestines, and saliva—is it finally excreted. The two major pathways of excretion are via the kidney into the urine and via the liver into feces. Table 17-1 gives a listing of excretion pathways, transport mechanisms, and examples of drugs.

Renal Excretion of Drugs

The most important organ for excretion is the kidney. The kidney measures 10–12 cm in length and 5–6 cm in width. It weighs 120–200 g. Its gross anatomy is seen in Figure 17-1.

The function of the kidney is the elimination of substances from blood to maintain the internal milieu. The actual unit where elimination (and reabsorption) takes place is the nephron. Each kidney has approximately 1 million nephrons or Malpighian bodies.

Each nephron unit consists of a capillary part and a tubular part. The capillary part is the glomerulus which is surrounded by the Bowman's capsule of connective tissue. The tubular part consists of the following components: the proximal convoluted tubule, the loop of Henle, and the distal convoluted tubule. The latter leads into the collecting duct which empties into the ureter. Arterial blood enters the glomerular capillary network, through an afferent arteriole. Since the intracapillary pressure is higher than the pressure in the tubular lumen, fluid containing most of the solutes found in plasma is mechanically filtered across the capillary walls and through pores of the adjacent epithelium of the Bowman's capsule into the lumen of the tubule. Arterial blood flows out of the glomerulus through an efferent arteriole which then divides to form a dense network of capillaries surrounding the tubular part of the nephron. Glomerular filtration is limited to solutes by their molecular size and shape. Long high molecular weight molecules are not freely filtered. Therefore, the filtrate in the normal kidney is practically free of proteins having a molecular weight of 60,000–70,000 or more. The molecular weights of a few representative proteins are as follows: gelatin = 35,000; egg albumin = 34,500; serum albumin = 67,500; serum globulin = 103,000. Albumin is found in

Table 17-1. Survey of Excretion Patterns

	EXCRETION PATTERN	
PATHWAY OF EXCRETION	**MECHANISM**	**EXAMPLES**
Urine	Glomerular filtration, active tubular secretion, passive diffusion	Most drugs in free (nonprotein bound) form, Salicylic acid ion, PAH, N-Methylnicotinamide, PAB, Penicillin, Sulfadimethylpyrimidine, Sulfaethylthiadiazole, Acetylsulfonamides, Organic mercuric diuretics, Chlorothiazide
Bile	Active transport, passive diffusion, pinocytosis	Quaternary ammonium compounds, Strychnine, Quinine, Digitoxin, Penicillin, Streptomycin, Tetracyclines
Intestines	Passive diffusion and unrecycled biliary secretion	Ionized organic acids, Doxycycline
Saliva	Passive diffusion and active transport	Penicillin, Tetracyclines and many other drugs, Thiamine, Desoxycholate, Ethanol, Ether
Lung	Passive diffusion	Camphor, Guaiacol, Ethereal oils, Ammonium chloride, iodides
Sweat	Passive diffusion	Weak organic acids and bases, Thiamine
Milk	Passive diffusion and active transport	Primarily weak organic bases, Less weak acids, Thyrostatics, Anesthetics, Anticoagulants, Erythromycin and other antibiotics

urine in nephritis, scarlet fever, pneumonia, sinusitis, streptococcal sore throat, and decaying teeth. Albuminuria depletes protein from the blood and leads to a decrease in colloidal osmotic pressure of plasma and, hence, results in edema.

The filtrate passes through the lumen of the proximal tubule, loop of Henle, and distal tubule and enters the collecting duct. During the passage, filtered molecules can diffuse or be actively transported back from the lumen into the blood by what is called urinary or renal reabsorption (urinary recycling). Also, molecules present in the capillary network surrounding the tubules can move passively or be actively transported (secreted) from the efferent blood capillaries into the tubules.

A schematic anatomic and functional diagram of the nephron unit is given in Figure 17-2.

The volume of each glomerulus is approximately 0.0042 mm³. About 25 percent of the volume of the glomerulus, i.e., approximately 0.001 mm³, is fil-

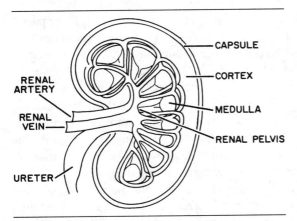

Figure 17-1. Schematic diagram of the human kidney.

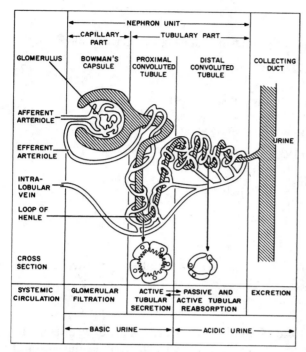

Figure 17-2. Schematic diagram of the structure of a nephron unit and its function.

tered per second. The normal renal blood flow is estimated at 1200 ml/min. This means that approximately 0.01 mm^3 blood flows through each glomerulus per second. This is approximately 2.5 times the glomerular volume. The glomeruli have a total filtration area of approximately 0.76 m^2. Both kidneys have a glomerular volume of approximately 8.4 ml and the filtration rate is about 2 ml per second. The total glomerular filtration rate in the healthy adult is approximately 130 ml/min which gives a total glomerular filtration of 187 liters of fluid per day, from which the renal distal tubuli will reabsorb approximately 185.5 liters while approximately 1.5 liters are excreted to form the urine.

The glomerular filtration is directly influenced by the blood flow through the kidney, which is neurally as well as humorally regulated. If the Na$^+$ content of the filtrate increases in the distal tubuli the kidney secretes the enzyme (protein) renin into the blood. Renin reacts with the α-globulin angiotensinogen in plasma from which angiotensin I is liberated and which is enzymatically transformed into angiotensin II. Angiotensin II causes a constriction of the *vasa afferentia* and, hence, leads to a diminished blood flow to the nephrons resulting in diminished urine formation. At the same time angiotensin leads to a secretion of aldosterone from the adrenal cortex. Aldosterone increases the reabsorption of sodium ions from the distal tubuli. The surplus of angiotensin II is inactivated by the plasma enzyme hypertensinase.

Glomerular Filtration of Drugs

Drugs are usually filtered through the glomerulus in a nonselective process if they are in free, non-protein bound form. If a drug is not bound to plasma protein it is filtered in the amount equal to:

$$F = C \cdot GFR \, [mg / min] \tag{1}$$

F   = amount of drug filtered through glomeruli [mg/min]
C   = drug concentration in plasma [mg/ml]
GFR = glomerular filtration rate = renal clearance [ml/min]

About 20 to 25 percent of the renal plasma flow is filtered into the tubular lumina.

Filtration of Drugs

The amount of any drug filtered through the glomeruli can be calculated as follows:

$$F = [(1-p) \cdot C] \cdot Cl_{creat.} \, [\text{mg}/\text{min}] \qquad (2)$$

F   = amount of drug filtered through glomeruli [mg/min]
C   = concentration of drug in plasma [mg/ml]
p   = fraction of drug bound to protein [fraction of 1]
$Cl_{creat.}$ = creatinine clearance [mg/min] (or $Cl_{in.}$)

$$FF = \frac{GFR}{RPF} = 0.20 \text{ to } 0.25 \qquad (3)$$

FF   = filtration fraction
RPF   = renal plasma flow

Any drug that lowers blood pressure or constricts renal arterioles will reduce the GFR.

Renal Clearance

The renal clearance for a drug is that volume of blood that is cleared of the drug during one minute via the kidneys. When the compound is filtered only by the glomerulus and not otherwise acted on by the kidney (inulin, creatinine), the clearance is also the glomerular filtration rate. The renal clearance or GFR in general is described by the following equation:

$$Cl_{ren.} = \frac{C_u \cdot V}{V} \, [\text{ml}/\text{min}] \qquad (4)$$

$Cl_{ren.}$ = renal clearance
C_u = concentration of drug in urine [mg/ml]
V   = volume of urine excreted [mg/min]
C   = concentration of drug (no protein binding present) in plasma [mg/ml] (at mid-point of urine collection period)

Compounds which are filtered through the glomeruli only are inulin and creatinine. They are used as test substances for the kidney function test to determine the glomerular filtration rate. In practice, usually the (endogenous) creatinine clearance is determined by collecting urine for exactly 24 hours and taking a blood sample at midpoint. The creatinine clearance is then calculated as follows:

$$Cl_{creat.} = \frac{C_u \cdot V \cdot 100}{C \cdot 1440} \, [\text{ml}/\text{min}] \qquad (5)$$

$Cl_{creat.}$ = observed creatinine clearance [ml/min]
C_u = creatinine concentration in urine [mg/ml]
V   = volume of urine excreted in 24 hr [ml]
C   = creatinine concentration in serum [mg/100 ml] (at midpoint of urine collection period)

The "normal" creatinine clearance in adults is approximately 120 [ml/min].

In case a drug is bound to protein the corrected renal clearance is calculated as follows:

$$Cl_{ren.\,corr.} = \frac{C_u \cdot V}{(1-p) \cdot C}[ml/min] \qquad (6)$$

$Cl_{ren.\,corr.}$ = corrected renal clearance [ml/min]
p = fraction of drug bound to protein [fraction of 1]
C_u = concentration of drug in urine [mg/ml]
V = volume of urine excreted [ml/min]
C = concentration of drug in plasma [mg/ml] (at midpoint of urine collection period)

Amount of Drug Excreted

The total amount of drug excreted via the kidney into urine is calculated according to the following equation:

$$E = C_u \cdot V[mg/min] \qquad (7)$$

E = amount of drug excreted via kidney [mg/min]
C_u = concentration of drug in urine [mg/ml]
V = volume of urine excreted [ml/min]

Tubular Transport of Drugs

Glomerular filtration is an essential part in the formation of urine. However, the final composition of urine actually excreted depends largely on the transport of solutes and water across the renal cells of the tubuli. It is the transfer from the lumina of the tubuli to the efferent capillaries and vice versa. The transport may be by passive diffusion or by active transport. In the case of passive diffusion, transfer in either direction depends on the principles of diffusion (concentration gradient, pH, pK_a, lipid solubility, etc.). It is assumed that only the unionized form of a drug can pass the membrane.

The urinary pH in man varies between pH 4.8 and pH 7.5 with an average value of pH 5.8.

Distribution ratio of the urinary concentration and the plasma concentration of *acidic* drugs R_a is:

$$R_a = \frac{1 + anti\log(pH_{urine} - pK_a)}{1 + anti\log(pH_{plasma} - pK_a)} \qquad (8)$$

Distribution ratio of the urinary concentration and the plasma concentration of a *basic* drug R_b is:

$$R_b = \frac{1 + anti\log(pK_a - pH_{urine})}{1 + anti\log(pK_a - pH_{plasma})} \qquad (9)$$

Table 17-2. pH Dependence of Drugs Excreted Into Urine (Renal Reabsorption)

CLEARANCE GREATER IN ACIDIC URINE	CLEARANCE GREATER IN ALKALINE URINE
Amphetamine	Amino acids
Chloroquine	Barbiturates
Codeine	Nalidixic acid
Imipramine	Nitrofurantoin
Levorphanol	Phenylbutazone
Mecamylamine	Probenecid
Mepacrine (Quinacrine)	Salicylic acid
Meperidine	Sulfonamides
Morphine	
Nicotine	
Procaine	
Quinine	

Renal reabsorption of weak electrolytes by passive diffusion can be influenced by changing the urinary pH. A significant change can be expected if the acidic drug has a pK_a between 3 and 7.5 and the basic drug a pK_a between 7 and 11. Some examples of pH-dependent drugs which are excreted into urine are listed in Table 17-2. In Table 17-3 drugs which may cause acidosis or alkalosis are listed.

In the case of active transport the general principles of this transport mechanism apply (carrier, against concentration or electrochemical gradient, saturable, competition, etc.). Active transport occurs from the efferent arterioles into the lumen of the tubuli (active secretion) and also from the tubuli back into the bloodstream (active reabsorption). Most active secretion occurs in the proximal tubuli. However secretion of hydrogen ions and ascorbic acid for acidification of urine occurs in the distal tubuli. Some drugs which are secreted by active transport are listed in Table 17-4.

Renal Plasma Flow and Blood Flow

p-Aminohippuric acid, PAH, is not only filtered through the glomerulus but is also actively secreted. The removal of PAH from arterial blood is 90 percent complete in a single circulation through the kidney. Using the clearance concept for PAH (filtration + active transport) we obtain the effective renal plasma flow:

Table 17-3. Drugs Causing Change of Urinary pH

CAUSE OF ACIDOSIS	CAUSE OF ALKALOSIS
Ammonium chloride	Antacids
Arginine HCl	Calcium carbonate
Ascorbic acid	Diuretics, mercurial
Aspirin	Diuretics, thiazides
Cyclamate	Sodium bicarbonate
Dimercaprol	Sodium glutamate
Lysine HCl	
Phenformin HCl	
Salicylates	

Table 17-4. Drugs Secreted by Active Transport into the Tubuli

ACIDS	BASES
Acetazolamide	Choline
Amino acids	Dihydromorphine
p-Aminohippuric acid	Dopamine
Ethacrynic acid	Histamine
Furosemide	Mepiperphenidol
Indomethacin	Methylnicotinamide
Mersalyl	Neostigmine
Penicillins	Quinine
Perabrodil	Tetraethylammonium
Phenol red	
Phenylbutazone	
Salicylates	
Thiazide	

$$\text{ERPF} = \frac{C_{u\,PAH} \cdot V}{C_{PAH}} [\text{ml/min}] \qquad (10)$$

ERPF = effective renal plasma flow [ml/min]
$C_{u\,PAH}$ = PAH concentration in urine [mg/ml]
C_{PAH} = PAH concentration in plasma [mg/ml]
V = urine volume excreted [ml/min]

ERPF is the volume of plasma cleared of PAH. Since the extraction of PAH is only 90 percent the actual renal plasma flow (RPF in ml/min) is:

$$\text{RPF} = \frac{\text{ERPF}}{0.9} [\text{ml/min}] \qquad (11)$$

Knowing the hematocrit ($\approx 45\%$) we can determine the renal blood flow:

$$\text{RBF} = \frac{\text{RPF}}{1-\text{H}} [\text{ml/min}] \qquad (12)$$

RBF = renal blood flow [ml/min]
H = hematocrit [fraction of 1]

Transport Maximum

The transport maximum tells the capacity of the kidney for active secretion using a test substance.

$$T_m = (Cl_{max.} - Cl_{creat.}) \cdot C \, [mg/min] \tag{13}$$

T_m = transport maximum for active secretion of drug (active transport) [mg/min]
$Cl_{max.}$ = maximum clearance by glomerular filtration and active transport, i.e., RPF of PAH or perabrodil [ml/min]
$Cl_{creat.}$ = renal clearance = GFR [ml/min] (often Cl_{in} is used)
C = concentration of drug in plasma used for Cl_{max}, i.e., PAH or perabrodil [mg/ml]

Active Secretion of Drugs

The amount of any drug secreted by active transport in the tubuli is calculated as follows:

$$AS = \text{excreted drug} - \text{filtered drug}$$

$$AS = (C_u \cdot V) - \left\{ Cl_{creat.} \cdot \left[(1-p) \cdot C\right] \right\} \left[mg/min \right] \tag{14}$$

AS = active secretion of drug [mg/min]
C_u = concentration of drug in urine [mg/ml]
V = urine volume excreted [ml/min]
$Cl_{creat.}$ = creatinine clearance [ml/min] (often Cl_{in} is used)
C = concentration of drug in plasma [mg/ml] (taken at midpoint of urine collection)

Drug Amount Reabsorbed

The amount of drug filtered through the glomerulus but reabsorbed from the tubuli into the bloodstream is calculated as follows:

$$RA = \text{filtered drug} - \text{excreted drug}$$

$$RA = \left\{ Cl_{creat.} \cdot \left[(1-p) \cdot C\right] \right\} - (C_u \cdot V) - [mg/min]$$

$$RA = \text{amount of drug reabsorbed [mg/min]} \tag{15}$$

Fraction of Drug Eliminated in Unchanged Form

The fraction of drug eliminated in urine in unchanged form (parent drug) can be calculated as follows:

$$F_{el} = \frac{k_u}{K} \tag{16}$$

$$F_{el} = \frac{Ae^{\infty}}{D \cdot f} \tag{17}$$

$$F_{el} = \frac{Cl_{ren.}}{Cl_{tot}} \tag{18}$$

F_{el} = fraction of drug eliminated in urine in unchanged form

k_u = rate constant for elimination of unchanged drug into urine [h^{-1}] (for determination of k_u, see chapter on Cumulative Urinary Excretion)

K = overall elimination rate constant (= k_{el}) [h^{-1}]

Ae^{∞} = amount of unchanged drug excreted into urine in infinite time [mg]

D = dose of drug administered [mg]

f = fraction of drug absorbed (for determination see Chapter 36, Bioavailability and Bioequivalence)

$Cl_{ren.}$ = renal clearance [ml/min]

Cl_{tot} = total clearance [ml/min]

Clearance Ratio

The clearance ratio is the ratio between the clearance of a particular drug to the renal clearance or GFR using inulin or creatinine:

$$Cl - R = \frac{Cl_{ren.}}{Cl_{creat.}}$$ (19)

$Cl - R$ = clearance ratio [fraction]

$Cl_{ren.}$ = clearance of drug [ml/min]

$Cl_{creat.}$ = creatinine clearance = GFR [ml/min] (often Cl_{in} is used)

Excretion Ratio

The excretion ratio considers the extent of protein binding of the drug under investigation. It is that fraction of free drug removed by glomerular filtration during one circulation through the kidney with respect to the GFR:

$$E - R = \frac{Cl_{ren.\ corr.}}{Cl_{creat.}}$$ (20)

$E - R$ = excretion ratio

Renal Excretion of Drugs and Metabolites

Many drugs are excreted via the kidney in unchanged form; however, many drugs are more or less excreted in the form of one or more metabolites. Determination of pharmacokinetic parameters of the parent molecule from urinary excretion studies is permissible only if at least 10 percent of the drug is excreted into urine in unchanged form. Table 17-5 lists some examples of drugs which are excreted via the kidney in unchanged or changed form.

Renal Clearance of Drugs

The renal clearance refers to the removal of drug from the apparent volume of distribution per unit of time. It is determined as follows:

Table 17-5. Renal Excretion of Drugs

Drugs Excreted in Unchanged Form	Barbital, digoxin, fluorescein, hexamethonium, kanamycin, streptomycin, gentamicin, vancomycin.
Drugs Excreted in Largely Unchanged Form ( ) = percent in unchanged form	Amphetamine (30), ampicillin (40), atropine (20–50), chloroguanide (40), guanethidine (50), neostigmine (40), phenformin (50), procainamide (50), penicillin G (60–80), carbenicillin (90), cephalothin (60–90), cephaloridine (70), tetracycline (60), oxytetracycline (70), chlortetracycline (20–35)
Drugs Excreted in Form of Inactive Metabolites	Phenacetin, isoniazid, chloramphenicol, morphine

$$Cl_{ren\ drug} = \frac{Ae^{\infty}}{AUC^{0\rightarrow\infty}}[ml/h] \tag{21}$$

$$Cl_{ren\ drug} = Cl_{tot} \cdot F_{el}[ml/h] \tag{22}$$

Serum Creatinine-Creatinine Clearance Relationship

Between the serum creatinine ($Ser_{creat.}$ [mg/100 ml]) and creatinine clearance [ml/min/1.73 m²] values exists a log-log linear relationship in the case of stabilized renal function. Hence, often the time-consuming determination of $Cl_{creat.}$ is not necessary; instead it can be estimated from the $Ser_{creat.}$ value. The normal $Cl_{creat.}$ depends on age and sex.

Factors Influencing Renal Clearance

Age

The renal clearance (measured as Cl_{in}), the renal plasma flow (determined as Cl_{PAH}), and the transport maximum (determined with PAH) are listed for different age groups in Table 17-6.

Age correction for $Cl_{creat.}$ can be made for elderly patients without renal failure according to Equations 17.23 and 17.24 for males and females, respectively:

Table 17-6. Influence of Age on Clearance

AGE	Cl_{in} [ml/min/1.73 m²]	Cl_{PAH} [ml/min/1.73 m²]	T_m [mg/min/1.73 m²]
1–10 days	15–45	20–125	5–60
1 month	30–60	100–400	15–60
6 months	50–100	400–500	25–70
1 year	80–120	500–600	25–70
1–70 years	120 (80–140)	500–700	35–60
70–80	70–110	250–450	30–50
80–90	45–85	200–400	20–40

$$Cl_{creat.\,aged\,male} = 120.7 - 0.988 \cdot (Age - 25)[ml/min] \qquad (23)$$

$$Cl_{creat.\,aged\,female} = 105.9 - 0.988 \cdot (Age - 25)[ml/min] \qquad (24)$$

The $Cl_{creat.}$ can also be estimated from $Ser_{creat.}$ for age beyond 25 years by the method of Cockcroft and Gault:

$$Cl_{creat.} = \frac{(140 - Age) \cdot BW}{72 \cdot Ser_{creat.}}[ml/min] \qquad (25)$$

Age = years
BW = body weight [kg] NOTE: In obese subjects use lean or ideal body weight.
$Ser_{creat.}$ = serum creatinine [mg/100 ml]

NOTE: To normalize clearance creatinine, divide into subject's surface area (see Equation 32.1).

Sex

Clearance is approximately 10 percent lower in females than in males.

Disease

In kidney diseases (nephritis, pyelonephritis, nephrosclerosis, and renal failure) and cardiac diseases (cardiac failure) the renal clearance is reduced. The creatinine clearance is a measure of extent of renal function as given in Table 17-7.

For dosing purposes in suspected renal failure, the elimination rate constant, k_{el}, must be corrected for renal failure, $k_{el\,r.f.}$, as given in Equation 17.26:

$$k_{el\,r.f.} = k_{el} \cdot \left\{ \left[\left(\frac{Cl_{creat.obs.corr.}}{120 - S} - 1 \right) \cdot F_{el} \right] + 1 \right\}[h^{-1}] \qquad (26)$$

$k_{el\,r.f.}$ = elimination rate constant of drug in renal failure [h^{-1}]
k_{el} = normal elimination rate constant of drug [h^{-1}]
$Cl_{creat.obs.corr.}$ = patient's creatinine clearance (for instance, as determined by Equation 17.25) corrected for 1.73 m^2
S = sex; males: S = 0; females: S = 12
F_{el} = fraction of drug eliminated in unchanged form in urine

NOTE: The closer F_{el} is to 1 the smaller will be $k_{el\,r.f.}$ with decreasing renal function.

Table 17-7. Clearance Values in Renal Failure

RENAL FUNCTION	CL$_{creat.}$
Normal	above 80
Slightly reduced	50–80
Mild renal failure	30–50
Moderate renal failure	10–30
Severe renal failure	< 5–10

It must be emphasized that the estimation of $Cl_{creat.}$ from $Ser_{creat.}$ *cannot* be done if one or more of the following situations are present:

a) acute or unstable kidney disease
b) very old age (>90)
c) during and after dialysis
d) severe uremia ($Ser_{creat.} > 8$ mg/100 ml)
e) disturbance of creatinine synthesis (systemic muscular disease, cachexia, weak general condition, long immobilization)
f) interference with creatinine assay by drugs
g) patients who are HIV-seropositive

In cases a through e, the $Cl_{creat.}$ must be determined as shown in Equation 17.4 or 17.5.

Pharmacogenetics of Drug-Metabolizing Enzymes and Transporters

The presence of drug-metabolizing enzymes and transporters in the cortex of the human kidney (located primarily in the renal tubular cells) can influence both the renal clearance and the total plasma clearance of selected xenobiotics that are substrates for these proteins. CYP3A5 is the predominant cytochrome P450 present in the kidneys and in humans; it is polymorphically expressed with a frequency distribution that is different between Caucasians and individuals of African origin (black Africans, African-Americans; see Chapter 39). A single-nucleotide polymorphism (A6986G) in the CYP3A5 gene distinguishes an expressor (*1) and a reduced-expressor (*3) allele and predicts CYP3A5 content in the small intestine, liver, and kidneys which, in turn, has been shown to be associated with the catalytic activity of this enzyme.

Specific drug transporters (OAT, OCT, OATP, and P-gp) are also found in the kidneys (see Chapter 6). Of these, P-glycoprotein (P-gp) appears to have the most important role with respect to regulating tubular secretion of substrates for this transporter. Given the apparent coordinate regulation between CYP3A and P-gp (Figure 6-13), enhanced renal clearance of selected substrates would be expected in patients with high levels of CYP3A5 and/or P-gp expression. As well, concomitant administration of compounds that inhibit either CYP3A5 (e.g., selected macrolide antibiotics, azole antifungal agents) or P-gp (e.g., quinidine, verapamil) would be expected to inhibit tubular secretion and thus reduce the renal clearance of drug substrates for these proteins.

Threshold of Substances Excreted into Urine

Many substances filtered through the glomeruli are reabsorbed from the tubuli by active transport as long as there are carriers available. When the concentration of the particular substance in blood rises above a given level, the tubuli cannot return all the substance back to the bloodstream and the substance then appears in urine. The blood level up to which the substance is returned to the bloodstream by active transport is called threshold.

An example is glucose. Up to about 300 mg glucose/100 ml blood the glucose filtered through the glomeruli is more or less completely reabsorbed (threshold level). Above this level glucose appears in urine in an amount directly proportional to the glucose concentration in blood. Below the threshold level the glucose clearance is zero.

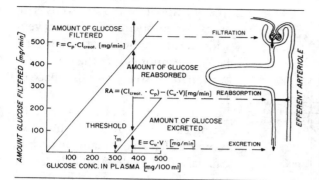

Figure 17-3. Schematic diagram for glomerular filtration, reabsorption, and secretion using glucose as example.

The tubular transport maximum and clearance for glucose are shown in Figure 17-3.

A schematic diagram of the activity of the nephron unit (glomerular filtration, active secretion, and reabsorption) with respect to the renal clearance of a compound, assuming normal kidney function, is given in Figure 17-4.

Biliary Excretion of Drugs

The liver is the largest organ in the adult man, weighs approximately 1.5 kg, and is situated to the right of the stomach. It is covered by connective tissue. The large transverse fissure (*porta hepatis*) on the visceral side (underside) divides the liver into a smaller left and a larger right lobe (*lobus sinister, lobus dexter*). The supporting connective tissue enters at the *porta* and branches extensively. Along with the branching connective tissue, the portal vein (*vena porta*), the hepatic artery (*arteria hepatica*), the bile duct (*ductus hepaticus*), and lymphatic vessels enter to transport material to and from the liver. The liver is supplied with blood coming from the intestines by the portal vein and with arterial blood from the circulation by the hepatic artery. The blood leaves the liver by hepatic veins which empty into the *vena cava*. The gross anatomy of the liver is seen in Figure 17-5.

The liver consists primarily of parenchymal cells which form plates. The plates are arranged in such a way that they form walls around continuous spaces or *lacunae*. Within the lacunae are the capillaries of the liver known as sinusoids. The liver capillaries differ from other capillaries in having larger pores, thus being more permeable for macromolecules (protein). The walls of the sinusoids are lined by Kupffer cells. Between the Kupffer cells and the parenchymal cells is a space, the space of Dissé. A schematic diagram of a liver lobule is seen in Figure 17-6 (see also Figure 3-1).

Blood entering the liver from the intestines by the portal vein enters the fine branches of the vein and finally reaches the sinusoids. Each fine branch of the portal vein is accompanied by fine branches of the hepatic artery with many anastomoses between the venous and arterial branches. The hepatic artery branches provide capillaries for the parenchymal cells and bile ducts and

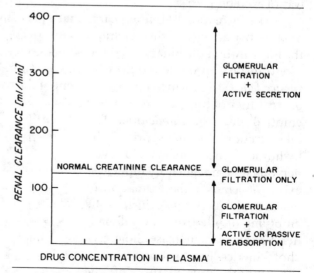

Figure 17-4. Schematic diagram indicating the types of renal processes involved (glomerular filtration, active secretion, and active and passive reabsorption) at a particular renal clearance.

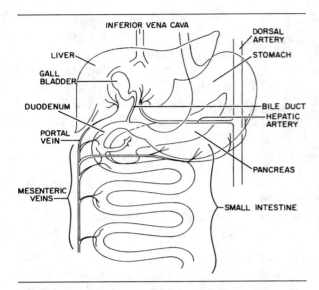

Figure 17-5. Schematic anatomical view of blood supply and drainage of the human liver.

finally empty into the sinusoids. The sinusoids empty into the central vein which leads to the hepatic vein. The latter one empties into the *vena cava*. Lymphatic vessels drain the space of Dissé.

The surfaces of two liver cells facing each other form a cylindrical lumen called bile canaliculi or bile capillaries. The bile canaliculi do not have walls but are formed by the cell membranes. Only the larger units, the bile ductules, have walls which combine to form the larger bile ducts. The liver cell is structured to carry out different functions, particularly metabolic and excretory tasks.

The side of the liver parenchymal cell facing the bloodstream has an extremely large surface area due to the presence of microvilli. However, the microvilli are not directly exposed to the bloodstream but separated from it by the layer of Kupffer cells which show a type of endothelial function. The cell has either one or two nuclei and a large number of mitochondria (2000 per cell) and lysosomes.

The liver acts as a blood pool and is able to compensate for fluctuations in blood pressure. However, its main functions are metabolism and energy production. The liver secretes the bile fluid into which drugs and their metabolites can be secreted thus becoming a pathway of excretion.

The formation of bile appears to take place in the canaliculi. Bile flow is the result of secretory activity of the hepatic cells lining the bile canaliculi. During the passage of the bile through the biliary duct free exchange of compounds to and from blood occurs. The transport into bile requires active secretion. The bile is stored in the gallbladder (*vesica fellea*) from which up to 90 percent of the water is reabsorbed. The liver produces 0.5 to 1 liter of bile per day which is emptied into the *duodenum*. The bile secretion is regulated principally by humoral mechanisms. However, nervous system regulatory influences exist. *Choleresis* is the formation of bile in the liver and *cholekinesis* is the emptying of bile from the gallbladder. (Choleretics increase choleresis, cholekinetics lead to contraction of the smooth musculature of the gallbladder and emptying of its contents.)

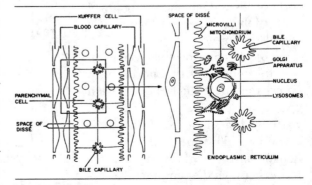

Figure 17-6. Schematic diagram of the structure of liver cells.

The magnitude of bile production depends on the type of food. Food rich in protein results in increased bile secretion, food rich in fat results in some increased secretion, and carbohydrates have hardly any influence.

Two hormones, secretin and cholecystokinin, are involved in the regulatory mechanism. Both are extracted from the duodenal mucosa, intestinally absorbed, and reach the liver via the bloodstream.

Drugs which are absorbed or directly introduced into the bloodstream enter the liver where they may undergo various metabolic changes. The further fate of the drug or its metabolites depends largely on their chemical and physical properties. If

Table 17-8. Biliary Excretion of Drugs

Drugs excreted in unchanged form	Cromoglycate, dichloromethotrexate, rifampin, fluorescein, penicillin, quaternary ammonium ions, mepiperphenidol
Drugs excreted at least partly as inactive metabolites	Indomethacin, taloximine, bromsulphalein, erythromycin, morphine, strychnine, quinine, steroid hormones, ouabain, digitoxin, digoxin, lanatoside C, scillaren A, chlorothiazide, thyroxine, stilbestrol, glutethimide, iodopanoic acid, chloramphenicol, estrone, estradiol, testosterone, norethynodrel, sulfonamides, phenacetin, isoniazid

they are secreted into the bile, they leave the systemic circulation and enter the small intestine from which the compounds are either excreted into the feces or they are reabsorbed into circulation. Often enzymatic reactions occur in the intestines which regenerate the parent molecule. In the case in which enterohepatic reabsorption occurs, it continues until further metabolism and renal excretion eliminate the drug from the body. The excretion rate of such compounds depends largely on the renal elimination of the metabolites.

Biliary excretion is of importance for drugs which are poorly absorbed from the intestines because they are completely or nearly completely ionized at the pH of the intestinal contents (primarily acids). Compounds which are ionized (anions) in blood and tissue fluid usually show biliary and renal excretion. It appears that there is a molecular weight threshold for polar drugs above which biliary excretion becomes significant (i.e., 5–10 percent of the amount of drug in the body). Above this threshold (approximately MW of 400–500) with increasing molecular weight, biliary excretion increases with a concomitant decrease in renal excretion. It is not known whether or not hepatic functions decline with age. However, it has been reported that the BSP (bromsulphalein) test shows abnormal results in patients aged 60 years or more. Sex differences occur in the excretion pattern of some compounds in animals but it is not known whether or not this also occurs in man.

Both organic acids and organic bases are secreted by active transport into bile. Secretion occurs against a concentration gradient until the transport maximum is reached. In Table 17-8 drugs which are secreted into the bile are listed.

Liver Function Test

Bromsulphalein (BSP) is used for determination of secretory function of the liver. Pathological data could be either due to damage of liver parenchymal cells or caused by icterus.

Test: 5 mg/kg BSP is administered IV. After 3 minutes and again after 45 minutes blood samples are taken and BSP is determined in serum:

$$\text{BSP retention} = \frac{\text{Extinction of 45 min sample}}{\text{Extinction of 3 min sample}} \cdot 100 \qquad (27)$$

No liver damage: up to 5 percent BSP retention
Mild liver damage: 5–25 percent BSP retention
Severe liver damage: 25–75 percent BSP retention
Very severe liver damage: 75–100 percent BSP retention

BSP Clearance

The BSP clearance may be used as a general test for liver function. However, the test indicates only the liver's capability for active transport and biliary excretion. A low BSP clearance may indicate reduced hepatic blood flow rate, lack of protein synthesis, reduced energy supply from ATP, or a competition for active transport, but it is not a test for metabolic capacity.

$$\text{Cl}_{hep} = \frac{v_i - v_u}{C} [\text{ml/min}] \qquad (28)$$

$$\text{Cl}_{hep} = \text{Cl}_{tot} - \text{Cl}_{ren} [\text{ml/min}] \qquad (29)$$

Cl_{hep} = hepatic clearance [ml/min]
Cl_{tot} = total clearance [ml/min]
Cl_{ren} = renal clearance [ml/min]
v_i = rate of infusion of BSP [mg/min]
v_u = rate of urinary excretion of BSP [mg/min]
C = BSP plasma concentration at midpoint of urine collection [mg/ml]

The hepatic clearance of drugs can be divided into two groups: flow limited and capacity limited. Whereas the BSP clearance (or propranolol or lidocaine clearance) gives an indication for liver blood flow, the capacity for Phase I and Phase II metabolism may be evaluated by the use of a test substance such as antipyrine, which shows a cytochrome P450-dependent biotransformation.

Salivary Excretion of Drugs

Drugs may pass from the circulatory system into the gastrointestinal tract by different routes. The major pathway is by biliary excretion. But drugs may also pass directly into the gastrointestinal tract from the bloodstream depending on the drug's pK_a and the environmental pH. Bases with pK_a values greater than 5 can pass into the stomach contents in high concentration whereas weak acids are found in minimal concentrations (experiments in the dog).

Additionally, drugs can enter the gastrointestinal tract by salivary excretion. The transport mechanism is primarily passive diffusion of the nonionized moiety. Hence, it depends on lipid solubility, pK_a, pH difference, and plasma protein binding. Also convective transport has been shown. For some drugs, active transport into saliva is assumed (i.e., lithium, penicillin, phenytoin). Proof of active secretion is the observation that probenecid reduces penicillin excretion into the saliva. Drugs which have been found to be excreted into saliva are listed in Table 17-9.

Table 17-9. Drugs Excreted in Saliva

DRUG	SALIVA/PLASMA RATIO
Acetaminophen	1.40
Acetazolamide	0.009
p-Aminohippurate	0.015
Aminopyrine	0.79
Amitriptyline	0.13
Amobarbital	0.35
Amphetamine	2.76
Antipyrine	0.92
Caffeine	0.55
Carbamazepine	0.26
Chloramphenicol	0.25
Cyclophosphamide	0.77
Diazepam	0.029
Digoxin	0.66
Erythromycin	0.21
Estriol	0.009
Ethosuximide	1.04
Isoniazid	1.02
Lidocaine	1.78
Lincomycin	0.086
Lithium	2.85
Methotrexate	0.042
Methylprednisolone	5.2
Metoprolol	2.9
Nitrazepam	0.057
Nortriptyline	0.14
Penicillin	0.015
Pentobarbital	0.42
Phenacetin	0.60
Phenobarbital	0.32
Phenytoin	0.11
Primidone	0.97
Procainamide	3.50
Propranolol	12.0
Quinidine	0.51
Salicylate	0.033
Streptomycin	0.15
Sulfacetamide	0.92
Sulfadiazine	0.31
Sulfadimidine	0.72
Sulfamerazine	0.32
Sulfamethoxazole	0.074
Sulfanilamide	0.87
Sulfapyridine	0.81
Sulfathiazole	0.23
Theophylline	0.75
Tolbutamide	0.012
Trimethoprim	1.26
Valproic Acid	0.06

In the case of weak electrolytes the saliva/plasma ratio can be predicted according to Equations 17.30 and 17.31:

$$R_{\text{saliva/plasma, acids}} = \frac{1+\text{antilog}\,(pH_{\text{saliva}} - pK_a)}{1+\text{antilog}\,(pH_{\text{plasma}} - pK_a)} \cdot \frac{f_{\text{plasma}}}{f_{\text{saliva}}} \qquad (30)$$

$$R_{\text{saliva/plasma, bases}} = \frac{1+\text{antilog}\,(pK_a - pH_{\text{saliva}})}{1+\text{antilog}\,(pK_a - pH_{\text{plasma}})} \cdot \frac{f_{\text{plasma}}}{f_{\text{saliva}}} \qquad (31)$$

f_{plasma} = free fraction of the total drug concentration in plasma
f_{saliva} = free fraction of the total drug concentration in saliva

In the case of "normal" pH values, i.e., plasma pH = 7.4 and saliva pH = 6.2 to 7.2, no correction for pH of saliva is necessary for acidic drugs with a pK_a greater than 8.5 nor for basic drugs with a pK_a of 5.5 or less. The saliva/plasma free drug concentration ratio will be less than unity for weak acids and will exceed unity for weak bases.

It has been suggested that the extent of protein binding could easily be determined by measurement of saliva and plasma concentration and correction for pK_a and pH.

The use of saliva concentrations can be a useful method for drug therapy monitoring because it is noninvasive, a large number of samples can be obtained, and it is particularly useful in ambulatory, pediatric, and geriatric patients.

The general saliva flow rate is approximately 0.6 ml/min. Saliva flow can be stimulated by chewing paraffin wax or Parafilm or by placing a few citric acid crystals into the mouth.

Mammary Excretion of Drugs

The question of mammary excretion of drugs arose with the pesticide residue problem and the use of antibiotics as admixtures with cattle food. Studies during the past two decades have revealed that many drugs pass into milk and may even attain a higher concentration in milk than in plasma. The transport mechanism is primarily by passive diffusion of the nonionized moiety. Extent of drug transfer into milk depends therefore on the drug's pK_a and the pH difference between milk and plasma, the amount of drug in maternal blood, and the lipid solubility of the nonionized drug. Since the pH of human milk is more acidic (pH 6.6) than the pH of plasma (pH 7.4) the milk-plasma ratio is higher for weak bases and lower for weak acids.

However, active transport for drug transport into milk has also been shown. Drugs may appear in milk in much higher concentrations if the nursing mother has decreased renal function.

Whenever possible, nursing mothers should not take any drugs. Mothers who must take antithyroid drugs, lithium, chloramphenicol, sulfonamides, and anticancer drugs should not nurse.

Special care has to be taken if lactating mothers are treated with bases of extremely narrow therapeutic index such as kanamycin, gentamicin, and streptomycin. Tetracyclines excreted into milk may lead to deposition of the drug in bones and teeth (discoloration of teeth). Sulfonamides, although acidic, are excreted into milk. The milk-plasma ratio is <1. However, since newborns have less albumin and cannot metabolize bilirubin, the latter may be displaced from its protein binding by sulfonamides resulting in hyperbilirubinemia and kernicterus. Some drugs which are excreted into milk are listed in Table 17-10.

Table 17-10. Drugs Appearing in Milk of Lactating Mothers

Allergens	Diazepam	Methimazole	Pyrilamine maleate
Aloe	Dicumarol	Methotrexate	Pyrimethamine
Alphaprodine	1,8-Dihydroxy-	Methotrimeprazine	Quinine sulfate
Ampicillin	anthraquinone	Methyprylon	Radiopharmaceuticals
Anticoagulants	Ergot alkaloids	Metronidazole	Reserpine
Antihistaminics	Erythromycin	Morphine	Rifampin
Aspirin	Ethanol	Nalidixic acid	Salicylic acid
Atropine	Ether	Nicotine	Scopolamine
Bethanechol	Ethyl	Nitrofurantoin	Sex hormones
chloride	biscoumacetate	Novobiocin	Sodium chloride
Bromides	Folic acid	Oral contraceptives	Sodium iodide
Caffeine	Gold	Oxyphenbutazone	Sodium salicylate
Calomel	Heroin	Penicillin	Streptomycin sulfate
Carbamazepine	Hexachlorobenzene	Pentobarbital	Sulfonamides
Cascara	Hydrochlorothiazide	Phenindione	Technetium
Chloral hydrate	Imipramine	Phenobarbital	(radioactive)
Chloramphenicol	Iodine[131]	Phenylbutazone	Tetracyclines
Chloroform	Isoniazid	Phenytoin	Theophylline
Chlorpromazine	Kanamycin	Potassium chloride	Thiouracil
Chlorthalidone	Lincomycin	Primidone	Thyrostatics
Colistin sulfate	Lithium carbonate	Propionyl	Thyroxine
Corticosteroids	Meperidine	erythromycin	Tolbutamide
Cyclophosphamide	Mephenesinic acid	lauryl sulfate	Triiodothyronine
Cycloserine	Mercury	Propoxyphene	Trimethoprim
Danthron	Methadone	Propylthiouracil	

For weak electrolytes (most drugs) which are excreted into milk by passive diffusion, the ratio between the milk and plasma concentrations can be calculated according to Equations 17.32 and 17

$$R_{\text{milk/plasma, acids}} = \frac{1 + \text{anti} \log (pH_{\text{milk}} - pK_a)}{1 + \text{anti} \log (pH_{\text{plasma}} - pK_a)} \qquad (32)$$

$$R_{\text{milk/plasma, bases}} = \frac{1 + \text{anti} \log (pK_a - pH_{\text{milk}})}{1 + \text{anti} \log (pK_a - pH_{\text{plasma}})} \qquad (33)$$

In order to estimate the amount of drug the infant might ingest with breast milk, Equation 17.34 can be used, assuming an average daily milk intake of 500 ml:

$$A_{\text{infant}} [\mu g/day] = C_{\text{av mother}}^{ss} \cdot R_{\text{milk/plasma}} \cdot 500 \qquad (34)$$

A_{infant} = amount of drug ingested by breast-fed infant [μg/day]

$C_{\text{av mother}}^{ss}$ = mean steady state drug concentration in maternal plasma [μg/ml]

$R_{\text{milk/plasma}}$ = ratio of drug concentrations between milk and maternal plasma

Table 17-11. Drugs Excreted into Sweat

DRUG	SWEAT/PLASMA RATIO
p-Aminohippuric acid	0.02
Sulfadiazine	0.11
Sulfanilamide	0.69
Sulfapyridine	0.58
Sulfathiazole	0.13
Urea	1.84

Excretion of Drugs into Sweat

Excretion of drugs into sweat follows passive diffusion of the nonionized moiety. Drugs which have been found to be excreted into sweat comprise the nonionized compounds alcohol, antipyrine and urea; weak acids such as sulfonamides, salicylic acid, and benzoic acid; weak bases such as thiamine; and metals such as iodine, bromine, lead, arsenic, mercury, and iron. Some sweat/plasma concentration ratios are listed in Table 17-11.

Excretion of Drugs into Expired Air

The excretion of gases via the lung is the inverted process of gas uptake. Excretion of less soluble anesthetics is high initially and declines rapidly to a lower level. The excretion of soluble gases is also high initially but then decreases gradually. In addition to gases, many volatile compounds are excreted via the lung, such as alcohol and ethereal oils. Some of the drugs excreted via the lung are listed in Table 17-12.

Genital Excretion

It has been shown that some drugs are excreted into prostate secretion. Several cases of malformations were reported which are believed to have occurred due to excretion of antineoplastic agents into seminal fluid. Drugs and metabolites also may be excreted into vaginal fluid. Quantitatively, genital excretion is a relatively unimportant route of clearance for most drugs.

Intestinal Excretion

Drugs may be excreted from systemic circulation into the small intestine, which has been verified for many drugs by their presence in the gut lumen after IV administration. The classical example is doxycycline which normally is excreted via the kidney. In renal failure, however, no dosage regimen adjustment is required because the drug is excreted intestinally as an alternate route.

Total Clearance Cl_{tot}, Hepatic Clearance Cl_{hep}, and Intrinsic Clearance Cl_{intr}

The total clearance characterizes the clearing of the hypothetical plasma volume of a drug per unit of time. This process comprises not only renal excretion but all other pathways of excretion including loss of drug (parent molecule) by metabolism. The total clearance is determined from blood level curves.

Table 17-12. Drugs Excreted via the Lung

DRUGS
Alcohol
Ammonium chloride
Anesthetics, gaseous
Camphor
Coumarin
Ethereal oils
Guaiacol
Iodides
Paraldehyde

For the open one-compartment model the total clearance is determined using the following equations:

$$Cl_{tot} = \frac{k_{el} \cdot V_d}{60} [ml/min]$$ (35)

$$Cl_{tot} = \frac{f \cdot f_{FPE} \cdot D}{AUC^{0 \to \infty}} [ml/min]$$ (36)

Cl_{tot}	=	total clearance [ml/min]
k_{el}	=	overall elimination rate constant [hr^{-1}]
V_d	=	volume of distribution [ml]
f	=	fraction of drug absorbed
f_{FPE}	=	fraction of drug reaching systemic circulation in presence of first-pass effect
$AUC^{0 \to \infty}$	=	area under the concentration-time curve from t = 0 to t = ∞ [(µg/ml) · h], multiplied by 60

For the open two-compartment model the total clearance is calculated according to the following equations:

$$Cl_{tot} = \frac{k_{13} \cdot V_c}{60} [ml/min]$$ (37)

$$Cl_{tot} = \frac{\beta \cdot V_{d\beta}}{60} [ml/min]$$ (38)

$$Cl_{tot} = \frac{f \cdot f_{FPE} \cdot D}{AUC^{0 \to \infty}} [ml/min]$$ (39)

k_{13}	=	elimination rate constant from central compartment [h^{-1}]
β	=	slow disposition rate constant [h^{-1}]
V_c	=	volume of distribution of central compartment [ml]
$V_{d\beta}$	=	volume of distribution during β-phase [ml]
f	=	fraction of drug absorbed
f_{FPE}	=	fraction of drug reaching systemic circulation in presence of first-pass effect
$AUC^{0 \to \infty}$	=	area under concentration-time curve from t = 0 to t = ∞ [(µg/ml) · h] multiplied by 60

Drugs can be cleared from the body by different pathways. The two most important organs are the kidney (Cl_{ren}) and the liver (Cl_{hep}). The other nonhepatic and nonrenal pathways (lung, skin, saliva, breast milk, etc.) are usually negligible. The sum of clearance pathways is the total (or systemic) clearance Cl_{tot}, which is the total volume of distribution totally cleared of drug per unit of time. Independent of any pharmacokinetic model the Cl_{tot} can be determined from the dose administered, D, the absolute bioavailability, f, and the total area under the blood concentration-time curve, $AUC^{0 \to \infty}$:

$$Cl_{tot} = \frac{D \cdot f}{AUC^{0 \to \infty}}$$ (40)

However, the clearance concept is more complex if a drug is bound to protein and is at least partially metabolized. At steady state, the total drug concentration is a function of dosing rate (dose size D/dosing interval τ) and Cl_{tot}:

$$C^{ss} = \frac{D/\tau}{Cl_{tot}} \tag{41}$$

The total drug concentration C is the ratio of free, unbound drug concentration, $f_u \cdot C$, and the free, unbound drug fraction, f_u:

$$C = \frac{f_u \cdot C}{f_u} \tag{42}$$

Assuming complete absorption, the fraction of drug not reaching systemic circulation is removed through either protein binding or first-pass metabolism (gut wall, mesenteric and portal blood, liver). The fraction thus "extracted" is called extraction ratio E. Hence, the fraction reaching systemic circulation, f_{FPE}, is:

$$f_{FPE} = 1 - E \tag{43}$$

E is determined from the concentrations of drug in arterial (C_a) and venous (C_v) blood perfusing the liver:

$$E = \frac{C_a - C_v}{C_a} \tag{44}$$

The extraction ratio of drugs may vary between 0 and 1. Drugs can be classified into those of low extraction ratio, $E < 0.3$, high extraction ratio, $E > 0.7$, and an intermediate group. Drugs of low E are diazepam, INH, phenytoin, theophylline, and warfarin. Drugs of high E are alprenolol, isoproterenol, lidocaine, meperidine, morphine, nitroglycerin, pentazocine, and propranolol. Aspirin and quinidine are of intermediate E. Knowing E and the liver blood flow, Q, one can calculate the *hepatic clearance*, Cl_{hep}:

$$Cl_{hep} = Q \cdot \frac{C_a - C_v}{C_a} = Q \cdot E \tag{45}$$

When blood flow to the liver is constant, Cl_{hep} equals the product of Q and E. However, one has to be aware that E is not a constant but changes with blood flow for drugs with low E as shown in Table 17-13.

Drugs of low E ($E < 0.3$) show a capacity-limited clearance, more or less independent of liver blood flow. The clearance is limited by the free fraction of drug; hence, these drugs are pharmacokinetically sensitive to changes in protein binding: displacement from binding; hypoproteinemia due to age, burns, malnutrition, or disease (renal impairment, liver damage, heart infarction); or hyperalbuminemia in psychiatric patients.

Drugs of high E ($E > 0.7$) show a liver blood flow-limited clearance, having more or less the same E independent of protein binding; hence, these drugs are pharmacokinetically insensitive to changes in protein binding.

Table 17-13. Influence of Change in Blood Flow on Total Clearance and Extraction Ratio

DRUG PROPERTY: EXTRACTION RATIO E	BLOOD FLOW	CHANGE IN:	
		EXTRACTION RATIO E	TOTAL CLEARANCE Cl_{tot}
Low	↑	↓	n.c.
E < 0.3	↓	↑	n.c.
High	↑	n.c.	↑
E > 0.7	↓	n.c.	↓

↑ = increase; ↓ = decrease; n.c. = no change

The liver's maximum capacity or the ability to remove a drug in the absence of flow limitations is called *intrinsic clearance*, Cl_{intr}. The Cl_{hep} is related to both liver blood flow, Q, and intrinsic clearance, Cl_{intr}:

$$Cl_{hep} = Q \cdot \left(\frac{Cl_{intr}}{Q + Cl_{intr}} \right) \qquad (46)$$

Cl_{intr} is directly related to E, and a change in plasma binding may influence Cl_{hep}. If the fraction of unbound drug, f_u, is considered, Equation 17.46 can be rewritten, substituting Cl_{intr} by $f_u \cdot Cl_{intr\ unbound}$:

$$Cl_{hep} = Q \cdot \left(\frac{f_u \cdot Cl_{intr\ unbound}}{Q + f_u \cdot Cl_{intr\ unbound}} \right) \qquad (47)$$

Since:

$$Cl_{tot} = f_u \cdot Cl_{intr} \qquad (48)$$

Equation 17.41 can be rewritten for total drug concentration:

$$C^{ss} = \frac{D/\tau}{f_u \cdot Cl_{intr}} \qquad (49)$$

and, hence, the free drug concentration is:

$$C^{ss} \cdot f_u = \frac{D/\tau}{Cl_{intr}} \qquad (50)$$

The influence of protein binding due to displacement from binding on pharmacokinetic parameters is shown in Table 17-14.

Inspection of Tables 17-13 and 17-14 reveals some important facts which can be summarized as follows:

- Change in liver blood flow will influence the rate of metabolism of drugs with high extraction ratios (E > 0.7). Increase in liver blood flow will increase hepatic and total clearance.

Table 17-14. Influence of Change in Protein Binding due to *Displacement (Increase in Free, Unbound Fraction f_u)* from Protein Binding on Apparent Volume of Distribution, V_d, Elimination Half-Life, $t_{1/2}$, Total Clearance, Cl_{tot}, Intrinsic Clearance, Cl_{intr}, Total Area Under the Curve, $AUC^{0 \to \infty}$, and Pharmacologic Response, R

DRUG PROPERTY: EXTRACTION RATIO E		CHANGE IN:						
	V_d	V_d	$t_{1/2}$	Cl_{tot}	Cl_{intr}	$AUC^{0 \to \infty}$	R
Low	Large	↑	↓	↑	n.c.	↓	?
E < 0.3	Small	n.c.	↓	↑	n.c.	↓	?
High	Large	↑	↑	n.c.	↓	n.c.	↑
E > 0.7	Small	n.c.	↑	n.c.	↓	n.c.	↑

↑ = increase; ↓ = decrease; n.c. = no change

- Change in liver blood flow will not influence drugs with low extraction ratios (E < 0.3).
- Change in protein binding of drugs with high extraction ratios (E > 0.7) will not influence total clearance.
- Decrease in protein binding increases the total clearance of drugs with low extraction ratios (E < 0.3).
- Decrease in protein binding does not influence the total clearance of drugs with high extraction ratios (E > 0.7). However, because the intrinsic clearance decreases, the free drug concentration increases; hence, pharmacodynamic response may increase.
- In the relationship between Cl_{tot}, V_d, and $t_{1/2}$, total clearance and volume of distribution are the independent variables and the elimination half-life is the dependent variable:

$$t_{1/2} = \frac{0.693 \cdot V_d}{Cl_{tot}} \tag{51}$$

For clinical applications, it is not feasible to collect a sufficient number of blood samples to either perform pharmacokinetic parameter calculations after curve-fitting or to calculate the AUC. Two methods can be used for estimating the total clearance from a single blood sample. If the bioavailability is not known, the clearance is Cl_{tot}/f.

Method I

Method I is based on a blood sample C(t) taken during the terminal phase, the literature value for V_d, and the body weight, BW:

$$Cl_{tot}/f = \left[\ln\left(\frac{D}{V_d/f} \right) - \ln C(t) \right] \cdot \frac{V_d/f}{t} \cdot BW \tag{52}$$

Method II

Method II is based on the postulate that in the absence of enzyme induction or enzyme inhibition, the total area under the curve after a single dose, $AUC^{0 \to \infty}$, is equal to the area under the curve during one dosing interval at steady state, $AUC^{\tau_n \to \tau_{n+1}}$. $AUC^{\tau_n \to \tau_{n+1}}$ can be obtained from the steady state concentration:

$$AUC^{\tau_n \to \tau_{n+1}} = C_{av}^{ss} \cdot \tau \tag{53}$$

Since $AUC^{\tau_n \to \tau_{n+1}} = AUC^{0 \to \infty}$:

$$Cl_{tot}/f = \frac{D}{AUC^{\tau_n \to \tau_{n+1}}} \tag{54}$$

or:

$$Cl_{tot}/f = \frac{D}{C_{av}^{ss} \cdot \tau} \tag{55}$$

If one wants to convert the total plasma clearance to blood clearance, Equation 17.56 can be used:

$$Cl_{tot\ blood} = \frac{Cl_{tot\ plasma}}{1 - Hematocrit} \tag{56}$$

For drugs bound to erythrocytes, Equation 17.57 is used:

$$Cl_{tot\ blood} = \frac{Cl_{tot\ plasma}}{\lambda} \tag{57}$$

where λ is the drug concentration ratio blood/plasma.

Extrarenal Clearance Cl$_{\text{extraren.}}$

Being able to calculate the total clearance from blood level curves and the renal clearance from blood and urine data, it is then possible to combine all other pathways of excretion, including metabolism, in one parameter, the extrarenal clearance which is the difference between the total and the renal clearance as given in Equation 17.58:

$$Cl_{extraren.} = Cl_{tot} - Cl_{ren.\ corr.} \, [ml/min] \tag{58}$$

The secretion of drug into bile, metabolism, excretion of drugs from blood directly into the intestines, and excretion via lung, skin, saliva, and milk are not included in the renal clearance but are included in the total clearance determination. The extrarenal clearance therefore gives a good estimate of the magnitude of metabolism or biliary excretion since the other components of the extrarenal clearance (excretion via lung, skin, saliva, and milk) are in general of subordinate importance.

Selected References

1. Abou-El-Makarem, M. M., Millburn, P., Smith, R. L. and Williams, R. T.: Biliary Excretion of Foreign Compounds: Species Differences in Biliary Excretion, *Biochem. J. 105*:1289 (1967).

2. Anderson, P. O.: Drugs and Breast Feeding—A Review, *Drug Intell. Clin. Pharm. 11*:208 (1977).

3. Beckett, A. H. M., Rowland, M. and Turner, P.: The Influence of Urinary pH on Excretion of Amphetamine, *Lancet 1*:303 (1965).

4. Cafruny, E. J.: Renal Pharmacology, *Annu. Rev. Pharmacol. 8*:131 (1968).

5. Danhof, M. and Breimer, D. D.: Therapeutic Drug Monitoring in Saliva, *Clin. Pharmacokinet. 3*:39 (1978).

6. Dossing, M., Poulsen, H., Andreasen, P. and Tigstrup, N.: A Simple Method for Determination of Antipyrine Clearance, *Clin. Pharmacol. Ther. 32*:392 (1982).

7. Dost, F. H.: *Grundlagen der Pharmakokinetik,* Georg Thieme Verlag, Stuttgart, 1968, pp. 35; 74.

8. Givens, R. C., Lin, Y. S., Dowling, A. L., Thummel, K. E., Lamba, J. K., Scheutz, E. G., Stewart, P. W. and Watkins, P. B.: CYP3A5 Genotype Predicts Renal CYP3A Activity and Blood Pressure in Healthy Adults. *J. Appl. Physiol. 95*:1297–1300 (2003).

9. Knowles, J. A.: Excretion of Drugs in Milk—A Review, *J. Pediatr. 66*:1068 (1965).

10. LaDu, B. N., Mandel, H. G. and Way, E. L.: *Fundamentals of Drug Metabolism and Drug Disposition,* Williams and Wilkins, Baltimore, 1971.

11. Lin, J. H. and Yamazaki, M.: Role of P-Glycoprotein in Pharmacokinetics: Clinical Implications. *Clin Pharmacokinet. 42*:59–98 (2003).

12. Milue, M. D., Scribner, B. H. and Crawford, M. A.: Nonionic Diffusion and the Excretion of Weak Acids and Bases, *Am. J. Med. 24*:709 (1958).

13. O'Brien, T. E.: Excretion of Drugs in Human Milk, *Am. J. Hosp. Pharm. 31*:844 (1974).

14. Ritschel, W. A.: *Angewandte Biopharmazie,* Wissenschaftliche Verlagsgesellschaft, Stuttgart, 1973, p. 162.

15. Ritschel, W. A. and Thompson, G. A.: Monitoring of Drug Concentrations in Saliva: a Non-Invasive Pharmacokinetic Method, *Methods Find. Exp. Clin. Pharmacol. 5*:511 (1983).

16. Rowland, M., Benet, L. Z. and Graham, G. G.: Clearance Concept in Pharmacokinetics, *J. Pharmacokinet. Biopharm. 1*:123 (1973).

17. Rowland, M. and Tozer, T. N.: Clearance and Renal Excretion. In *Clinical Pharmacokinetics: Concepts and Applications,* Lea and Febiger, Philadelphia, 1980, pp. 48–64.

18. Stowe, C. M. and Plaa, G. L.: Extrarenal Excretion of Drugs and Chemicals, *Annu. Rev. Pharmacol. 8*:337 (1968).

19. Thayson, J. H. and Schwartz, I. L.: The Permeability of Human Sweat Glands to a Series of Sulfonamide Compounds, *J. Exp. Med. 98*:261 (1953).

20. Wagner, J. G.: *Biopharmaceutics and Relevant Pharmacokinetics,* Drug Intelligence Publications. Hamilton, Ill., 1971, pp. 247, 260.

21. Wandell, M. and Wilcox-Thole, W. L.: Protein Binding and Free Drug Concentrations. In: *Applied Clinical Pharmacokinetics,* Mungall, D. R., Editor, Raven Press, New York, 1983, pp. 17–48.

22. Weiner, I. M.: Mechanisms of Drug Absorption and Excretion: The Renal Excretion of Drugs and Related Compounds, *Annu. Rev. Pharmacol. 7*:39 (1967).

23. West, J. R., Smith, H. W. and Casis, H.: Glomerular Filtration Rate, Effective Renal Blood Flow, and Maximal Tubular Excretory Capacity, *J. Pediatr. 32*:10 (1948).

18

Urinary and Biliary Recycling

Urinary Recycling

Lipid soluble, unionized drugs can be reabsorbed from the tubuli by passive diffusion. The factors involved include pK_a, pH, and lipid/water partition coefficient of which the latter is the predominant mechanism of reabsorption. Organic ions can be reabsorbed to some extent from the tubuli by active transport. The factors involved relate to the carriers present and competitive inhibition.

Consequences for Urinary Recycling by Passive Diffusion

In acidic urine, acidic drugs are more unionized, hence reabsorbed → increase in $t_{1/2}$, whereas basic drugs are more ionized, hence not reabsorbed → decrease in $t_{1/2}$. In basic urine, acidic drugs are more ionized, hence not reabsorbed → decrease in $t_{1/2}$, whereas basic drugs are more unionized, hence reabsorbed → increase in $t_{1/2}$.

Food (rhubarb → acidic; sauerkraut → acidic; citrus fruits → acidic; milk and milk products → basic) and drugs (acidifiers such as ammonium chloride, aspirin, phenformin hydrochloride; alkalinizers such as calcium carbonate, mercurial diuretics, ethacrynic acid, sodium bicarbonate, sodium glutamate) may change urinary pH and hence increase or decrease elimination rate of drugs.

Decreased recycling increases the elimination rate constant and decreases $t_{1/2}$; hence it shortens duration of pharmacologic response and lowers the therapeutic concentration in the body. Increased recycling decreases the elimination rate constant and increases $t_{1/2}$; hence blood levels rise and persist longer. Thus, there is danger of toxicity in multiple dosing.

Any change in the normal excretion pattern may demand a change of dose size and dose regimen.

Biliary Recycling

Drugs entering the bile must be considered as drugs administered perorally. Upon emptying of the bile into the duodenum, the drugs may be reabsorbed by one of the absorption mechanisms into the portal circulation and returned to the liver from where they are re-excreted into bile. Recycling is possible for drugs excreted into bile in unchanged form and for metabolites if they are either absorbed or modified by the gut flora, particularly after splitting of conjugates.

Biliary recycling (or enterohepatic reabsorption) is influenced by:

- Rate of excretion of drug into the bile;
- Form of drug which is excreted into the bile;
- Function of gut flora;
- Gallbladder function;
- Type of food intake (protein and fat increase bile flow); and
- Rate of loss of drug with feces.

Drugs which have been found to take part in biliary recycling are: digitoxin, rifamycin, stilbestrol, glutethimide, chloramphenicol, indomethacin, morphine, and rigomycin.

Consequences for Biliary Recycling

Blood level curves of drugs that undergo biliary recycling show fluctuations in the plasma concentration versus time profile that may manifest as multiple peaks and/or a longer apparent elimination half-life. Consequently, differences in the bioavailability, apparent volume of distribution, and/or clearance of a given compound may result. It is generally recognized that the extent of biliary (and enterohepatic) recycling is not only associated with drugs (choleretics) and nutrients (fat) that stimulate bile flow but also that it is highly variable between individuals. Part of this variability is thought to reside with the interindividual differences in the expression of transporters that can impact biliary drug secretion/excretion (e.g., MRP2, MRP3, P-glycoprotein; see Chapter 6), especially those that have functionally significant genetic polymorphisms. Finally, it should be recognized that alterations in bioavailability of drugs that undergo enterohepatic recycling also result from intestinal reabsorption which may be rate limited by both gut wall efflux mediated by P-glycoprotein and also gut-wall metabolism.

Selected References

1. Abou-El-Makarem, M. M., Millburn, P., Smith, R. L. and Williams, R. T.: Biliary Excretion of Foreign Compounds: Species Differences in Biliary Excretion, *Biochem. J.* 105:1289 (1967).

2. Beckett, A. H., Boyes, R. N. and Tucker, G. T.: Use of Analogue Computer to Examine the Quantitative Relation Between Urinary pH and Kidney Reabsorption of Drugs Partially Ionized at Physiological pH, *J. Pharm. Pharmacol.* 20:269 (1968).

3. Roberts, M. S., Magnusson, B. M., Burczynski, F. J. and Weiss, M.: Enterohepatic Circulation: Physiological, Pharmacokinetic and Clinical Implications. *Clin. Pharmacokinet.* 41:751–790 (2002).

4. Wilkinson, G. R. and Beckett, A. H.: Absorption, Metabolism and Excretion of Ephedrines in Man I: The Influence of Urinary pH and Urine Volume Output, *J. Pharmacol. Exp. Ther.* 162:139 (1968).

5. Yesair, D. W., Callahan, M., Remington, L. and Kensler, C. J.: Role of Entero-Hepatic Cycle in Indomethacin on its Metabolism, Distribution in Tissues and its Excretion by Rats, Dogs and Monkeys, *Biochem. Pharmacol.* 19:1579 (1970).

19

Cumulative Urinary Excretion

Cumulative urinary excretion is often used in pharmacokinetic and clinical studies in man and animals to learn about the disposition of the drug and to determine the elimination rate constant k_{el}, the absorption rate constant k_a, the fraction of drug absorbed f, the percent of drug absorbed, the ultimate amount of drug absorbed, and the extent of bioavailability (EBA) of a drug.

In a cumulative urinary excretion study, urine is collected upon administration of a drug product until the unchanged drug is more or less excreted from the body (at least $7 \cdot t_{1/2}$ when > 99 percent of the drug is eliminated). In each urine sample of a collecting period, the drug concentration per ml is determined. Upon multiplication by the volume of urine excreted during a collecting period, the amount of unchanged drug excreted is obtained. By plotting the cumulative (additive) amounts of drug excreted for each collecting period versus time (collecting intervals) on numeric graph paper, a cumulative urinary excretion versus time plot is obtained (Figure 19-1).

For a urinary excretion study based upon single dose administration to be suitable for pharmacokinetic evaluation, the following prerequisites must be met:

- The drug under investigation must be excreted via the kidney in a fraction of at least 10 percent in the form of unchanged drug.
- "Water-loading" is done in order to provoke diuresis and in order to obtain a sufficient number of urine samples during the first hours after administration, which is necessary for determination of the absorption and distribution phases. For water-loading, 400 ml of water is taken after overnight fasting one hour before the experiment, and 200 ml of water is taken at the time of administration of the drug product, followed by 200 ml given in hourly intervals for the next four hours.
- Immediately before administration of the drug, the bladder is emptied completely. A sample of urine is kept as a blank (for chemical, physical, or microbiological analysis).
- Total bladder emptying at each sampling is necessary. If the bladder is not completely emptied, the amount of drug remaining in the urine would falsely be added to the next sample and incorrect pharmacokinetic data would result. Because of the need for complete bladder emptying, adults between 20 and 40 years of age should be used. With

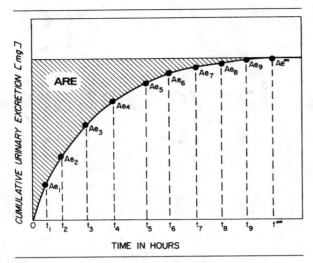

Figure 19-1. Numeric plot of cumulative amount of drug excreted in urine versus time.

Ae index = cumulative amount of drug excreted
Ae^∞ = amount of drug excreted in infinite time
t index = sampling times
t^∞ = time when all drug is excreted
ARE = amount of drug remaining to be excreted

increasing age, muscle contractability is weakened.

- For each urine sample obtained, the exact time should be noted and the volume of urine excreted [ml] should be read.
- If the urine is not immediately analyzed for its drug concentration, a small sample of 20 to 50 ml is stabilized and immediately frozen and kept in the freezer until analysis is performed.
- It is essential that all urine samples be collected. If only one urine sample is lost the entire experiment is invalidated.
- Urine must be collected until practically all of the unchanged drug is excreted. Therefore, urine collection shall be done for at least 7 to 10 elimination half-lives (after 7 and 10 half-lives, 99.2 and 99.9 percent, respectively, of the drug is excreted).

In case only the fraction of drug absorbed f or the extent of bioavailability EBA is studied, the total volume of urine excreted within 7 to 10 half-lives can be pooled and the total amount of unchanged drug excreted in infinite time Ae^∞ can be determined in the pooled sample.

In case the pharmacokinetics of metabolites which are excreted via the kidney are to be studied, the same prerequisites apply as already outlined.

The sampling times T, urine volumes of sampling periods V, and drug concentrations in urine C_u of each sample are entered in Table 19-1. The amount excreted during each sampling period Ae_i is determined by multiplying the drug concentration in urine C_u with the corresponding urine volume V, as given for sample number 1 as follows:

$$Ae_{i1} = C_{u1} \cdot V_1 [mg] \tag{1}$$

The cumulative amount of drug excreted up to time T is the sum of amounts of drug excreted ΣAe_i during that time T.

The midpoint time, $t_{midp.}$, between two sampling times is calculated according to Equation 19.2:

$$t_{midp.} = \frac{t_{n+1} + t_{n-1}}{2} \tag{2}$$

Table 19-1. Table for Cumulative Urinary Excretion Studies

SAMPLE NUMBER	T [hrs]	C_u [mg/ml]	V [ml]	Ae_i [mg]	Ae [mg]	$t_{midp.}$ [hrs]	dAe/dt [mg/hr]	$\dfrac{1}{k_{e1}} \cdot \dfrac{dAe}{dt}$	$A_T(f)$ [mg]	PERCENT OF DRUG ABSORBED*
1	t_1	C_{u1}	V_1	Ae_{i1}	Ae_1	$(t_2 + 0)/2$	$\dfrac{Ae_2 - 0}{t_2 - 0}$		$A_T(f)_1$	$A_T(f)_1/A_T(f)_{AS}$
2	t_2	C_{u2}	V_2	Ae_{i2}	Ae_2	$(t_3 + t_1)/2$	$\dfrac{Ae_3 - Ae_1}{t_3 - t_1}$		$A_T(f)_2$	$A_T(f)_2/A_T(f)_{AS}$
3	t_2	C_{u3}	V_3	Ae_{i3}	Ae_3	$(t_4 + t_2)/2$	$\dfrac{Ae_4 - Ae_2}{t_4 - t_2}$		$A_T(f)_3$	$A_T(f)_3/A_T(f)_{AS}$
4	t_4	C_{u4}	V_4	Ae_{i4}	Ae_4	$(t_5 + t_3)/2$	$\dfrac{Ae_5 - Ae_3}{t_5 - t_3}$		$A_T(f)_4$	$A_T(f)_4/A_T(f)_{AS}$
5	t_5	C_{u5}	V_5	Ae_{i5}	Ae_5	$(t_6 + t_4)/2$	$\dfrac{Ae_6 - Ae_4}{t_6 - t_4}$		$A_T(f)_5$	$A_T(f)_5/A_T(f)_{AS}$
6	t_6	C_{u6}	V_6	Ae_{i6}	Ae_6	$(t_7 + t_5)/2$	$\dfrac{Ae_7 - Ae_5}{t_7 - t_5}$		$A_T(f)_6$	$A_T(f)_6/A_T(f)_{AS}$
→	→	→	→	→	→	→	→	→	$\rightarrow \Big\}$**	→

*Value is multiplied by 100   **Take average value

T = sampling time; C_u = drug concentration in urine sample; V = urine volume excreted per sampling interval; Ae_i = amount of drug excreted per sampling interval; Ae = cumulative amount of drug excreted; $t_{midp.}$ = midpoint time between two sampling intervals; dAe/dt = excretion rate of sampling interval; k_{el} = elimination rate constant; $A_T(f)$ = cumulative amount of drug absorbed; $A_T(f)_{AS}$ = total amount of drug absorbed.

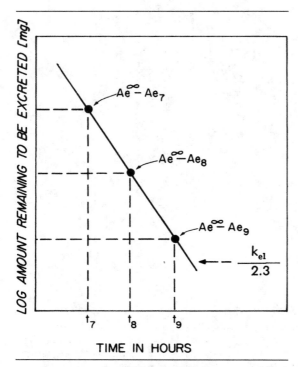

Figure 19-2. Semilog ARE—time plot for determination of the elimination rate constant from urinary excretion data (symbols see text).

The excretion rate dAe/dt is determined by calculating the amount of drug excreted at the midpoint between two sampling intervals divided by the corresponding time at the midpoint.

In order to calculate the data for the last three columns in Table 19-1 we must first determine the overall elimination rate constant k_{el} (or β).

k_{el} (or β) is determined by the ARE (amount of drug remaining to be excreted) method. For this purpose we use an ARE plot as shown in Figure 19-2. The last few (terminal) points of cumulative amounts of drug excreted, Ae, are subtracted from the total amount excreted in infinite time, Ae^{∞} (when all drug is excreted the cumulative urinary excretion curve runs asymptotic (parallel) to the abscissa) and are plotted on semilog paper versus time. The slope of the curve gives the elimination rate constant k_{el} (or β):

$$k_{el} = \frac{\ln(Ae^{\infty} - Ae_7) - \ln(Ae^{\infty} - Ae_9)}{t_9 - t_7} [hr^{-1}] \qquad (3)$$

Upon multiplication of the excretion rate, dAe/dt, for each sampling period by the reciprocal value of the elimination rate constant k_{el}, and adding the cumulative amount excreted, Ae, up to that sampling time one obtains the amount of drug absorbed up to that time $A_T(f)$:

$$A_T(f) = \frac{1}{k_{el}} \cdot \frac{dAe}{dt} + Ae \, [mg] \qquad (4)$$

As soon as all of the drug is absorbed, successive values will stay more or less constant (characterized by ** in Table 19-1). The average of the asymptotic values gives the total amount absorbed $A_T(f)_{AS}$.

Percent of drug absorbed up to a particular sampling time is calculated according to Equation 19.5:

$$\text{Percent Drug Absorbed} = \frac{A_T(f)}{A_T(f)_{AS}} \cdot 100 \qquad (5)$$

However, it should be pointed out that percent of drug absorbed is not that percentage of drug absorbed from a given amount of drug, but the percentage of drug absorbed of the amount of drug ultimately absorbed. (In other words, if for instance only 80 mg is absorbed from a given dose size of 100 mg then percent absorbed refers to the percentage of drug absorbed from these 80 mg at a particular time.)

The absorption rate constant k_a can be determined from a plot of log $(1 - A_T(f)/A_T(f)_{AS})$ versus time as shown in Figure 19-3. There is also another possibility for determination of the absorption rate constant and the elimination rate constant. If one plots log excretion rate versus midpoint sampling time, a curve is obtained which matches perfectly the corresponding blood level curve in both its course and shape. The log excretion rate versus midpoint sampling time curve (see Figure 19-4) can be treated like a blood level curve for obtaining k_a and k_{el}.

Knowing the amount excreted Ae, the distribution coefficient Δ', the frac-

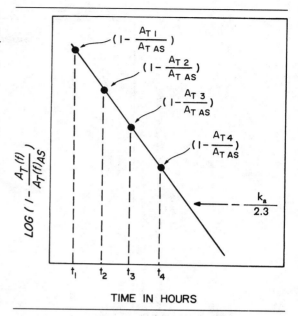

Figure 19-3. Semilog plot of (1 − fraction absorbed) versus time for determination of the absorption rate constant from urinary excretion data (symbols see text).

tion absorbed f, the absorption rate constant k_a, and the elimination rate constant k_{el}, one can actually calculate the theoretical blood level curve using the equations as outlined in the discussion on single dose administration. This represents a translation of urinary excretion data into blood level data.

Precise and reliable data on the absorption rate constant, elimination rate constant, and translation of urinary excretion data into a blood level curve will be obtained only if the drug is cleared exclusively from the body via the kidney in unchanged form, or if the drug is partly metabolized in such a manner that the metabolites can be recovered from urine and subjected to a procedure as outlined above. This method is not applicable if appreciable amounts of drug are cleared from the body by extrarenal pathways.

To summarize the treatment of cumulative urinary excretion data, Figure 19-5 shows the models for intravascular IV and extravascular EV routes of administration on which the evaluation is based and as outlined in the schematic diagrams of Figures 19-6 through 19-9.

Cumulative Urinary Excretion—Time Plot

Figure 19-6 shows the cumulative amount-time plot after IV (left-hand side) and EV (right-hand side) administration. The amounts are plotted versus time on numeric graph paper. IV:

$$\text{Intercept} = D \cdot \frac{k_u}{k_{el}}$$

(6)

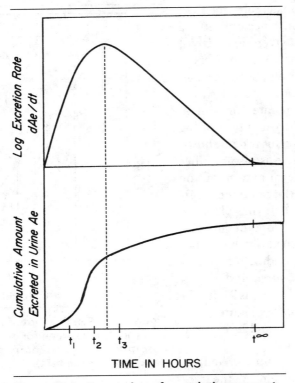

Figure 19-4. Conversion of cumulative amount of drug excreted in urine versus time into log excretion rate versus midpoint time plot. The latter one is an image of the corresponding blood level versus time curve.

$$k_u = \frac{\text{Intercept} \cdot k_{el}}{D} \tag{7}$$

$$Ae(t) = \frac{k_u}{k_{el}} \cdot D \cdot (1 - e^{-k_{el} \cdot t}) \tag{8}$$

$$F_{el} = \frac{\text{Intercept}}{D} \tag{9}$$

EV:

$$\text{Intercept} = D \cdot f \cdot \frac{k_u}{k_{el}} \tag{10}$$

$$k_u = \frac{\text{Intercept} \cdot k_{el}}{D \cdot f} \tag{11}$$

$$Ae(t) = \frac{k_u \cdot k_a}{k_{el}} \cdot D \cdot f \cdot \left[\frac{1}{k_a} + \frac{e^{-k_{el} \cdot t}}{k_{el} - k_a} - \frac{k_{el} \cdot e^{-k_a \cdot t}}{k_a \cdot (k_{el} - k_a)} \right] \tag{12}$$

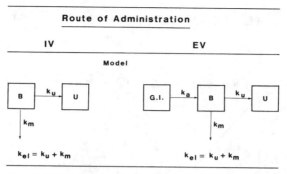

Figure 19-5. Box diagram model for IV and EV route of administration. B = body; U = urine; G.I. = gastrointestinal tract; k_{el} = elimination rate constant; k_a = absorption rate constant; k_u = rate of appearance of unchanged drug in urine; k_m = rate of metabolism.

$$F_{el} = \frac{\text{Intercept}}{D \cdot f} \tag{13}$$

Ae(t) = amount of unchanged drug eliminated in urine at time t.

Excretion Rate—Midpoint Time Plot

Figure 19-7 shows a schematic plot of log excretion rate, dAe/dt, versus midpoint time (for calculating midpoint time see Equation 19.2) for IV (left-hand side) and EV (right-hand side) administration.
IV:

$$\text{Intercept} = k_u \cdot D \tag{14}$$

$$k_u = \frac{\text{Intercept}}{D} \tag{15}$$

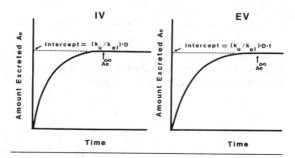

Figure 19-6. Schematic diagram of a urinary excretion-time plot.

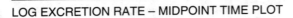

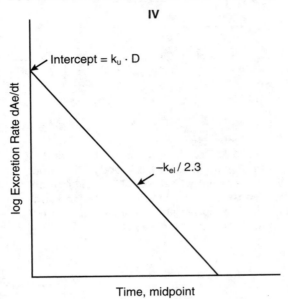

LOG EXCRETION RATE – MIDPOINT TIME PLOT

IV

Intercept = $k_u \cdot D$

$-k_{el} / 2.3$

log Excretion Rate dAe/dt

Time, midpoint

EV

Intercept = $(k_u \cdot k_a / (k_a - k_{el})) \cdot D \cdot f$

$-k_{el} / 2.3$

$-k_a / 2.3$

log Excretion Rate dAe/dt

Time, midpoint

Figure 19-7. Schematic diagram of a log excretion rate versus midpoint time plot.

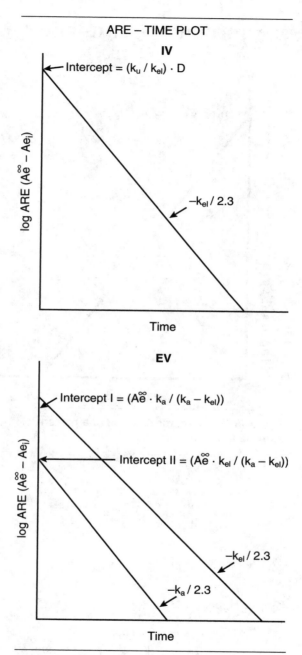

Figure 19-8. Schematic diagram of a log ARE-time plot.

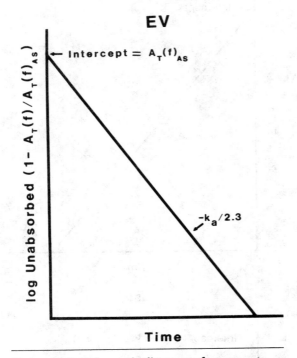

% ABSORBED - TIME PLOT

EV

Figure 19-9. Schematic diagram of a percent absorbed-time plot.

$$\frac{dAe}{dt} = k_u \cdot D \cdot e^{-k_{el} \cdot t} \tag{16}$$

$$F_{el} = \frac{k_u}{k_{el}} \tag{17}$$

k_{el} can be obtained from the slope.

EV:

$$\text{Intercept} = \left(\frac{k_u \cdot k_a}{k_a - k_{el}}\right) \cdot D \cdot f \tag{18}$$

$$k_u = \frac{\text{Intercept} \cdot (k_a - k_{el})}{k_a \cdot D \cdot f} \tag{19}$$

$$\frac{dAe}{dt} = \frac{k_u \cdot k_a}{k_a - k_{el}} \cdot D \cdot f \cdot (e^{-k_{el} \cdot t} - e^{-k_a \cdot t}) \tag{20}$$

$$F_{el} = \frac{Intercept}{k_{el} \cdot D \cdot f} \tag{21}$$

k_a and k_{el} can be obtained from the slopes.

ARE—Time Plot

Figure 19-8 shows a schematic diagram of log amount to be excreted, ARE, versus time plot for IV (left-hand side) and EV (right-hand side) administration.

IV:

$$Intercept = \frac{k_u}{k_{el}} \cdot D \tag{22}$$

$$k_u = \frac{Intercept \cdot k_{el}}{D} \tag{23}$$

$$Ae^{\infty} - Ae_i(t) = Ae^{\infty} \cdot e^{-k_{el} \cdot t} \tag{24}$$

$$F_{el} = \frac{Intercept}{D} \tag{25}$$

k_{el} can be obtained from the slope.

EV:

$$Intercept\ I = \frac{Ae^{\infty} \cdot k_a}{k_a - k_{el}} \tag{26}$$

$$Intercept\ II = \frac{Ae^{\infty} \cdot k_{el}}{k_a - k_{el}} \tag{27}$$

$$Ae^{\infty} - Ae_i(t) = \frac{Ae^{\infty}}{k_a - k_{el}} \cdot (k_a \cdot e^{-k_{el} \cdot t} - k_e \cdot e^{-k_a \cdot t}) \tag{28}$$

k_a and k_{el} can be obtained from the slopes.

Percent Absorbed—Time Plot

Figure 19-9 shows a percent absorbed-time plot with the $\log(1 - A_T(f)/A_T(f)_{AS})$ on the ordinate. For calculation of this term consult Table 19-1.

EV:

$$Intercept = A_T(f)_{AS} \tag{29}$$

$$\%\ Absorbed = A_T(f)_{AS} \cdot e^{-k_a \cdot t} \tag{30}$$

k_a can be obtained from the slope.

Evaluation of the urinary excretion data discussed above applies for disposition following a one-compartment model. Although it is mathematically possible to determine pharmacokinetic parameters from urinary excretion data for drugs following multicompartment models, it is usually not feasible because of difficulties in obtaining frequent urine samples within short periods of time, particularly in the beginning, to characterize the distribution phase.

If a drug is partly eliminated in unchanged form and partly by nonrenal (usually hepatic) pathways, the rate constant for nonrenal elimination, k_{nr} (usually by hepatic metabolism) can be calculated using Equation 19.31:

$$k_{nr} = k_{el} - k_u \, [h^{-1}] \tag{31}$$

If other nonrenal pathways than metabolism are involved, the rate constant for metabolism k_m can be obtained from one of the plots discussed above for the metabolite. The nonrenal (sweat, saliva, milk) elimination rate constant k_{nr} is then calculated by Equation 19.32:

$$k_{nr} = k_{el} - k_u - k_m \, [h^{-1}] \tag{32}$$

Selected References

1. Wagner, J. G. and Nelson, E.: The Kinetic Analysis of Blood Levels and Urinary Excretion in the Absorptive Phases After Single Doses of Drugs, *J. Pharm. Sci.* 53:1392 (1964).
2. Wagner, J. G. and Northam, J. I.: Lag Time Before Essentially Constant Urinary Excretion Rate is Attained, *J. Pharm. Sci.* 57:994 (1968).

20

Area Under the Blood Level-Time Curve

The area under the blood level-time curve (AUC) is a measure of quantity of drug in the body. If one knows the AUC for a given dose size upon IV administration of a drug, the fraction of drug absorbed (f) (absolute bioavailability) upon extravascular administration can be calculated from the AUC obtained by the latter route. Similarly the extent of relative bioavailability (EBA) can be determined by comparing the AUC of a test dosage form with that of a standard. In both cases one has to use complete areas, i.e., from zero to infinite time until all of the unchanged drug is eliminated from the body.

Estimates on the relative magnitude of the AUC can be obtained by either of the following two methods: counting or weighing.

Counting Method. Plot the blood level data versus time on numeric graph paper and count the number of squares enclosed by the blood level curve.

Weighing Method. Plot the blood level data versus time on numeric graph paper, cut out the area enclosed by the blood level curve and the coordinates and weigh the cuttings on an analytical balance.

Exact calculation of the AUC is done by either one of the following two methods: trapezoidal rule or blood level equations.

Trapezoidal Rule. The trapezoidal rule is used if no curve-fitting has been done for a set of blood level data, if the blood level curve is not smooth, or if no pharmacokinetic data have been determined. It is not necessary to know whether the open one- or two-compartment model applies.

AUC upon Intravascular Injection

In the case of intravascular administration, the AUC from time zero to the last blood level point determined is composed of trapezoids only. The remaining area is calculated by dividing the last blood level point by k_{el} or β under the assumption that this point is beyond the absorptive and distributive phases on the terminal slope of the blood level-time curve.

Figure 20-1 shows a schematic drawing of an intravascular blood level-time curve with the terminology used in the following equations:

$$AUC^{o \to t_x} = \left\{ \left[\frac{C_1 + C_2}{2} \cdot (t_2 - t_1) \right] + \left[\frac{C_2 + C_3}{2} \cdot (t_3 - t_2) \right] \right.$$
$$+ \left[\frac{C_3 + C_4}{2} \cdot (t_4 - t_3) \right] + \left[\frac{C_4 + C_5}{2} \cdot (t_5 - t_4) \right]$$
$$\left. + \left[\frac{C_5 + C_x}{2} \cdot (t_x - t_5) \right] \right\} \left[(\mu g/ml) \cdot h \right] \qquad (1)$$

To determine the remaining or rest area (method of corresponding areas by Dost), the last 3 or 4 blood level points are plotted versus time on semilog paper and the rate constant of the slope (k_{el} or β) is calculated (see Chapter 15, Determination of Rate Constants). The last blood sample concentration C_x (which must be in the terminal phase) as predicted from curve fitting divided by k_{el} or β is the rest area:

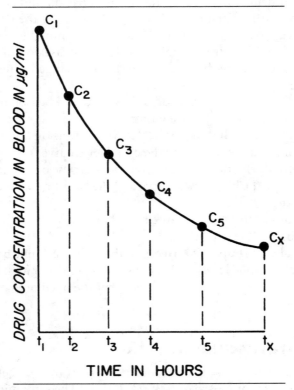

Figure 20-1. Determination of area under the curve AUC upon intravascular route of administration using the trapezoidal rule (compartment model independent).

$$\text{AUC}^{t_x \to \infty} = \frac{C_x}{k_{el} \text{ or } \beta}[(\mu g/ml) \cdot h] \tag{2}$$

$$\text{AUC}^{0 \to \infty} = \text{AUC}^{0 \to t_x} + \text{AUC}^{t_x \to \infty}[(\mu g/ml) \cdot h] \tag{3}$$

AUC upon Extravascular Route of Administration

In the case of extravascular route of administration, the AUC from time zero to the last blood level point determined is composed of one triangle followed by trapezoids.

Figure 20-2 illustrates the treatment of an extravascular blood level curve for the determination of AUC with the terminology used in the following equation:

$$
\begin{aligned}
\text{AUC}^{0 \to t} = &\left\{ \left(\frac{C_1 \cdot t_1}{2} \right) + \left[\frac{C_1 + C_2}{2} \cdot (t_2 - t_1) \right] \right. \\
&+ \left[\frac{C_2 + C_3}{2} \cdot (t_3 - t_2) \right] + \left[\frac{C_3 + C_4}{2} \cdot (t_4 - t_3) \right] \\
&+ \left[\frac{C_4 + C_5}{2} \cdot (t_5 - t_4) \right] + \left[\frac{C_5 + C_6}{2} \cdot (t_6 - t_5) \right] \\
&\left. + \left[\frac{C_6 + C_x}{2} \cdot (t_x - t_6) \right] \right\} [(\mu g/ml) \cdot h]
\end{aligned}
\tag{4}
$$

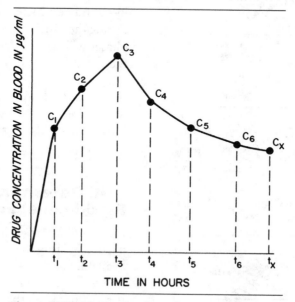

Figure 20-2. Determination of area under the curve AUC upon extravascular route of administration using the trapezoidal rule (compartment model independent).

To determine the remaining or residual area (method of corresponding areas by Dost), the apparent terminal elimination rate constant (k_{el}) is calculated from curve fitting (e.g., curve stripping or weighted least squares nonlinear regression) or simple linear regression of the concentration vs. time points which comprise the apparent terminal elimination phase. The residual area is then approximated according to Equation 20.5 as follows:

$$AUC^{t_x \to \infty} = C_x / k_{el} [(\mu g/ml) \cdot h] \tag{5}$$

where t_x represents the time corresponding to the last observed blood level concentration on the terminal phase (C_x). The area under the curve from time zero to infinity can then be determined by summation as reflected in Equation 20.6:

$$AUC^{0 \to \infty} = AUC^{0 \to t_x} + AUC^{t_x \to \infty} [(\mu g/ml) \cdot h] \tag{6}$$

In those instances where the measured drug concentrations on the terminal phase are scattered (Figure 20-3), applying Equation 20.5 to the determination of the residual area can produce significant differences based upon whether the actual value of C_x is significantly different from (i.e., above or below) the value of C_x estimated from the fitting procedure (Figure 20-3). In this instance, it is preferable to use the value of C_x estimated from the curve fit used to calculate the apparent terminal elimination rate constant in Equations 20.5 and 20.6 for the determination of the residual and total AUC, respectively.

The procedure discussed above is known as the *linear trapezoidal rule*. The more concentration-time data available, the more accurate the estimate of the AUC will be. Scarcity of concentration-time data during the absorption phase and around the peak time will result in an underestimate, and scarcity of data during the distribution and elimination phases will result in an overestimate of the actual AUC as shown in Figure 20-4.

Some prefer to use the *logarithmic trapezoidal rule* for the declining phase of the blood level-time curve, employing ln C instead of C for that portion of the curve.

AUC Determination from Blood Level Equations

If the general blood level equation of a particular drug in a certain dose size is available, or if a blood level curve can be well fitted and the intercepts with the ordinate and the rate constants are known, the AUC can be calculated according to the equations given in Table 20-1.

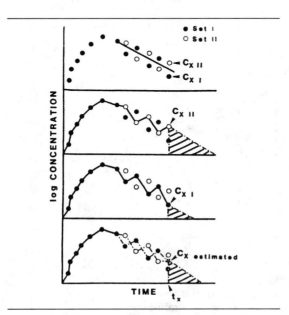

Figure 20-3. Determination of residual AUC using observed versus estimated C_x.

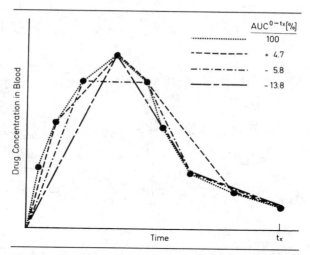

Figure 20-4. Schematic presentation of overestimation and underestimation of AUC due to scarcity of concentration-time data.

For the open one-compartment model, intravascular route of administration, the $AUC^{0 \to \infty}$ as given in Equation 20.12 can be calculated from the dose size D, the elimination rate constant k_{el}, and the volume of distribution V_d, since:

$$B = C(0) = \frac{D}{V_d} [\mu g/ml] \tag{11}$$

and, hence:

$$AUC^{0 \to \infty} = \frac{B}{k_{el}} = \frac{D}{k_{el} \cdot V_d} [(\mu g/ml) \cdot h] \tag{12}$$

For the open one-compartment model, extravascular route of administration, the $AUC^{0 \to \infty}$ can be calculated similarly according to Equation 20.13:

$$AUC^{0 \to \infty} = \frac{D \cdot f}{k_{el} \cdot V_d} \tag{13}$$

where f is the fraction of drug absorbed.

Compartment model independent, the $AUC^{0 \to \infty}$ can be calculated via the total clearance, Cl_{tot}:

$$AUC^{0 \to \infty} = \frac{D \cdot f}{Cl_{tot}} \tag{14}$$

AUC as Test for Dose Dependency, First-Pass Effect, Enzyme Induction, or Enzyme Inhibition

Tests for nonlinearity between AUC and dose size for dose dependency and first-pass effect are carried out by evaluation of the AUCs obtained upon administration of single doses with increasing dose size. A straight line through the origin indicates absence of dose

Table 20-1. Calculation of AUC from Zero to Infinite Time from General Blood Level Equations

COMPARTMENT MODEL	GRAPH AND TERMINOLOGY	GENERAL BLOOD LEVEL EQUATION [µg/ml]	AREA UNDER BLOOD LEVEL VS TIME CURVE AUC [(µg/ml)·h]	
Open one, Intravascular		$C(t) = B \cdot e^{-k_{el} \cdot t}$	$AUC^{0 \to \infty} = \dfrac{B}{k_{el}}$	Eq. 20.7
Open one, Extravascular		$C(t) = B \cdot e^{-k_{el} \cdot t} - A \cdot e^{-k_a \cdot t}$	$AUC^{0 \to \infty} = \dfrac{B}{k_{el}} - \dfrac{A}{k_a}$	Eq. 20.8
Open two, Intravascular		$C(t) = B \cdot e^{-\beta \cdot t} + A \cdot e^{-\alpha \cdot t}$	$AUC^{0 \to \infty} = \dfrac{B}{\beta} + \dfrac{A}{\alpha}$	Eq. 20.9
Open two, Extravascular		$C(t) = B \cdot e^{-\beta \cdot t} + A \cdot e^{-\alpha \cdot t}$ $- C(0) \cdot e^{-k_a \cdot t}$	$AUC^{0 \to \infty} = \dfrac{B}{\beta} + \dfrac{A}{\alpha} - \dfrac{C(0)}{k_a}$	Eq. 20.10

dependency. If saturation of metabolism, of renal elimination, or of transport to periph-eral tissues occurs, the line starts at the origin as a straight line, but then increases curvi-linear (concave) as saturation starts. If a drug exhibits first-pass effect, the AUCs of small doses may be negligible or small; hence the curve may start to the right of the origin, but then increases curvilinear (concave) and continues as a straight line, once the first-pass is saturated.

Upon multiple dosing with equal dose sizes in equal dosing intervals ($\tau < 3 \cdot t_{1/2}$), accumulation occurs. The shorter τ, the more pronounced is the accumulation. In absence of any dose dependency, the AUC after the first dose, $AUC^{0 \to \infty}$ (considered as a single dose) will be equal to the AUC during *one dosing interval*, $AUC^{\tau_n \to \tau_{n+1}}$ at *steady state* as shown in Figure 20-5.

In case enzyme systems become saturated upon multiple dosing:

$$AUC^{\tau_n \to \tau_{n+1}} > AUC^{0 \to \infty}$$

Then the steady state blood levels will be higher than predicted. The ratio is:

$$AUC^{0 \to \infty} / AUC^{\tau_n \to \tau_{n+1}} < 1$$

If enzyme systems become induced upon multiple dosing: $AUC^{0 \to \infty} > AUC^{\tau_n \to \tau_{n+1}}$.

Then the steady state blood levels will be lower than predicted. The ratio is: $AUC^{0 \to \infty} / AUC^{\tau_n \to \tau_{n+1}} > 1$.

The results of AUC evaluation for nonlinearity are summarized in Figure 20-6.

Prediction of C_{av}^{ss} from Single Dose AUC

In absence of dose dependency, first-pass effect, enzyme induction, or enzyme inhibition, the $AUC^{0 \to \infty}$ of a single dose is equal to the AUC for any dosing interval at steady state, $AUC^{\tau_n \to \tau_{n+1}}$ if equal dose sizes are used.

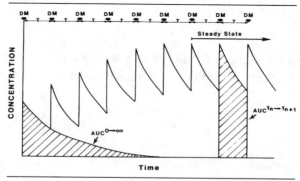

Figure 20-5. Schematic diagram showing equality of the total AUC after the first dose and the AUC during any dosing interval at steady state upon multiple dosing.

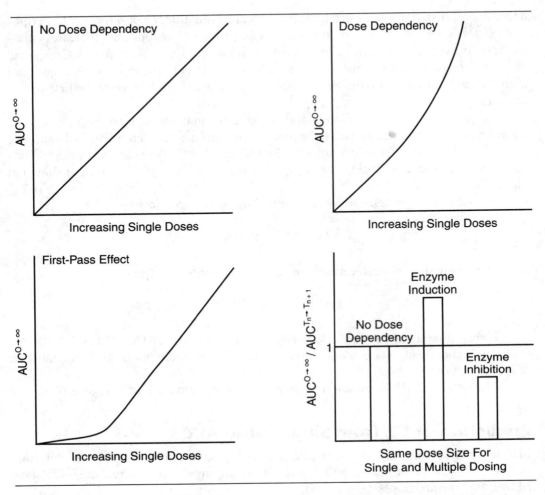

Figure 20-6. Schematic representation of AUC evaluation upon single and multiple dosing for dose dependency, first-pass effect, enzyme induction, and enzyme inhibition.

Since steady concentration, C_{av}^{ss}, is given by the ratio of $AUC^{\tau_n \to \tau_{n+1}}$ and the dosing interval τ, C_{av}^{ss} can be obtained from the total single dose area, AUC_{SD}:

$$C_{av}^{ss} = \frac{AUC_{SD}}{\tau} \tag{15}$$

In case a different dose size is used for multiple dosing, Equation 20.16 is used:

$$C_{av}^{ss} = \frac{AUC_{SD} \cdot (D_{MD}/D_{SD})}{\tau} \tag{16}$$

where D_{MD} and D_{SD} are the dose sizes for multiple and single doses, respectively.

AUC Determination in Michaelis-Menten Kinetics

From drug concentration-time data the $AUC^{0 \to t_x}$ is determined by the trapezoidal rule (see Equation 20.1), and the $AUC^{t_x \to \infty}$ by Equation 20.17:

$$AUC^{t_x \to \infty} = \frac{V_d \cdot C_x}{V_{max}} \cdot \left(\frac{C_x}{2} + K_m \right) \tag{17}$$

For the IV or PO route of administration with instant absorption, the total area under the curve after a bolus dose, $AUC^{0 \to \infty}_{bolus}$, and after constant rate input (controlled release or infusion), $AUC^{0 \to \infty}_{zero\text{-}order}$, can be calculated by Equations 20.18 and 20.19, respectively:

$$AUC^{0 \to \infty}_{bolus} = \frac{D}{V_{max}} \cdot \left(\frac{D}{2 \cdot V_d} + K_m \right) \tag{18}$$

$$AUC^{0 \to \infty}_{zero\ order} = \frac{K_m \cdot D}{V_{max} - R^\circ} - \left(\frac{1}{V_{max} - R^\circ} - \frac{1}{V_{max}} \right) \cdot \left(\frac{C_x}{2} K_m \right) \tag{19}$$

where D is the dose size, V_{max} is the theoretical maximum rate of the process, K_m is the Michaelis-Menten constant, V_d is the volume of distribution, R° is the zero-order infusion rate or zero-order release rate, and C_x is the last blood sample taken.

Under multiple dose conditions, the AUC within a dosing interval at steady state, $AUC^{\tau_n \to \tau_{n+1}}$ is:

$$AUC^{\tau_n \to \tau_{n+1}} = \frac{D}{V_{max}} \cdot \left(\frac{D}{2V_d} + C^{ss}_{min} + K_m \right) \tag{20}$$

Selected References

1. Dost, F. H.: *Grundlagen der Pharmakokinetik,* Georg Thieme Verlag, Stuttgart, 1968, p. 156.

2. Jusko, W. J.: Pharmacokinetics of Capacity-Limited Systems, *J. Clin. Pharmacol.* 29:488–493 (1989).

3. Sokolnikoff, I. S. and Sokolnikoff, S.: *Higher Mathematics for Engineers and Physicists,* 2nd Ed., McGraw-Hill, New York, 1941, p. 555.

4. Wagner, J. G.: Propranolol: Pooled Michaelis-Menten Parameters and the Effect of Input Rate on Bioavailability, *Clin. Pharmacol. Ther.* 37:481–487 (1985).

5. Wagner, J. G.: *Fundamentals of Clinical Pharmacology,* Drug Intelligence Publications, Hamilton, Ill., 1975, p. 175.

21

Pharmacokinetics of Single Dose Administration

We open this chapter with five general remarks:

1. For determination of correct pharmacokinetic parameters from blood level curves, sampling should be continued for at least 3, or better 5, elimination half-lives.
2. There should be at least 3 blood level points during the absorptive phase, about 3 in the region of the peak, at least 3 during the distributive phase (in the open two-compartment model) and at least 3 during the elimination phase.
3. For determination of factor f (fraction of drug absorbed), the drug must be given IV for comparison.
4. If urinary cumulative excretion curves are used to determine pharmacokinetic parameters, sampling should be continued for at least 7, or better 10, elimination half-lives.
5. A given blood level curve can be translated to any other dose size or any other body weight via the parameter Δ' (distribution coefficient) under the assumption that:

   - No dose-dependent pharmacokinetics is involved.
   - No change in urinary excretion (change of urinary pH; change in creatinine clearance) is involved.
   - The translation is for a patient of normal body stature.
   - The translation is not valid for children or edematous, obese, or aged patients.

Open One-Compartment Model

General Concept

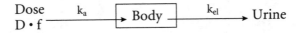

$$\text{Dose} \atop D \cdot f \xrightarrow{\;k_a\;} \boxed{\text{Body}} \xrightarrow{\;k_{el}\;} \text{Urine}$$

RAPID INTRAVASCULAR ADMINISTRATION, ASSUMING ALL OR MOST DRUG IS ELIMINATED IN UNCHANGED FORM

$$D_B \xrightarrow{\;k_{el}\;} Ae$$

D_B = amount of drug in body
Ae = amount of drug excreted into urine
k_{el} = elimination rate constant

$$C(t) = C(0) \cdot e^{-k_{el} \cdot t} [\mu g/ml] \tag{1}$$

$$C(t) = \frac{D}{V_d} \cdot e^{-k_{el} \cdot t} [\mu g/ml] \tag{2}$$

$C(t)$ = drug concentration in blood, plasma, or serum at time t [$\mu g/ml$]
$C(0)$ = drug concentration in blood, plasma, or serum at time zero [$\mu g/ml$]
D = dose [μg]
k_{el} = elimination rate constant [h^{-1}]
t = time [h]

$$k_{el} = \frac{\ln C_1 - \ln C_2}{t_2 - t_1} [h^{-1}] \tag{3}$$

$\ln C_1, \ln C_2$ = any two drug concentrations on the monoexponential declining
line [$\mu g/ml$]
t_1, t_2 = time corresponding to $\ln C_1$ and $\ln C_2$ [h]

$$t_{1/2} = \frac{0.693}{k_{el}} [h] \tag{4}$$

$t_{1/2}$ = elimination half-life [h]

$$V_d = \frac{D}{C(0)} [ml] \tag{5}$$

V_d = volume of distribution [ml]
D = dose [μg]

$$V_{d\,area} = \frac{D}{k_{el} \cdot AUC} [ml] \tag{6}$$

$V_{d\,area}$ = volume of distribution from clearance method [ml]
AUC = area under blood level curve [($\mu g/ml$) $\cdot$ h]

$$Ae(t) = \frac{C(0) \cdot V_d \cdot k_u}{k_{el}} \cdot (1 - e^{-k_{el} \cdot t}) [\mu g] \tag{7}$$

$Ae(t)$ = amount of drug excreted into urine until time t [μg]
k_u = rate constant for excretion of unchanged drug via kidney into urine
k_{el} = elimination rate constant

RAPID INTRAVASCULAR ADMINISTRATION, ASSUMING A CONSIDERABLY LARGE AMOUNT OF DRUG IS ELIMINATED IN FORM OF A METABOLITE

$$
\begin{array}{ccc}
 & M_B & \xrightarrow{\ k_2\ } M_u \\
k_1 \nearrow & & \\
D_B & \xrightarrow{\ k_3\ } & Ae
\end{array}
$$

D_B = amount of drug in body
Ae = amount of drug excreted into urine
M_B = amount of metabolite in body
M_u = amount of metabolite excreted into urine
k_1 = rate constant of formation of metabolite (biotransformation of drug) in body
k_2 = rate constant of elimination of metabolite
k_3 = rate constant of elimination of unchanged drug

$$K = k_1 + k_3 \, [h^{-1}] \tag{8}$$

K = overall elimination rate constant $[hr^{-1}]$ (determined as rate of loss of unchanged drug in body from monoexponential declining line)

$$K = \frac{\ln C_1 - \ln C_2}{t_2 - t_1} [h^{-1}] \tag{9}$$

k_3 = determined from a plot of cumulative urinary excretion of unchanged drug versus time using ARE method (see Chapter 19.)
k_2 = determined from blood level data of the metabolite or from a plot of cumulative urinary excretion of metabolite versus time using ARE method
k_1 = determined by back-feathering from a blood level curve of the metabolite, or having determined K and k_3 from Eq. 21.8

$$C(t) = C(0) \cdot e^{-K \cdot t} [\mu g/ml] \tag{10}$$

$$C(t) = \frac{D}{V_d} \cdot e^{-K \cdot t} [\mu g/ml] \tag{11}$$

$$t_{1/2} = \frac{0.693}{K} [h] \tag{12}$$

$$V_{d\ area} = \frac{D}{K \cdot AUC} [ml] \tag{13}$$

$$M(t) = \frac{C(0) \cdot k_1}{k_2 - K} \cdot (e^{-K \cdot t} - e^{-k_2 \cdot t}) [\mu g/ml] \tag{14}$$

$M(t)$ = metabolite concentration in blood, plasma, or serum at time t $[\mu g/ml]$

$$Ae(t) = \frac{C(0) \cdot V_d \cdot k_3}{K} \cdot (1 - e^{-K \cdot t}) \, [\mu g] \tag{15}$$

$Ae(t)$ = amount of drug excreted into urine at time t $[\mu g]$

$$M_u(t) = \frac{C(0) \cdot V_d \cdot k_1}{K \cdot (k_2 - K)} \cdot [k_2 \cdot (1 - e^{-K \cdot t}) - K \cdot (1 - e^{-k_2 \cdot t})] \, [\mu g] \tag{16}$$

$M_u(t)$ = amount of metabolite excreted into urine at t $[\mu g]$

EXTRAVASCULAR ADMINISTRATION, ALL OR MOST OF THE DRUG IS ELIMINATED IN UNCHANGED FORM

$$D \cdot f \xrightarrow{k_a} D_B \xrightarrow{k_{el}} Ae$$

f = fraction of administered dose which is absorbed

$$C(t) = B \cdot e^{-k_{el} \cdot t} - A \cdot e^{-k_a \cdot t} \, [\mu g/ml] \tag{17}$$

$$C(t) = \frac{D \cdot f}{V_d} \cdot \frac{k_a}{k_a - k_{el}} \cdot (e^{-k_{el} \cdot t} - e^{-k_a \cdot t}) \, [\mu g/ml] \tag{18}$$

B = determined graphically as intercept of back-extrapolated monoexponential declining line with the ordinate $[\mu g/ml]$

A = determined graphically as intercept of monoexponential line obtained from ln C_{diff} points by back-feathering or residual method, with the ordinate $[\mu g/ml]$

$$k_{el} = \frac{\ln C_1 - \ln C_2}{t_2 - t_1} \, [h^{-1}] \tag{19}$$

$$k_a = \frac{\ln C_{1\,diff} - \ln C_{2\,diff}}{t_2 - t_1} \, [h^{-1}] \tag{20}$$

k_u = rate of urinary excretion of unchanged drug $[h^{-1}]$

ln $C_{1\,diff}$ = differences between the actual blood, plasma, or serum concentrations during

ln $C_{2\,diff}$ the absorptive phase at time t_1 and t_2 and the back-extrapolated monoexponential declining line

$$t_{1/2} = \frac{0.693}{k_{el}} \, [h] \tag{21}$$

$$V_d = \frac{D \cdot f}{B} \cdot \frac{k_a}{k_a - k_{el}} \, [ml] \tag{22}$$

$$V_{d\,area} = \frac{D \cdot f}{k_{el} - AUC} \, [ml] \tag{23}$$

$$Ae(t) = \frac{D \cdot f \cdot k_a \cdot k_u}{k_{el}} \cdot \left[\frac{1}{k_a} + \frac{e^{-k_{el} \cdot t}}{k_a - k_{el}} - \frac{k_{el} \cdot e^{-k_a \cdot t}}{k_a \cdot (k_{el} - k_a)} \right] [\mu g] \tag{24}$$

$Ae(t)$ = amount of drug excreted into urine until time t [μg]

EXTRAVASCULAR ADMINISTRATION, ASSUMING A CONSIDERABLY LARGE AMOUNT OF DRUG IS ELIMINATED IN FORM OF A METABOLITE

$$K = k_1 + k_3 [h^{-1}] \tag{25}$$

$$C(t) = \frac{D \cdot f}{V_d} \cdot \left(\frac{k_a}{k_a - K} \right) \cdot (e^{-K \cdot t} - e^{-k_a \cdot t}) [\mu g/ml] \tag{26}$$

$$\frac{D \cdot f}{V_d} = C(0) = B [\mu g/ml] \tag{27}$$

K = overall elimination rate constant [h⁻¹], determined as given in Eq. 21.9
k_a = absorption rate constant, determined by back-featuring as given in Eq. 21.20
k_3 = determined from a plot of cumulative urinary excretion of unchanged drug versus time using ARE method
k_2 = determined from blood level data of the metabolite or from a plot of cumulative urinary excretion of metabolite versus time using ARE method
k_1 = determined by back-featuring from a blood level curve of the metabolite, or having determined K and k_3 from Eq. 21.8

$$t_{1/2} = \frac{0.693}{K} [h] \tag{28}$$

$$V_d = \frac{D \cdot f}{B} \cdot \left(\frac{k_a}{k_a - K} \right) [ml] \tag{29}$$

$$V_{d\,area} = \frac{D \cdot f}{K \cdot AUC} [ml] \tag{30}$$

$$M(t) = \frac{D \cdot f}{V_d} \cdot k_a \cdot k_1 \cdot \left\{ \left[\frac{e^{-K \cdot t}}{(k_a - K) \cdot (k_2 - K)} - \frac{e^{-k_a \cdot t}}{(k_a - K) \cdot (k_2 - k_a)} \right] \right.$$
$$\left. + \frac{e^{-k_2 \cdot t}}{(k_2 - k_a) \cdot (k_2 - K)} \right\} [\mu g/ml] \tag{31}$$

$M(t)$ = metabolite concentration in blood, plasma, or serum [μg/ml]

$$Ae(t) = D \cdot f \cdot \frac{k_3}{K} \cdot \left[1 - \frac{1}{k_a - K} \cdot (k_a \cdot e^{-K \cdot t} - K \cdot e^{-k_a \cdot t}) \right] [\mu g] \qquad (32)$$

Ae(t) = amount of unchanged drug excreted into urine at time t [mg]

$$M_u(t) = D \cdot f \cdot \frac{k_1}{K} \cdot \left\{ 1 - \left[\frac{k_a \cdot k_2 \cdot e^{-K_a \cdot t}}{(k_a - K) \cdot (k_2 - K)} \right. \right.$$
$$\left. \left. - \frac{k_2 \cdot K \cdot e^{-k_a \cdot t}}{(k_a - K) \cdot (k_2 - k_a)} + \frac{k_a \cdot K \cdot e^{-k_2 \cdot t}}{(k_2 - k_a) \cdot (k_2 - K)} \right] \right\} [\mu g] \qquad (33)$$

$M_u(t)$ = amount of metabolite excreted into urine at time t [mg]

Open Two-Compartment Model

General Concept

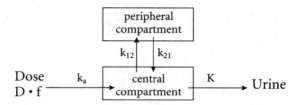

RAPID INTRAVASCULAR ADMINISTRATION, ASSUMING ALL OR MOST OF THE DRUG IS ELIMINATED IN UNCHANGED FORM

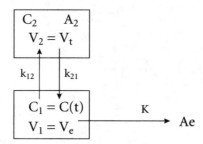

C_1 = drug concentration in central compartment = C(t)
V_1 = volume of central compartment = V_c (plasma volume)
C_2 = drug concentration in peripheral compartment
A_2 = amount of drug in peripheral compartment
V_2 = volume of peripheral compartment = V_t (tissue volume)
k_{12} = distribution rate constant for transfer of drug from central to peripheral compartment
k_{21} = distribution rate constant for transfer of drug from peripheral to central compartment
K = overall elimination rate constant
Ae = amount of drug excreted into urine

$$C(t) = B \cdot e^{-\beta \cdot t} + A \cdot e^{-\alpha \cdot t} [\mu g/ml] \qquad (34)$$

$$C(t) = \frac{D}{V_c \cdot (\alpha - \beta)} \cdot [(k_{21} - \beta) \cdot e^{\beta \cdot t} - (k_{21} - \alpha) \cdot e^{-\alpha \cdot t}] \, [\mu g/ml] \tag{35}$$

B = intercept of back-extrapolated monoexponential declining line with the ordinate [µg/ml]

β = slope of monoexponential declining line (hybrid constant) [h^{-1}]

$$\beta = \frac{\ln C_1 - \ln C_2}{t_2 - t_1} \, [h^{-1}] \tag{36}$$

α = slope of monoexponential concentration line (hybrid constant) [h^{-1}]

$$\alpha = \frac{\ln C_{1\,diff} - \ln C_{2\,diff}}{t_2 - t_1} \, [h^{-1}] \tag{37}$$

$\ln C_{1\,diff}$ = differences between actual blood, plasma, or serum concentrations at time t_1 and
$\ln C_{2\,diff}$ t_2 and back-extrapolated monoexponential β slope [µg/ml] (back-feathering)
A   = intercept of monoexponential α line with ordinate [µg/ml]

$$C(0) = B + A \, [\mu g/ml] \tag{38}$$

$$k_{12} = \frac{A \cdot B \cdot (\beta - \alpha)^2}{C(0) \cdot (A \cdot \beta + B \cdot \alpha)} \, [h^{-1}] \tag{39}$$

$$k_{21} = \frac{A \cdot \beta + B \cdot \alpha}{C(0)} \, [h^{-1}] \tag{40}$$

$$k_{13} = \frac{C(0)}{A/\alpha + B/\beta} \, [h^{-1}] \tag{41}$$

k_{13} = elimination rate constant of drug [h^{-1}]

$$t_{1/2\alpha} = \frac{0.693}{\alpha} \, [h] \tag{42}$$

$t_{1/2\alpha}$ = α phase half-life [h]

$$t_{1/2\beta} = \frac{0.693}{\beta} \, [h] \tag{43}$$

$t_{1/2\beta}$ = β phase half-life considered as elimination half-life [h]

$$V_c = \frac{D}{C(0)} \, [ml] \tag{44}$$

$$V_{d\,ss} = V_c + V_t \, [ml] \tag{45}$$

$V_{d\ ss}$ = volume of distribution at steady state [ml]

$$V_{d\ ss} = \frac{k_{12} + k_{21}}{k_{21}} \cdot V_c\,[\text{ml}] \qquad (46)$$

$$B = \frac{D \cdot (k_{21} \cdot \beta)}{V_c \cdot (\alpha - \beta)}\,[\mu g/\text{ml}] \qquad (47)$$

$$V_{d\ extrap} = \frac{D}{B} = \frac{V_c \cdot (\alpha - \beta)}{(k_{21} - \beta)}\,[\text{ml}] \qquad (48)$$

$V_{d\ extrap}$ = extrapolated volume of distribution [ml] (least precise method)

$$V_{d\ area} = V_{d\ ss} + \frac{k_{13} - \beta}{k_{21}} \cdot V_c\,[\text{ml}] \qquad (49)$$

$V_{d\ area}$ = volume of distribution according to area or clearance method [ml]

$$A_2(t) = \frac{D \cdot k_{12}}{(\alpha - \beta)} \cdot (e^{-\beta \cdot t} - e^{\alpha \cdot t})\,[\mu g] \qquad (50)$$

$A_2(t)$ = amount of drug in peripheral compartment [μg]

EXTRAVASCULAR ADMINISTRATION, ASSUMING ALL OR MOST OF THE DRUG IS ELIMINATED IN UNCHANGED FORM

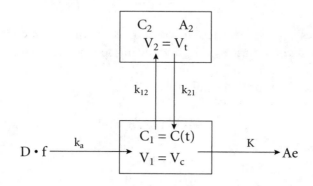

f = fraction of administered dose which is absorbed
k_a = absorption rate constant
C_1 = drug concentration in central department = C(t)
V_1 = volume of central compartment = V_c (plasma volume)
C_2 = drug concentration in peripheral compartment
A_2 = amount of drug in peripheral compartment
V_2 = volume of peripheral compartment = V_t (tissue volume)
k_{12} = distribution rate constant for transfer of drug from central to peripheral compartment
k_{21} = distribution rate constant for transfer of drug from peripheral to central compartment

K = overall elimination rate constant
Ae = amount of drug excreted into urine

$$C(t) = B \cdot e^{-\beta \cdot t} + A \cdot e^{-\alpha \cdot t} - C(0) \cdot e^{-k_a \cdot t} [\mu g/ml] \tag{51}$$

B = intercept of back-extrapolated monoexponential declining line with the ordinate [μg/ml]
β = slope of monoexponential declining line (hybrid constant) [h⁻¹]

$$\beta = \frac{\ln C_1 - \ln C_2}{t_2 - t_1} [h^{-1}] \tag{52}$$

α = slope of monoexponential distribution line (hybrid constant) [h⁻¹]

$$\alpha = \frac{\ln C_{1\,diff} - \ln C_{2\,diff}}{t_2 - t_1} [h^{-1}] \tag{53}$$

$\ln C_{1\,diff}$ = differences between the actual blood, plasma, or serum concentrations of the
$\ln C_{2\,diff}$ *postabsorptive* phase at time t_1 and t_2 and the back-extrapolated monoexponential β slope (μg/ml) (back-feathering)
A   = intercept of monoexponential α line with ordinate [μg/ml]
k_a = absorption rate constant, obtained by back-feathering [h⁻¹]

$$k_a = \frac{\ln C_{a_1} - \ln C_{a_2}}{t_2 - t_1} [h^{-1}] \tag{54}$$

$\ln C_{a1}$ = differences between the actual blood, plasma, or serum concentrations of the
$\ln C_{a2}$ *absorptive phase* at time t_1 and t_2 and the monoexponential α slope [μg/ml] (back-feathering)
C(0) = intercept of k_a slope with ordinate [μg/ml]

$$C = C(0) = B + A[\mu g/ml] \tag{55}$$

$$k_{12} = \frac{A \cdot B \cdot (\beta - \alpha)^2}{C(0) \cdot (A \cdot \beta + B \cdot \alpha)} [h^{-1}] \tag{56}$$

$$k_{21} = \frac{A \cdot \beta + B \cdot \alpha}{C(0)} [h^{-1}] \tag{57}$$

$$k_{13} = \frac{C(0)}{A/\alpha + B/\beta - C(0)/k_a} [h^{-1}] \tag{58}$$

$$t_{1/2\alpha} = \frac{0.693}{\alpha} [h] \tag{59}$$

$$t_{1/2\beta} = \frac{0.693}{\beta}[h] \tag{60}$$

$$V_c = \frac{D \cdot f \cdot k_a \cdot (k_{21} - k_a)}{-C(0) \cdot (\beta - k_a) \cdot (\alpha - k_a)}[ml] \tag{61}$$

$$V_{d\ ss} = V_c + V_t[ml] \tag{62}$$

$$V_{d\ ss} = \frac{k_{12} + k_{21}}{k_{21}} \cdot V_c[ml] \tag{63}$$

$$V_{d\ extrap} = \frac{V_c \cdot (\alpha - \beta)}{(k_{21} - \beta)}[ml] \tag{64}$$

$$V_{d\ area} = V_{d\ ss} + \frac{k_{13} - \beta}{k_{21}} \cdot V_c[ml] \tag{65}$$

$$C(t) = \frac{D \cdot f \cdot k_a}{V_c} \cdot \left\{ \left[\frac{k_{21} - \alpha}{(k_a - \alpha) \cdot (\beta - \alpha)} \right] \cdot e^{-\alpha \cdot t} \right.$$
$$+ \left[\frac{k_{21} - \beta}{(k_a - \beta) \cdot (\alpha - \beta)} \right] \cdot e^{-\beta \cdot t} + \left[\frac{k_{21} - k_a}{(\alpha - k_a) \cdot (\beta - k_a)} \right]$$
$$\left. \cdot e^{-k_a \cdot t} \right\}[\mu g/ml] \tag{66}$$

$$A_2(t) = D \cdot f \cdot k_a \cdot k_{12} \cdot \left[\frac{e^{-\alpha \cdot t}}{(k_a - \alpha) \cdot (\beta - \alpha)} \right.$$
$$+ \left[\frac{e^{-\beta \cdot t}}{(k_a - \beta) \cdot (\alpha - \beta)} \right] + \left[\frac{e^{-k_a \cdot t}}{(\alpha - k_a) \cdot (\beta - k_a)} \right][\mu g] \tag{67}$$

Flip-Flop Model

A flip-flop model results if the rate of absorption or the microconstants of distribution are slower than the rate of elimination. Figure 21-1 shows a diagram of the flip-flop model where, after extravascular administration, the ascending portion of the curve is the elimination phase and the terminal portion of the curve is the absorption phase; intravascular and extravascular curves are compared. The slope of the extravascular concentration-time plot, which is comparable to the elimination phase of the IV plot, is the elimination process.

Examples of flip-flop models are sometimes observed upon topical or rectal route of administration where the absorption is slower than the elimination. The concentration-time curve upon IM procaine penicillin G is also a flip-flop model, because the dissolution of the procaine penicillin and appearance of penicillin G in blood takes longer than its elimination.

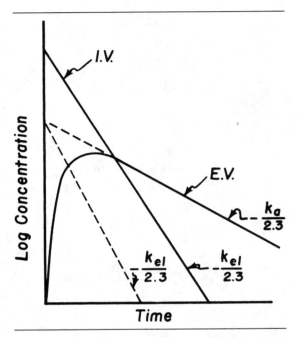

Figure 21-1. Schematic diagram demonstrating a flip-flop model. Upon IV administration the elimination rate constant k_{el} is obtained. Upon backfeathering of the fast ascending part of the curve with the slow terminal phase of the concentration-time curve upon extravascular administration, EV, a rate constant is obtained being identical to the k_{el} upon IV dosing; hence, the ascending part of the EV curve shows the drug's elimination phase, and the terminal portion characterizes the absorption phase.

Flip-flop models are often observed for metabolite concentration-time curves, because the metabolite may be eliminated more quickly than formed.

Model with Equal k_a and k_{el}

In the model where k_a is equal or close to k_{el}, absorption continues throughout the elimination phase and the terminal slope of the log concentration-time curve is not linear. Hence, it cannot be used to determine a proper rate constant. Further, the method of residuals (back-feathering) cannot be used.

In such a case t_{max} and C_{max}, the peak time and peak concentration, are read from the graph. The $AUC^{0 \to \infty}$ is calculated by the linear trapezoidal rule, whereby the last concentration should be close to zero.

When $k_a = k_{el} = k$, the drug concentration in the body is:

$$C(t) = \frac{D \cdot f \cdot k \cdot t \cdot e^{-k \cdot t}}{V_d} \qquad (68)$$

and:

$$t_{max} = \frac{1}{k} \tag{69}$$

$$C_{max} = \frac{D \cdot f}{V_d \cdot e} \tag{70}$$

where e is the base of the natural logarithm = 2.718. The product $t_{max} \cdot C_{max}$ is equal to $AUC^{o \rightarrow \infty}/e$:

$$t_{max} \cdot C_{max} = \frac{D \cdot f}{k \cdot V_d \cdot e} = \frac{D \cdot f}{Cl_{tot} \cdot e} = \frac{AUC^{o \rightarrow \infty}}{e} \tag{71}$$

Hence, whenever $t_{max} \cdot C_{max}$ equals AUC/e, the rate constants for absorption and elimination are equal:

$$k = k_a = k_{el} = \frac{1}{t_{max}} \tag{72}$$

and the relevant pharmacokinetic parameters can be calculated from Equation 21.68 or 21.71.

Regression Model for Equal k_a and k_{el}

If one plots the ln of C/t versus t, for a one-compartment model with equal k_a and k_{el}, the intercept on the ordinate is $(f \cdot D \cdot k)/V_d$, and the slope is k (where $k = k_a = k_{el}$). After estimating k by regression, V_d can be calculated:

$$V_d = \frac{D \cdot f \cdot k}{Intercept} \tag{73}$$

Selected References

1. Bialer, M.: A Simple Method for Determining Whether Absorption and Elimination Rate Constants Are Equal in the One-Compartment Open Model with First-Order Processes, *J. Pharmacokinet. Biopharm.* 8:111 (1980).

2. Byron, P. R. and Notari, E.: Clinical Analysis of the "Flip-Flop" Phenomenon in the Two-Compartment Pharmacokinetic Model, *J. Pharm. Sci.* 65:1140 (1976).

3. Doluisio, J. T. and Dittert, L. W.: Pharmaceutical Parameters, *Am. J. Pharm. Ed.* 32:895 (1968).

4. Dost, F. H.: *Grundlagen der Pharmakokinetik.* Georg Thieme Verlag, Stuttgart, 1968, p. 36.

5. Garrett, E. R.: Theoretische Pharmakokinetik. In *Klinische Pharmakologie und Pharmakotherapie.* Kuemmerle, H. P., Garrett, E. R. and Spitzy, K. H., editors. Urban and Schwarzenberg, Munich-Berlin-Vienna, 1973, p. 27.

6. Hoke, J. F. and Ravis, W. R.: A Simple Method for Obtaining the Rate Constant for a One Compartment Absorption Model when KA = KE. *Pharm. Res.* 5:S226 (1988).

7. Rescino, A. and Segre, G.: *Drug and Tracer Kinetics,* Blaisdell, Waltham, Mass., 1966.

8. Ritschel, W. A.: Fundamentals of Pharmacokinetics. In: *Methods of Clinical Pharmacology,* Kuemmerle, H. P., Ed. Urban and Schwarzenberg, Munich-Vienna-Baltimore, 1978, pp. 133–166.

9. Ritts, D. S.: *A Critical Primer—The Mathematical Approach to Physiological Problems,* M.I.T. Press, Cambridge, Mass., 1967, p. 120.

10. Wagner, J. G.: *Biopharmaceutics and Relevant Pharmacokinetics,* Drug Intelligence Publications, Hamilton, Ill. 1971, p. 292.

22

Pharmacokinetics of Multiple Dosing

It is generally recognized that the drug concentration in blood, plasma, or serum of many drugs must be maintained above a certain minimum concentration throughout the course of therapy to ensure clinical effectiveness. Some such drugs are, for instance, the antibiotics, anticoagulants, cytostatics, antidiabetics, hormones, coronary dilators, etc. However, sometimes fluctuations between high and low levels are preferred, as has been suggested, for instance, for penicillin.

If a drug is administered in fixed doses and at fixed intervals, accumulation occurs if drug intake exceeds elimination. Knowing the accumulation of drugs in the body, it is possible to calculate the dosage regimen, i.e., the necessary dose size and the necessary dosing interval to maintain a definite minimum or therapeutic drug concentration.

General Concepts

1. Subsequent doses are administered before the previously given dose is totally eliminated, thus resulting in accumulation. Noticeable accumulation will be seen only if $\tau < 3 \cdot t_{1/2}$. After $3 \cdot t_{1/2}$ the trough concentration after the first dose is about 10 percent of the first peak concentration.
2. All dose sizes are equal; loading dose and maintenance dose have the same amount of drug.
3. The dosing intervals are equal throughout the course of therapy.
4. Upon multiple dosing, the blood-, plasma-, or serum-level curves increase (accumulate) to an asymptotic value. The reason the accumulating curve levels off in an asymptotic value is that the term $e^{-k_{el} \cdot \tau}$ is always smaller than 1.0.
5. In these pharmacokinetic considerations it is assumed that all pharmacokinetic parameters remain constant during the entire course of therapy. Factors which would lead to a deviation of the actual blood level from the calculated one are the following:
   • Change in urinary excretion (change of urinary pH; change in creatinine clearance);
   • Change in hepatic clearance (liver disease, saturation of metabolic pathways);

- Enzyme induction and enzyme inhibition; and
- Dose dependent pharmacokinetics.

6. The following multiple dose administration equations are based on the open one-compartment model. However, one can also use these equations for drugs following the open two-compartment model, if k_{el} is substituted by β and $C(0)$ by B. This approximation is especially useful in dose size and dosing interval calculation. This simplification will yield a usable approximation since it is based on the amount of drug still in the body when the following dose is given. At that time, the persisting blood level is in the monoexponential declining phase. However, only C_{min}^{ss} will be accurate whereas C_{max}^{ss} will always result in an underestimation.

Accumulation of the average amount of drug in the body during any dosing interval at steady state ($V_{dss} \cdot C_{av}^{ss}$), less the average amount of drug unabsorbed after a single dose, will be better predicted the closer the ratio $V_{dss}/V_{d\beta}$ is to unity. If $V_{dss}/V_{d\beta}$ is very small, treatment by the one-compartment will result in overestimation of accumulation ratio. In this case a correction factor $V_{dss}/V_{d\beta} \cdot (1/\beta \cdot \tau)$ is indicated.

The following factors should be recognized in multiple dosing:

$$\text{Persistence factor: } e^{-k_{el} \cdot \circledR}$$

$$\text{Loss factor: } 1 - e^{-k_{el} \cdot \circledR}$$

$$\text{Accumulation factor: } \frac{1}{1 - e^{-k_{el} \cdot \circledR}}$$

Intravenous Constant Rate Infusion

Intravenous infusion at constant (zero-order) rate can be considered as multiple dosing with infinitely small dosing intervals. It takes 5 elimination half-lives until steady state (approximately 95% of it) is reached. Therefore, for therapeutic purposes it is essential to administer an IV loading dose in order to immediately reach steady state. Once steady state is obtained, IV constant rate infusion is the most accurate method of dosing to reach and maintain a required therapeutic concentration. Only with IV infusion are the steady state concentrations identical during the course of therapy, i.e., $C_{av}^{ss} = C_{max}^{ss} = C_{min}^{ss}$, or, in other words, no fluctuations are occurring. However, a sinus wave-like fluctuation may be observed for some drugs in a 24 hour cycle due to changes in some pharmacokinetic parameters by circadian rhythms.

An IV constant rate of infusion without a loading dose starts at time zero and zero concentration in a curvilinear (convex) fashion and leads to an asymptotic curve at steady state. The magnitude of the steady state concentration is a function of the infusion rate (R^o) and the total clearance (Cl_{tot}). Increasing R^o will increase the steady state level, but the time to reach steady state remains unchanged ($\sim 5 \cdot t_{1/2}$). With decreasing renal and/or hepatic function (longer $t_{1/2}$) and unchanged R^o, the steady state concentration increases and the time to reach steady state will be prolonged.

After termination of the infusion, the drug concentration-time curve declines in the same fashion as after IV push injections (Figure 22-1).

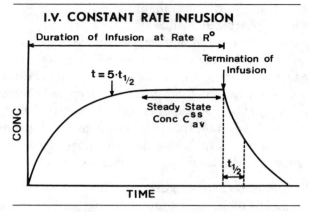

Figure 22-1. Blood concentration versus time curve
upon IV infusion at constant rate.
R° = zero-order rate of infusion
$t_{1/2}$ = elimination half-life
t = approaching steady state at $5 \cdot t_{1/2}$

One-Compartment Open Model

During the time of infusion, t_i, the drug concentration is given by Equation 22.1:

$$C(t) = \frac{R^\circ}{V_d \cdot k_{el}} \cdot (1 - e^{-k_{el} \cdot t_i})$$ (1)

After the infusion is terminated the drug concentration can be calculated by Equation 22.2:

$$C(t) = \frac{R^\circ}{V_d \cdot k_{el}} \cdot (1 - e^{-k_{el} \cdot t_i}) \cdot e^{-k_{el} \cdot (t - t_i)}$$ (2)

$C(t)$ = drug concentration in blood, plasma, or serum [µg/ml]
R° = zero-order infusion rate [µg/h]
V_d = volume of distribution [ml]
k_{el} = overall elimination rate constant [h⁻¹]
t_i = time (duration) of infusion [h]
t = total time since start of infusion [h]

Short-Term Infusion

A short-term infusion is when the duration of infusion or infusion time is $t_i < 5 \cdot t_{1/2}$. In this case, steady state is not reached. For pharmacokinetic evaluation only two blood samples are needed: one at the moment the infusion is terminated, C_{max} (not C_{max}^{ss}), and one at any later time, C_{min} (not C_{min}^{ss}), as shown in Figure 22-2.

SHORT - TERM INFUSION

SS NOT REACHED

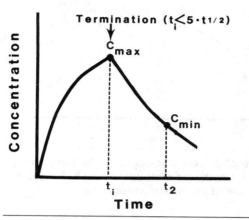

Figure 22-2. Schematic diagram for short-term infusion.

$$k_{el} = \frac{\ln C_{max} - \ln C_{min}}{t_2 - t_1} [h^{-1}] \tag{3}$$

$$V_d = \frac{R^{\circ}}{k_{el}} \cdot \frac{(1 - e^{k_{el} \cdot t_i}) \cdot (1 - e^{k_{el} \cdot (t - t_i)})}{C_{max} - C_{min}} [ml] \tag{4}$$

$$Cl_{tot} = V_d \cdot k_{el} [ml/h] \tag{5}$$

Equations 22.1 and 22.2 apply also for short-term infusion to characterize the course of the blood level-time curve.

If enough blood samples are taken to permit calculation of the total area under the curve, $AUC^{0 \to \infty}$, Equation 22.6 can be used to calculate V_d:

$$V_d = \frac{D}{AUC^{0 \to \infty} \cdot k_{el}} [ml] \tag{6}$$

Long-Term Infusion

A long-term infusion is when the duration of infusion or infusion time exceeds $5 \cdot t_{1/2}$. In this case steady state is reached. For pharmacokinetic evaluation two approaches, each of them requiring only two blood samples, can be used: Method A, during infusion and Method B, after termination, as shown in Figure 22-3.

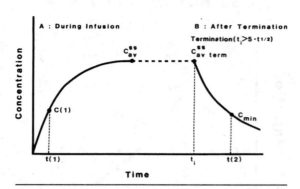

Figure 22-3. Schematic diagram for long-term infusion with two methods, A and B, for determination of pharmacokinetic parameters.

Method A: During Infusion

Two blood samples are taken, one during the ascending part of the curve, say after 0.5 to $1.5 \cdot t_{1/2}$, and one after steady state is reached, i.e., after $5 \cdot t_{1/2}$.

Since:

$$C_{av}^{ss} = \frac{R^\circ}{V_d \cdot k_{el}} = \frac{R^\circ}{Cl_{tot}} \; [\mu g/ml] \qquad (7)$$

the total clearance can be calculated:

$$C_{tot} = \frac{R^\circ}{C_{av}^{ss}} \; [ml/h] \qquad (8)$$

$$k_{el} = \frac{\ln\left(1 - \dfrac{C(1) \cdot Cl_{tot}}{R^\circ}\right)}{t(1)} [h^{-1}] \qquad (9)$$

$$V_d = \frac{Cl_{tot}}{k_{el}} [ml] \qquad (10)$$

Method B: After Termination

Two blood samples are taken, one at the moment of termination of the infusion, $C_{av\ term}^{ss}$, and one at any later time, C_{min}. Then:

$$k_{el} = \frac{\ln C^{ss}_{av\ term} - \ln C_{min}}{t(2) - t_1} [h^{-1}] \tag{11}$$

$$V_d = \frac{R^\circ}{C^{ss}_{av} \cdot k_{el}} [ml] \tag{12}$$

Equations 22.1 and 22.2 apply also for long-term infusion to characterize the course of the blood level-time curve.

Two-Compartment Open Model

The drug concentration-time curve for an infusion according to the two-compartment open model can be expressed by Equation 22.13:

$$C(t) = \frac{R^\circ \cdot (k_{21} - \alpha) \cdot (1 - e^{-\alpha \cdot t_i})}{V_c \cdot \alpha \cdot (\alpha - \beta)} \cdot e^{-\alpha \cdot t}$$
$$+ \frac{R^\circ \cdot (\beta - k_{21}) \cdot (1 - e^{-\beta \cdot t_i})}{V_c \cdot \beta \cdot (\alpha - \beta)} \cdot e^{-\beta \cdot t} [\mu g/ml] \tag{13}$$

$C(t)$ = drug concentration during or after termination of infusion [$\mu g/ml$]
R° = zero-order infusion rate [$\mu g/h$]
α = fast disposition rate constant [h^{-1}]
β = slow disposition rate constant [h^{-1}]
k_{21} = distribution rate constant for transfer from central to the peripheral compartment [h^{-1}]
t_i = infusion time [h]
t = total time since start of infusion [h]

Using the postinfusion declining portion of a blood level-time curve and applying the back-feathering technique in a way as discussed in Chapter 21 for the two-compartment open model, the rate constants β and α are the same whether they are obtained from a postinfusion curve or a single dose IV push curve. However, the intercepts of the exponential terms are different and the differences increase as the infusion time lengthens. Since the intercepts can be used to calculate pharmacokinetic parameters, correction has to be made.

Corrected intercept A′:

$$A' = \frac{A \cdot (1 - e^{-\alpha \cdot t_i})}{\alpha \cdot t_i} [\mu g/ml] \tag{14}$$

Corrected intercept B′:

$$B' = \frac{B \cdot (1 - e^{-\beta \cdot t_i})}{\beta \cdot t_i} [\mu g/ml] \tag{15}$$

where A and B are the intercepts obtained from back-feathering of the postinfusion curve to the time the infusion was terminated at t_i.

Intravascular Multiple Dose Administration

If a second IV dose is given at a time interval which is longer than the time required to eliminate the previous dose (theoretically 10 elimination half-lives) a series of single doses will be obtained (upper part of Figure 22-4). If the dosing interval is shorter than the time required for total elimination of the drug (practically $\tau < 3 \cdot t_{1/2}$), an accumulation curve is obtained (lower part of Figure 22-4).

However, the accumulation curve does not increase indefinitely, but levels off to a plateau depending on the elimination half-life of the drug and the dosing interval. The reason for obtaining a plateau is that the accumulating drug concentration is multiplied for each dosing interval by the persistence factor $e^{-k_{el} \cdot \tau}$, which is always <1. Therefore, accumulation of a drug in the body is not a specific property of any drug, but solely a question of the dos-

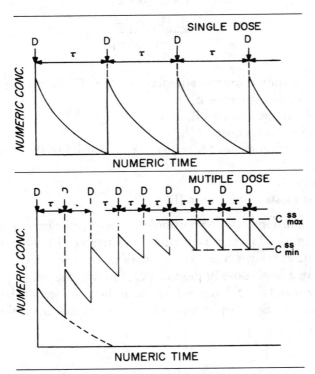

Figure 22-4. Blood level versus time curves upon intravascular single dose (top) and multiple dose (bottom) administration (open one-compartment model).

D	=	dose size
τ	=	dosing interval
C^{ss}_{max}	=	maximum blood level at plateau
C^{ss}_{min}	=	minimum blood level at plateau

ing interval. The longer the elimination half-life and the shorter the dosing interval the higher will be the accumulation:

$$C_{max}^{ss} = \frac{C(0)}{1-e^{-k_{el} \cdot \tau}} [\mu g/ml] \tag{16}$$

C_{max}^{ss} = maximum drug concentration in blood, plasma, or serum in multiple dosing at steady state [μg/ml]
$C(0)$ = initial drug concentration in blood, plasma, or serum after first dose [μg/ml]
k_{el} = overall elimination rate constant [h⁻¹]
τ = dosing interval [hr]

$$C_{min}^{ss} = \frac{C(0) \cdot e^{-k_{el} \cdot \tau}}{1-e^{-k_{el} \cdot \tau}}$$

$$= C_{max}^{ss} \cdot e^{-k_{el} \cdot \tau} [\mu g/ml] \tag{17}$$

$$C_{av}^{ss} = \frac{D}{V_d \cdot k_{el} \cdot \tau} [\mu g/ml] \tag{18}$$

C_{min}^{ss} = minimum drug concentration in blood, plasma, or serum in multiple dosing at steady state [μg/ml]
C_{av}^{ss} = average (mean) drug concentration in blood, plasma, or serum in multiple dosing [μg/ml]
V_d = volume of distribution [ml]
D = dose size [μg]

Accumulation of Individual IV Doses

$$r = e^{-k_{el} \cdot \tau} \tag{19}$$

r = persistence factor

$$\text{maximum after 1 dose: } C_{max\,1} = C(0) [\mu g/ml] \tag{20}$$

$$\text{minimum after 1 dose: } C_{min\,1} = C(0) \cdot r [\mu g/ml] \tag{21}$$

$$\text{maximum after 2 doses: } C_{max\,2} = C_{min\,1} + C(0) [\mu g/ml] \tag{22}$$

$$\text{minimum after 2 doses: } C_{min\,2} = C_{max\,2} \cdot r [\mu g/ml] \tag{23}$$

$$\text{maximum after 3 doses: } C_{max\,3} = C_{min\,2} + C(0) [\mu g/ml] \tag{24}$$

$$\text{minimum after 3 doses: } C_{min\,3} = C_{max\,3} \cdot r [\mu g/ml] \tag{25}$$

$$\text{maximum after n doses: } C_{max\,n} = C_{min\,(n-1)} + C(0) [\mu g/ml] \tag{26}$$

$$\text{minimum after n doses: } C_{\min n} = C_{\max n} \cdot r \; [\mu g/ml] \tag{27}$$

The accumulation of individual doses to steady state is shown in Figure 22-5. Note that the $AUC^{0 \to \infty}$ after the first dose (single dose) is equal to the $AUC^{\tau_n \to \tau_{n+1}}$ at steady state in the absence of dose dependency, enzyme induction, or enzyme inhibition:

$$\tau = \frac{1}{k_{el}} \cdot \ln\left(1 + \frac{C(0)}{C_{\min}^{ss}}\right) [h] \tag{28}$$

τ = desired dosing interval to maintain a therapeutic concentration [h]
$C_{\min}^{ss}$ = minimum drug concentration during any dosing interval at steady state [$\mu g/ml$]

Extravascular Multiple Dose Administration

Here, the situation is similar to that with the IV route of administration. If the dosing interval τ is shorter than the time required for elimination we obtain an accumulation curve as seen in Figure 22-6.

The longer the elimination half-life and the shorter the dosing interval, the higher will be the accumulation and the higher the plateau level, as seen in Figure 22-7. The shorter the dosing interval, the smaller will be the fluctuation between $C_{\max}^{ss}$ and $C_{\min}^{ss}$.

There are several methods for calculation of $C_{\max}^{ss}$ and $C_{\min}^{ss}$. The first is very precise; however, one must know all the pharmacokinetic parameters: namely, C(0) after a single dose, k_a and k_{el}, and one has to calculate the time to reach the plateau. The equations for Method A are Equations 22.29 to 22.31.

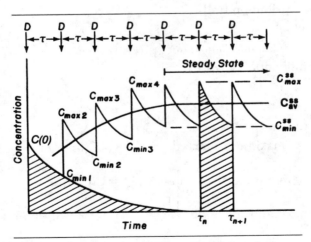

Figure 22-5. Blood level versus time curve to demonstrate accumulation to steady state (open one-compartment model).

D   = dose size
τ = dosing interval
C_{av}^{ss} = mean steady state blood concentration
$C_{\max}^{ss}$ = maximum steady state blood concentration
$C_{\min}^{ss}$ = minimum steady state blood concentration

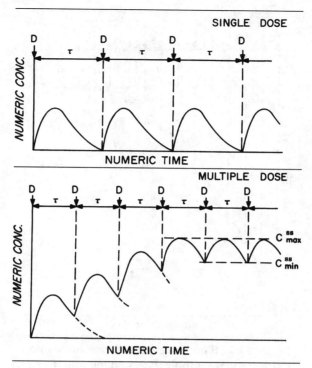

Figure 22-6. Blood level versus time curves upon extravascular single dose (top) and multiple dose (bottom) administration (open one-compartment model).

D = dose size

τ = dosing interval

C_{max}^{ss} = maximum blood level at plateau

C_{min}^{ss} = minimum blood level at plateau

Method A (Dost)

$$C_{max}^{ss} = \frac{C(0) \cdot k_a}{k_a - k_{el}} \cdot \left[\frac{e^{-k_{el} \cdot t_{max}^{ss}}}{1 - e^{-k_{el} \cdot \tau}} - \frac{e^{-k_a \cdot t_{max}^{ss}}}{1 - e^{-k_a \cdot \tau}} \right] [\mu g/ml] \qquad (29)$$

$$t_{max}^{ss} = \frac{1}{k_a - k_{el}} \cdot \ln \left[\frac{k_a \cdot (1 - e^{-k_{el} \cdot \tau})}{k_{el} \cdot (1 - e^{-k_a \cdot \tau})} \right] [\mu g/ml] \qquad (30)$$

$$C_{max}^{ss} = \frac{C(0) \cdot k_a}{k_a - k_{el}} \cdot \left(\frac{1}{1 - e^{-k_{el} \cdot \tau}} - \frac{1}{1 - e^{-k_a \cdot \tau}} \right) [\mu g/ml] \qquad (31)$$

k_a = absorption rate constant [h⁻¹]

k_{el} = elimination rate constant [h⁻¹]

C_{max}^{ss} = maximum drug concentration in blood, plasma, or serum in multiple dosing at steady state [µg/ml]

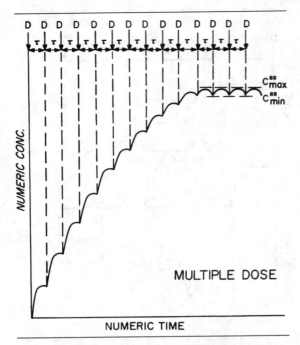

Figure 22-7. Blood level versus time curve upon extravascular multiple dose administration showing large accumulation due to short dosing interval τ.
Note: The shorter τ the higher accumulation and the fewer fluctuations between C_{max}^{ss} and C_{min}^{ss}.
D = **dose size**
τ = **dosing interval**
C_{max}^{ss} = **maximum blood level at plateau**
C_{min}^{ss} = **minimum blood level at plateau**

C_{min}^{ss} = minimum drug concentration in the blood, plasma, or serum in multiple dosing at steady state [μg/ml]
$C(0)$ = back-extrapolated hypothetical $C(0) = B$ (intercept)
t_{max}^{ss} = time to maximum concentration after n doses [h]

Method B (Doluisio and Dittert)

The second method is a simplification where one needs to know $C(0)$ after a single dose (obtained from a graph), the time to reach the peak, and k_{el}; knowing also k_a, one can calculate the peak time. However, there may be a difference in C_{max}^{ss} between the calculated and the value actually found. This is because the peak concentration is calculated as the concentration on the back-extrapolated monoexponential line from the graphically determined $C(0)$ at the time of the peak. Usually the actual peak concentration does not lie on the monoexponential slope, as seen from the schematic in Figure 22-8 and C_{max}^{ss} is therefore an overestimation:

$$C_{max}^{ss} = \frac{C(0) \cdot e^{-k_{el} \cdot t_{max}}}{1 - e^{-k_{el} \cdot \tau}} \ [\mu g/ml] \tag{32}$$

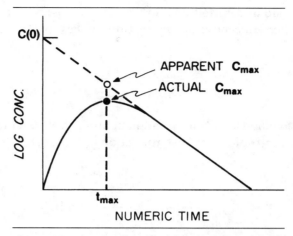

Figure 22-8. Demonstration for deviation of the apparent peak height from the actual peak height C_{max} if C_{max} is calculated using C(0), k_{el}, and t_{max} according to equation: C(t) = C(0) · $e^{-k_{el} \cdot t_{max}}$, an artifact to be used if k_a is not available.

Note: The more pronounced the peak the less difference between the apparent and the actual C_{max}.

$$t_{max} = \frac{2.303}{k_a - k_{el}} \cdot \log \frac{k}{k_{el}} \, [h] \tag{33}$$

$$C_{min}^{ss} = \frac{C(0) \cdot e^{-k_{el} \cdot \tau}}{1 - e^{-k_{el} \cdot \tau}} \, [\mu g/ml] \tag{34}$$

t_{max} = time to reach the peak after first dose [h]

Method C (Ritschel)

The third method is applicable for approximation if only a limited amount of pharmacokinetic information is available. Often one finds in the medical literature only two or three blood level data for a given patient. In this case a graphical estimation is not possible.

Method C may however be used under the following assumptions:

- The drug's performance in the blood is treated as an open one-compartment model.
- The highest of the available blood level points is considered as the actual peak, thus indicating the peak time, or a literature value is used for t_{max}.
- The last of the available blood level points is considered to be on the monoexponential declining line.
- The patient has a normal elimination pattern, i.e., no renal or hepatic failure, since the k_{el} value is taken from the literature or calculated from an elimination half-life compilation according to $k_{el} = 0.693/t_{1/2}$. In the case of renal dysfunction a correction must be made.

What has been said under Method B in respect to a possible difference between the actual and the calculated concentration at peak time applies also to Method C:

$$C(0) = \frac{C_{px}}{e^{-k_{el} \cdot t_x}} \; [\mu g/ml] \tag{35}$$

C_{px} = last determined blood level concentration upon single dose administration $[\mu g/ml]$
t_x = time from administration until determination of $C_{px}[h]$

$$C_{max}^{ss} = \frac{\dfrac{C_{px}}{e^{-k_{el} \cdot t_x}} \cdot e^{-k_{el} \cdot t_{max}}}{1 - e^{-k_{el} \cdot \tau}} \; [\mu g/ml] \tag{36}$$

$$C_{min}^{ss} = \frac{\dfrac{C_{px}}{e^{-k_{el} \cdot t_x}} \cdot e^{-k_{el} \cdot \tau}}{1 - e^{-k_{el} \cdot \tau}} \; [\mu g/ml] \tag{37}$$

If one wants to calculate the drug concentration C_{av}^{ss} of the average or mean blood level curve, Equation 22.38 can be used:

$$C_{av}^{ss} = \frac{D \cdot f}{V_d \cdot k_{el} \cdot \tau} \; [\mu g/ml] \tag{38}$$

However, Equation 22.38 should not be used for dose size and dosage regimen calculation for bacteriostatic antimicrobials and highly toxic drugs because we do not get any information on the fluctuations between C_{max}^{ss} and C_{min}^{ss}. Although C_{av}^{ss} may be above the required minimum effective concentration, the actual drug concentration may undercut the MEC for a certain time period per dosing interval as seen from Figure 22-9.

Method D (Schumacher)

The fourth method, or superposition method, is based on the finding that the blood concentration versus time profile for each successive dose of a multiple dose regimen may be superimposed on the blood concentration of drug remaining at the end of the dosage interval, just prior to administration of the next dose. The maximum and minimum drug concentration in blood, plasma, or serum, C_{max}^{ss} and C_{min}^{ss}, achieved at steady state can be obtained from single dose parameters as given in Equations 22.39 and 22.40:

$$C_{max}^{ss} = C_{max} + \frac{C_\tau \cdot 10^{-0.3 \cdot t_{max}/t_{1/2}}}{1 - 10^{-0.3 \cdot \tau/t_{1/2}}}$$

$$= C_{max} + \frac{C_\tau \cdot 10^{-0.43 \cdot k_{el} \cdot t_{max}}}{1 - 10^{-0.43 \cdot k_{el} \cdot \tau}} \; [\mu g/ml] \tag{39}$$

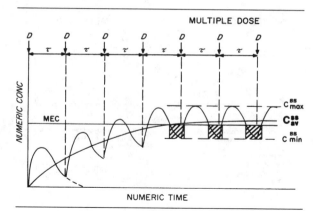

Figure 22-9. Blood level versus time curve upon multiple dose extravascular route of administration resulting in C_{max}^{ss} and C_{min}^{ss} at the plateau and average blood level curve C_{av}^{ss}. If it is necessary to maintain a minimum effective concentration MEC and dose size D or dosing interval τ calculations are based on the C_{av}^{ss} equations, the actual blood level curve will undercut the MEC line for a considerable period of time, depending on the elimination half-life and the dosing interval. If the blood level curve undercuts the MEC (shaded area) the patient is unprotected.

$$C_{min}^{ss} = C_\tau + \frac{C_\tau \cdot 10^{-0.3 \cdot \tau/t_{1/2}}}{1 - 10^{-0.3 \cdot \tau/t_{1/2}}}$$

$$= C_\tau + \frac{C_\tau \cdot 10^{-0.43 \cdot k_{el} \cdot \tau}}{1 - 10^{-0.43 \cdot k_{el} \cdot \tau}} \ [\mu g/ml] \qquad (40)$$

C_{max} = drug concentration at peak time after single dose [μg/ml]
C_τ = drug concentration of single dose just prior to administration of following dose (at end of dosing interval) [μg/ml]
t_{max} = time to reach the peak after first dose [h]

Situations for appropriate use of Methods A (Dost), B (Doluisio and Dittert), C (Ritschel), and D (Schumacher) to predict steady state blood levels from data following administration of a single dose are illustrated in Figure 22-10.

Considerations for the Open Two-Compartment Model

We have said that dose size and dose interval calculations are based on the open one-compartment model even if an open two-compartment model would apply. This can be done since each succeeding dose is given when the drug concentration of the previous dose is in the monoexponential elimination phase. Instead of C(0), we use the intercept B of the back-extrapolated monoexponential slope with the ordinate and, instead of k_{el}, we use β.

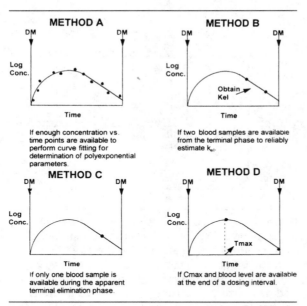

Figure 22-10. Example of when to use Method A (Eqs. 22.29–22.31), Method B (Eqs. 22.32–22.34), Method C (Eqs. 22.35–22.38), and Method D (Eqs. 22.39 and 22.40) for the evaluation of steady state blood levels from data obtained after a single dose. All methods assume that representative blood levels are obtained within a fixed dosing interval where maintenance doses (DM) of a fixed amount are given.

The C_{min}^{ss} thus determined will be the true value. However, the C_{max}^{ss} will be an underestimation since the peak used in calculation is an artifact, at least intravascularly, as seen from Figure 22-11. Extravascularly, the difference might not be that large depending on the distribution rate constants.

If literature data are available for a drug following a two-compartment model after intravascular administration, such as α, β, V_c, and Cl_{tot}, one can calculate the intercept B:

$$k_{13} = \frac{Cl_{tot}}{V_c}[h^{-1}] \tag{41}$$

$$k_{21} = \frac{\alpha \cdot \beta}{k_{13}}[h^{-1}] \tag{42}$$

$$B = \frac{D \cdot (k_{21} - \beta)}{V_c \cdot (\alpha - \beta)}[\mu g/ml] \tag{43}$$

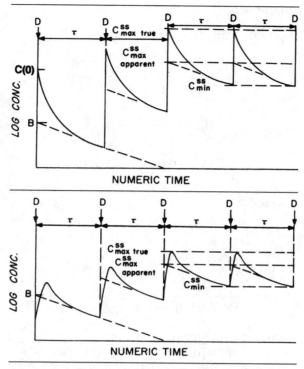

Figure 22-11. Blood level versus time curves for multiple dosing upon intravascular (top) and extravascular (bottom) route of administration. Although the open two-compartment model applies C_{min}^{ss} can be calculated using the equations for the open one-compartment model under the assumption that subsequent doses are given when the blood level of the previous dose has reached the β-phase. However, C_{max}^{ss} will always be an artifact.

Knowing C_{min}^{ss} for the two-compartment model C_{max}^{ss} can be established according to Equation 22.44:

$$C_{max}^{ss} = C_{min}^{ss} + \frac{D}{\Delta_c' \cdot BW} \; [\mu g/ml] \tag{44}$$

D   = dose size [μg]
Δ_c' = distribution coefficient for central compartment volume of distribution [ml/g]
BW = body weight [g]

If one wants to calculate the actual drug concentration in blood at any time upon multiple dosing, Equations 22.45 and 22.46 can be used.

Open Two-Compartment Model

Rapid intravenous injection:

$$C(t)_n = \frac{D}{V_c(\alpha-\beta)} \cdot \left[\left(\frac{1-e^{-n\cdot\beta\cdot\tau}}{1-e^{-\beta\cdot\tau}}\right)\right.$$
$$\cdot(k_{21}-\beta)\cdot e^{-\beta\cdot t} - \left(\frac{1-e^{-n\cdot\alpha\cdot\tau}}{1-e^{-\alpha\cdot\tau}}\right)$$
$$\left.\cdot(k_{21}-\alpha)\cdot e^{-\alpha\cdot t}\right][\mu g/ml] \qquad (45)$$

Extravascular administration:

$$C(t)_n = \frac{D\cdot f\cdot k_a}{V_c} \cdot \left[\left(\frac{1-e^{-n\cdot\alpha\cdot\tau}}{1-e^{-\alpha\cdot\tau}}\right)\right.$$
$$\cdot\left(\frac{k_{21}-\alpha}{(k_a-\alpha)\cdot(\beta-\alpha)}\right)\cdot e^{-\alpha\cdot t} + \left(\frac{1-e^{-n\cdot\beta\cdot\tau}}{1-e^{-\alpha\cdot\tau}}\right)$$
$$\cdot\left(\frac{k_{21}-\beta}{(k_a-\beta)\cdot(\alpha-\beta)}\right)\cdot e^{-\beta\cdot t} + \left(\frac{1-e^{-n\cdot k_a\cdot\tau}}{1-e^{-k_a\cdot\tau}}\right)$$
$$\left.\cdot\left(\frac{k_{21}-k_a}{(\alpha-k_a)\cdot(\beta-k_a)}\right)\cdot e^{-k_a\cdot t}\right][\mu g/ml] \qquad (46)$$

$C(t)_n$ = drug concentration after n th dose [μg/ml]
D = dose administered [μg]
f = fraction of dose absorbed [fraction of 1]
V_c = volume of central compartment [ml]
n = number of doses given
τ = dosing interval [h]
t = time after dose administration [h]
k_a = absorption rate constant [h^{-1}]
k_{21} = distribution rate constant for back transport from peripheral to central compartment [h^{-1}]
α = slope of monoexponential distribution line (hybrid constant) [h^{-1}]
β = slope of monoexponential terminal line (hybrid constant) [h^{-1}]

Mean Steady State Concentration

The mean steady state concentration C_{av}^{ss} is not the arithmetic mean between C_{max}^{ss} and C_{min}^{ss} but the mean of the integrated drug concentration-time curve. C_{av}^{ss} was originally derived for the one-compartment open model as given in Equation 22.47:

$$C_{av}^{ss} = \frac{D\cdot f}{V_d\cdot k_{el}\cdot\tau}[\mu g/ml] \qquad (47)$$

However, C_{av}^{ss} can be calculated as a compartment model independent parameter from the area under the concentration-time curve for a complete dosing interval at steady state, $AUC^{\tau_n \to \tau_{n+1}}$:

$$C_{av}^{ss} = \frac{AUC^{\tau_n \to \tau_{n+1}}}{\tau} \, [\mu g/ml] \tag{48}$$

Fluctuation at Steady State

The extent of fluctuation at steady state between C_{max}^{ss} and C_{min}^{ss} after intravenous administration is given by the drug's elimination half-life and the dosing interval. The longer the elimination half-life and the shorter the dosing interval the less will be the fluctuation.

The percent fluctuation can be calculated according to Equation 22.49:

$$\% \, \text{Fluctuation} = (1 - e^{-k_{el} \cdot \tau}) \cdot 100 \tag{49}$$

Relationship between IV Constant Rate Infusion, IV Push, and Extravascular Administration

Let us assume a drug is given to the same subject once as an IV constant rate infusion (top panel in Figure 22-12), once as IV push injection (second panel in Figure 22-12), and once extravascularly (PO, IM, SC, Rectal, etc.) whereby the drug is completely bioavailable (third panel of Figure 22-12). For IV and EV identical dose sizes in identical dosing intervals are used. For IV constant rate infusion, the total dose infused is equal to the sum of all doses given by IV push or extravascularly, and the duration of infusion TI is equal to the sum of all IV push or EV dosing intervals. No saturation kinetics, enzyme induction, or enzyme inhibition is present.

The IV constant rate infusion will result in accumulation to a steady state concentration C^{ss}. Since the input is at constant rate, no fluctuations occur (top panel of Figure 22-12).

Upon IV push multiple dosing, the steady state concentrations will

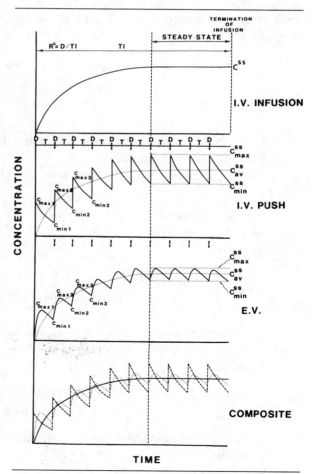

Figure 22-12. Relationship between IV constant rate infusion, IV push, and extravascular administration.

fluctuate between C_{max}^{ss} and C_{min}^{ss}. The theoretical mean steady state concentration C_{av}^{ss} will be the same as if the drug were given by IV constant rate infusion (second panel of Figure 22-12).

Upon EV multiple dosing, the steady state concentrations will fluctuate between C_{max}^{ss} and C_{min}^{ss}. Note, however, that the fluctuation is less after EV than after IV. The mean steady state concentration C_{av}^{ss} will be the same as if the drug were given by IV constant rate infusion (third panel of Figure 22-12).

A composite of the three routes of administration is given in the bottom panel of Figure 22-12.

Prediction of Steady State Blood Levels in Drug-Naive Patients

For those drugs which do not exhibit pronounced Michaelis-Menten kinetics and/or are subject to enzyme induction or inhibition (which is the case for most drugs), the AUC after a single dose extrapolated to infinity ($AUC_{SD}^{0\to\infty}$) is equal to the AUC at steady state for multiple dosing ($AUC_{MD}^{\tau_n\to\tau_{n+1}}$). This equality is true only when fixed doses of a drug are administered at equally spaced dosing intervals and no changes in the disposition characteristics of the drug occur during multiple dosing. When these assumptions are met, the mean steady state concentration (C_{av}^{ss}) can be determined as denoted in Equations 22.50 and 22.51:

$$C_{av}^{ss} = (AUC_{MD}^{\tau_n\to\tau_{n+1}})/\tau \tag{50}$$

$$C_{av}^{ss} = (AUC_{SD}^{0\to\infty})/\tau \tag{51}$$

Accordingly, one can predict the C_{av}^{ss} for any dosage regimen based on the aforementioned assumptions and thus estimate the expected peak and trough plasma concentrations (C_{max}^{ss} and C_{min}^{ss}) at steady state. This procedure is illustrated as follows using the example of ibuprofen.

1. Obtain the pertinent, age-appropriate pharmacokinetic parameters of a drug (see Appendix or other reference sources):
Example:

$$t_{1/2} = 2.2\,h \quad \lambda_z = 0.318\,h^{-1} \quad V_d = 0.1\,L/kg$$

$$F = 10 \quad \text{Therapeutic Range} = 5 \text{ to } 50\,\mu g/ml$$

2. Obtain pertinent patient demographic parameters and select a dose size (D) and dosing interval (τ) for initiation of therapy:
Example:

$$\text{Body Weight (BW)} = 59\,kg$$

$$D = 400\,mg \quad \tau = 8\,hr$$

3. Estimate the achievable plasma concentration (C[0]) following a single dose:
Example:

$$C[0] = (D \cdot F)/(V_d \cdot BW) = \frac{400{,}000\,\mu g/ml \cdot 1}{0.1\,ml/g \cdot 59{,}000\,g} = 67.8\,\mu g/ml \tag{52}$$

4. Estimate $AUC_{SD}^{0\to\infty}$ as follows:
Example:

$$AUC_{SD}^{0\to\infty} = C[0]/k_{el} = \frac{67.8\,\mu g/ml}{0.318\,h^{-1}} = 213.2\,[(\mu g/ml)\cdot h] \tag{53}$$

5. Estimate C_{av}^{ss} as follows:
Example:

$$C_{av}^{ss} = \frac{AUC_{SD}^{0\to\infty}}{\tau} = \frac{213.2\,[(\mu g/ml)\cdot h]}{8h} = 26.7\,\mu g/ml \tag{54}$$

6. Estimate the fluctuation of the blood level at steady state (FL) as follows:
Example:

$$FL = [1 - e^{-(k_{el}\cdot\tau)}]\cdot 100 = [1 - e^{-(0.318\cdot 8)}]\cdot 100 = 92.1\% \tag{55}$$

7. Estimate the fluctuation around $C_{av}^{ss}(FL_{av})$ as follows:
Example:

$$FL_{av} = FL/2 = 92.1/2 = 46.0\% \tag{56}$$

8. Estimate C_{max}^{ss} and C_{min}^{ss} by using C_{av}^{ss} to "adjust" FL_{av} as follows:
Example:

As 46% of $C_{av}^{ss} = 12.3$; therefore:

$$C_{max}^{ss} = C_{av}^{ss} + FL_{av} = 26.7 + 12.3 = 39.0\,\mu g/ml \tag{57}$$

$$C_{min}^{ss} = C_{av}^{ss} - FL_{av} = 26.7 - 12.3 = 14.4\,\mu g/ml \tag{58}$$

Selected References

1. Doluisio, J. T. and Dittert, C. W.: Influence of Repetitive Dosing of Tetracycline on Biological Half-Life in Serum, *Clin. Pharmacol. Ther. 10*:690 (1969).

2. Dost, F. H.: *Grundlagen der Pharmakokinetik,* Georg Thieme Verlag, Stuttgart, 1968, p. 169.

3. Loo, J. C. K. and Riegelman, S.: Assessment of Pharmacokinetic Constants from Postinfusion Blood Curves Obtained After I.V. Infusion. *J. Pharm. Sci. 59*:53 (1970).

4. Ritschel, W. A.: Dose Size and Dosing Interval Determination, *Arzneim. Forsch. 25*:1442 (1975).

5. Ritschel, W. A.: Pharmacokinetics of Multiple Dosing, Dose Size and Dosing Interval, *Pharm. Ind. 38*:82 (1976).

6. Schumacher, G. E.: Practical Pharmacokinetic Techniques for Drug Consultation and Evaluation I: Use of Dosage Regimen Calculations, *Am. J. Hosp. Pharm. 29*:474 (1972).

7. Wagner, J. G.: *Biopharmaceutics and Relevant Pharmacokinetics,* Drug Intelligence Publications, Hamilton, Ill. 1971, pp. 22; 242; 270; and 292.

8. Wagner, J. G.: Significance of Ratios of Different Volumes of Distribution in Pharmacokinetics, *Biopharm. Drug Dispos. 4*:263 (1983).

23

Compartment Model Independent Analysis

The compartment model concept is imperative for understanding the principles of pharmacokinetics. However, in recent years the compartment model free or compartment model independent analysis has gained increasing attention and application. The reason may be found in the fact that the human body is in reality a multimillion-compartment model, but the most sophisticated kinetic multicompartment model may have only very few compartments, in which the microconstants are mathematical artifacts. Another reason is the realization that for clinical application of pharmacokinetics it is neither possible to obtain a large number of blood samples to properly characterize a multicompartmental concentration-time course, nor is it necessary, because dosage regimen design and dosage regimen adjustment require only a few parameters.

Compartment model independent analysis is based on the terminal rate constant, λ_z, the total area under the curve, AUC, and the dose administered, D. Primary parameters derived are the total clearance, CL, the elimination half-life, $t_{1/2}$, and the apparent volume of distribution, V_z. These parameters are called "robust" because they are determined via the AUC and are thus not very sensitive to small changes in concentration-time data.

The AUC ($_0\int^t$ Cdt) is the area under the statistical zero moment (concentration · time). If the concentration-time data are again multiplied by time (concentration · time · time) ($_0\int^t$ tCdt), the area under the first statistical moment is obtained, which in essence is the center of gravity of the area under the curve.

Note that the new ACCP nomenclature is used in the following discussion to underline the fact that this procedure is *model independent*. The terminal disposition rate constant will be called λ_z regardless of compartment model. The apparent volume is called V_z to point out that this is determined via the model independent area method.

Procedure for Model Independent Analysis
Terminal Rate Constant λ_z and Half-Life $t_{1/2}$

Plot concentration-time data on semilog paper. Identify the last concentration-time points which constitute the monoexponential, *terminal* slope. Use least square method (see

Chapter 34, Curve Fitting), or select any two concentration-time points $C(1)$, $t(1)$ and $C(2)$, $t(2)$ on the terminal straight line:

$$\lambda_z = \frac{\ln C(1) - \ln C(2)}{t(2) - t(1)} [h^{-1}] \tag{1}$$

$$t_{1/2} = \frac{0.693}{\lambda_z} [h] \tag{2}$$

Total Area Under the Curve AUC

The *total* AUC requires the entire area from zero to infinity. For EV administration, the first concentration-time data set will be 0,0. For IV administration it is advisable to collect the first blood sample soon after one blood circulation time which is 1.5 to 3 min. Such an early drug concentration-time point may be used as the zero-time concentration. If such an early blood sample is not available, one should back-extrapolate the curve to the ordinate to obtain an estimate on the fictitious $C(0)$.

The AUC is determined, as discussed in Chapter 20, in two steps via the linear trapezoidal rule from $t = 0$ to the last sampling time t_x.

$$AUC^{0 \to t_x} = \sum \left(\frac{C_n + C_{n+1}}{2} \right) \cdot (t_{n+1} - t_n) [(\mu g/ml)h] \tag{3}$$

and for the remaining area:

$$AUC^{t_x \to \infty} = \frac{C_x}{\lambda_z} [(\mu g/ml)h] \tag{4}$$

The total AUC is:

$$AUC = AUC^{0 \to t_x} + AUC^{t_x \to \infty} [(\mu g/ml)h] \tag{5}$$

Area Under the First Moment Curve AUMC

This is again done in two steps, namely for $t = 0$ to t_{last} or t_x:

$$AUMC^{0 \to t_x} = \sum \left(\frac{C_n + C_{n+1}}{2} \right) \cdot (t_{n+1} - t_n) \cdot \left(\frac{t_{n+1} + t_n}{2} \right) \tag{6}$$

and for the remaining area under the moment curve:

$$AUMC^{t_x \to \infty} = \frac{t_x \cdot C_x}{\lambda_z} + \frac{C_x}{\lambda_z^2} [(\mu g/ml)h^2] \tag{7}$$

The total AUMC is:

$$AUMC = AUMC^{0 \to t_x} + AUMC^{t_x \to \infty} [(\mu g/ml)h^2] \tag{8}$$

$$t_{1/2} = \ln 2 \cdot (AUMC^{0 \to \infty} / AUC^{0 \to \infty}) \tag{9}$$

Total Clearance CL

$$\text{For IV} \quad CL = D/AUC [ml/h] \tag{10}$$

$$\text{For EV} \quad CL/f = D/AUC [ml/h] \tag{11}$$

Apparent Volume of Distribution V_z

$$\text{For IV} \quad V_z = D/(AUC \cdot \lambda_z) [ml] \tag{12}$$

$$V_{d\,ss} = CL \cdot (AUMC^{0 \to \infty} / AUC^{0 \to \infty}) \tag{13}$$

$$\text{For EV} \quad V_z/f = D/(AUC \cdot \lambda_z) [ml] \tag{14}$$

$$V_{d\,ss}/f = CL \cdot (AUMC^{0 \to \infty} / AUC^{0 \to \infty}) \tag{15}$$

The V_z is usually normalized for body weight BW [g], giving the distribution coefficient Δ':

$$\text{For IV} \quad \Delta' = V_z/BW[ml/g] \text{ or } [1/kg] \tag{16}$$

$$\text{For EV} \quad \Delta'/f = V_z/BW[ml/g] \text{ or } [1/kg] \tag{17}$$

Mean Residence Time MRT and Variance of Residence Time VRT

The mean residence time is the time corresponding to the time (average time) the number of molecules absorbed reside in the body, or the time when 63.2 percent of an intravenous dose has been eliminated:

$$MRT = \frac{AUMC}{AUC}[h] \tag{18}$$

$$VRT = \frac{AUMC}{AUC} - MRT^2 \tag{19}$$

For the one-compartment model, one may calculate MRT and VRT simply as follows:
For IV:

$$\text{Push:} \quad MRT = \frac{1}{\lambda_z}[h] \tag{20}$$

$$VRT = \frac{1}{\lambda_z^2} \tag{21}$$

$$\text{Infusion: } MRT = \frac{t_i}{2} + \frac{1}{\lambda_z}[h] \tag{22}$$

$$VRT = \frac{t_i^2}{4} + \frac{1}{\lambda_z^2} \tag{23}$$

where t_i = duration of infusion

$$\text{For EV: } MRT = \frac{1}{k_a} + \frac{1}{\lambda_z}[h] \tag{24}$$

$$VRT = \frac{1}{k_a^2} + \frac{1}{\lambda_2^2} \tag{25}$$

Volume of Distribution at Steady State V_{ss}

For IV:

$$\text{Push: } V_{ss} = D \cdot \frac{AUMC}{AUC^2}[ml] \tag{26}$$

$$\text{Infusion: } V_{ss} = D \cdot \frac{AUMC}{AUC^2} - \frac{t_i \cdot D}{2 \cdot AUC}[ml] \tag{27}$$

For EV:

$$V_{ss} = D \cdot f \cdot \frac{AUMC}{AUC^2} - \frac{D \cdot f}{k_a \cdot AUC}[ml] \tag{28}$$

Rate of Absorption k_a

If one determines MRT according to Equation 23.18 then k_a can be obtained independent of compartment model from IV and EV data:

$$k_a = (MRT_{EV} - MRT_{IV})^{-1}[h^{-1}] \tag{29}$$

However, if one assumes a one-compartment model, where MRT for IV is $1/\lambda_z$ (see Equation 23.20), then k_a can be obtained as follows:

$$k_a = \left(MRT_{EV} - \frac{1}{\lambda_z}\right)^{-1}[h^{-1}] \tag{30}$$

Two other methods should be mentioned here to obtain an estimate of k_a:

C_{max}—Area Method

$$k_a = \frac{C_{max}}{AUC^{t_{max} \to \infty} - C_{max}/\lambda_z}[h^{-1}] \qquad (31)$$

Absorption Time Method

Under the assumption that at time zero upon EV administration 100 percent is unabsorbed, and that at the time when the actual blood level-time curve after the peak is just distinguishable before entering the distribution phase or the terminal phase only 1 percent is unabsorbed, k_a can be estimated from the absorption time t_a, assuming first-order kinetics. For graphically determining t_a see Figure 23-1.

$$k_a = \frac{4.61}{t_a}[h^{-1}] \qquad (32)$$

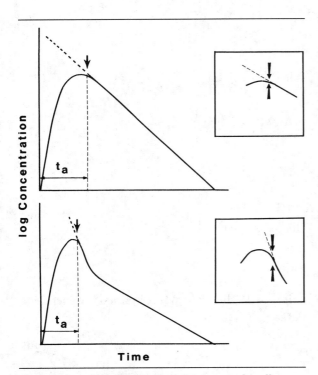

Figure 23-1. Schematic diagram to graphically determine time of absorption t_a. The insets demonstrate that one should find the time when the actual blood level curve is still distinguishable from the terminal phase (top) or the distribution phase (bottom).

Formulation Specific Applications

It is possible to conceptualize compartment model independent pharmacokinetics by examining it in the context of the LADMER "model." This is accomplished by relating the mean times for disintegration (MDisT), dissolution (MDT), absorption (MAT), and disposition (i.e., distribution, metabolism, and excretion) as reflected by the mean residence time (MRT) to the specific drug formulation administered. This approach is illustrated in Figure 23-2.

Steady State Concentration

The mean steady state concentration, C_{av}^{ss}, is the ratio of the AUC at steady state during any dosing interval, $AUC^{\tau_n \to \tau_{n+1}}$ and the dosing interval, τ.

In absence of dose dependency, $AUC^{\tau_n \to \tau_{n+1}}$ equals the total area under the curve of a single dose of same size, AUC_{SD}. Hence, C_{av}^{ss} can be predicted from AUC_{SD} and the proposed τ:

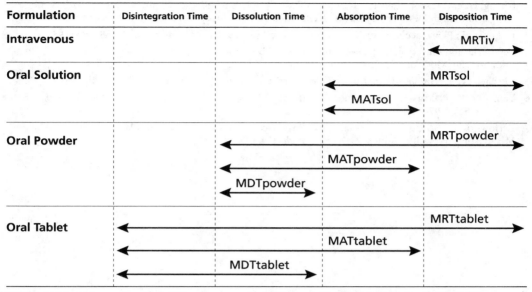

Figure 23-2. Schematic depiction of compartment model independent drug disposition. Abbreviations include: MRT, mean residence time; MAT, mean absorption time; and MDT, mean dissolution time, which, in the case of oral tablets, includes the mean disintegration time.

$$C_{av}^{ss} = \frac{AUC_{SD}}{\tau} \tag{33}$$

In case of different sizes for single (D_{SD}) and multiple dosing (D_{MD}), Equation 23.34 is used:

$$C_{av}^{ss} = \frac{AUC_{SD} \cdot (D_{MD}/D_{SD})}{\tau} \tag{34}$$

Mean Residence Time (MRT) for Michaelis-Menten or Nonlinear Drugs

$$MRT = \frac{V_z \cdot AUC}{D_{bolus}} \tag{35}$$

$$\text{or } MRT = \frac{V_z}{V_{max}} \cdot \left(\frac{D_{bolus}}{2\,V_z} + K_m \right) \tag{36}$$

where V_{max} is the maximum velocity of process, K_m is the Michaelis-Menten constant, and D_{bolus} is the instantly absorbed dose.

Selected References

1. Benet, L. Z. and Galeazzi, R. L.: Noncompartmental Determination of the Steady-State Volume of Distribution, *J. Pharm. Sci.* 68:1071 (1979).

2. Cheng, H. and Jusko, W.: Mean Residence Time Concepts for Pharmacokinetic Systems with Nonlinear Drug Elimination Described by the Michaelis-Menten Equation, *Pharmacol Res. 5*:156–164 (1988).

3. Jusko, W. J.: Pharmacokinetics of Capacity-Limited Systems, *J. Clin. Pharmacol. 29*:488–493 (1989).

4. Perrier, D. and Mayersohn, M.: Noncompartmental Determination of the Steady-State Volume of Distribution for Any Mode of Administration, *J. Pharm. Sci. 71*:372 (1982).

5. Ritschel, W. A.: *Graphic Approach to Clinical Pharmacokinetics*, J. R. Prous, Barcelona, 1983, pp. 24–25.

6. Yamaoka, K., Nakagawa, T. and Uno, T.: Statistical Moments in Pharmacokinetics, *J. Pharmacokinet. Biopharm. 6*:547 (1978).

7. Zerfowski, M., Schlegel, P. and Maier, H.: Pharmacokinetics of Cefotiam in Plasma, Parotid Saliva and Mixed Saliva in Healthy Adults, *Arzneim.-Forsch./Drug Res. 41*:257–259 (1991).

24

Pediatric Pharmacokinetics

The principles of biopharmaceutics and pharmacokinetics are based on a number of aspects of physiology. Accordingly, the process of development has been shown to impact upon each of the "phases" of drug disposition (e.g., absorption, distribution, metabolism, and excretion) and, in some instances, on drug effect (e.g., response) as well. A better understanding of the various physiological variables regulating and determining the fate of drugs in the body and their pharmacologic effects has, in many instances, dramatically improved both the safety and efficacy of drug therapy for neonates, infants, children, and adolescents. This understanding has largely resulted from data which have accumulated over the last 20 years and have resulted not only from guided clinical experience in pediatric drug therapy (e.g., application of therapeutic drug monitoring and clinical pharmacokinetics) but, most importantly, from carefully conducted pediatric clinical trials of both old and new drugs.

Development, *per se*, represents a continuum of biologic events that enable adaptation, somatic growth, neurobehavioral maturation, and eventually reproduction. The impact of development on the pharmacokinetics of a given drug is determined, to a great degree, upon age-related changes in body composition (e.g., body water spaces, circulating plasma protein concentrations) and the acquisition of function of organs and organ-systems which are important in determining drug metabolism (e.g., the liver) and excretion (e.g., the kidney). While it is often convenient to classify pediatric patients on the basis of postnatal age for the provision of drug therapy (e.g., neonate ≤ 1 month of age; infant = 1 to 24 months of age; children = 2 years to 12 years of age; and adolescents = 12 to 18 years of age), it is important to recognize that the changes in physiology which characterize development may not correspond to these age-defined "breakpoints" and also are not linearly related to age. In fact, the most dramatic changes in drug disposition occur during the first 18 months of life where the acquisition of organ function is most dynamic. Additionally, it is important to note that the pharmacokinetics of a given drug may be altered in pediatric patients consequent to intrinsic (e.g., gender, genotype, ethnicity, inherited diseases) and/or extrinsic (e.g., acquired disease states, xenobiotic exposure, diet) factors which may occur during the first two decades of life.

Selection of an appropriate drug dose for a neonate, infant, child, or adolescent not only requires an understanding of the basic pharmacokinetic and pharmacodynamic properties of a given compound but also how the process of development might impact upon each facet of drug disposition. Accordingly, it is most useful to conceptualize pediatric pharmacokinetics by examining the impact of development on those physiological variables which govern drug absorption, distribution, metabolism, and excretion.

Drug Absorption

The rate and extent of gastrointestinal (GI) absorption is primarily dependent upon pH dependent passive diffusion and motility of the stomach and small intestine, both of which control transit time. In term (i.e., fully mature) neonates, the gastric pH ranges from 6 to 8 at birth and drops to 2 to 3 within the first few hours. After the first 24 hours of extrauterine life, the gastric pH increases to approximately 6 to 7 consequent to immaturity of the parietal cells. A relative state of achlorhydria remains until adult values for gastric pH are reached at 20 to 30 months of age.

In the neonate, GI transit time is prolonged consequent to reduced motility and peristalsis. Gastric emptying is both irregular and erratic, and only partially dependent upon feeding. Gastric emptying rates approximate adult values by 6 to 8 months of age. During infancy, intestinal transit time is generally reduced relative to adult values consequent to increased intestinal motility. In the neonate and young infant, additional factors may play a role in intestinal drug absorption. These include relative immaturity of the intestinal mucosa leading to increased permeability, immature biliary function, high levels of β-glucuronidase activity, and variable microbial colonization.

The developmental changes in GI function/structure in the newborn period and early infancy produce alterations in drug absorption which are quite predictable. In general, the oral bioavailability of acid-labile compounds (e.g., beta-lactam antibiotics) is increased while that of weak organic acids (e.g., phenobarbital, phenytoin) is decreased. For orally administered drugs with limited water solubility (e.g., phenytoin, carbamazepine), the rate of absorption (i.e., t_{max}) can be dramatically altered consequent to changes in GI motility. In older infants with more rapid rates of intestinal drug transit, reductions in residence time for some drugs (e.g., phenytoin) and/or drug formulations (e.g., sustained-release theophylline) can reduce the extent of absorption (i.e., decreased bioavailability).

In the newborn and young infant, both rectal and percutaneous absorption is highly efficient for properly formulated drug products. The bioavailability of many drugs administered by the rectal route (e.g., diazepam, acetaminophen) is increased not only consequent to efficient translocation across the rectal mucosa but also reduced presystemic drug clearance produced by immaturity of many drug metabolizing enzymes in the liver. Both the rate and extent of percutaneous drug absorption is increased consequent to a thinner and more well hydrated stratum corneum in the young infant. As a consequence, systemic toxicity can be seen with percutaneous application of some drugs (e.g., diphenhydramine, lidocaine, corticosteroids, hexachlorophene) to seemingly small areas of the skin during the first 8 to 12 months of life.

In contrast to older infants and children, the rate of bioavailability for drugs administered by the intramuscular route may be altered (i.e., delayed t_{max}) in the neonate. This developmental pharmacokinetic alteration is the consequence of relatively low muscular blood flow in the first few days of life, the relative inefficiency of muscular contractions (useful in dispersing an IM drug dose), and an increased percentage of water per unit of muscle mass. Generally, intramuscular absorption of drugs in the neonate is slow and erratic with the rate dependent upon the physicochemical properties of the drug and on the maturational stage of the newborn infant.

Developmental differences in drug absorption between neonates, infants, and older children are summarized in Table 24-1. It must be recognized that the data contained therein reflect developmental differences which might be expected in healthy infants and children. Certain conditions/disease states which might modify the function and/or structure of the absorptive surface area(s), GI motility, and/or systemic blood flow can further impact upon either the rate or extent of absorption for extravascularly administered drugs in pediatric patients.

Plasma Protein Binding and Drug Distribution

During development, marked changes in body composition occur. Alterations in the total body water (TBW), extracellular water (ECW), and body fat "pools" are illustrated in Figure 24-1.

The most dynamic changes occur in the first year of life with the exception of total body fat which in males is reduced by approximately 50% between 10 and 20 years of life. In females, this reduction is not as dramatic, decreasing from approximately 28 to 25% during this same period. It is also important to note that adipose tissue of the neonate may contain as much as 57% water and 35% lipids, whereas values in the adult approach 26.3% and 71.7%, respec-

Table 24-1. Summary of Drug Absorption in Neonates, Infants, and Children

	NEONATE	INFANTS	CHILDREN
Physiological Alteration			
Gastric Emptying Time	Irregular	Increased	Slightly increased
Gastric pH	>5	4 to 2	Normal (2–3)
Intestinal Motility	Reduced	Increased	Slightly increased
Intestinal Surface Area	Reduced	Near adult	Adult pattern
Microbial Colonization	Reduced	Near adult	Adult pattern
Biliary Function	Immature	Near adult	Adult pattern
Muscular Blood Flow	Reduced	Increased	Adult pattern
Skin Permeability	Increased	Increased	Near adult pattern
Possible Pharmacokinetic Consequences			
Oral Absorption	Erratic—reduced	↑ rate	Near adult pattern
IM Absorption	Variable	Increased	Adult pattern
Percutaneous Absorption	Increased	Increased	Near adult pattern
Rectal Absorption	Very efficient	Efficient	Near adult pattern
Presystemic Clearance	< adult	> adult	> adult (↑ rate)

Direction of alteration given relative to expected normal adult pattern
Adapted from Morselli, P. L. (1983)

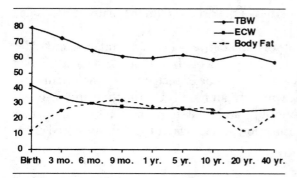

Figure 24-1. Developmental changes in body water and fat content. Abbreviations include: TBW, total body water; ECW, extracellular body water. Data represent mean values for males. Adapted from Friis-Hansen (1983)

tively. Finally, despite the fact that body fat content during the first three months of life is low relative to the other periods of development, the lipid content of the developing central nervous system is quite high, thus having potential adverse implications for the localization of lipophilic compounds (e.g., propranolol) administered early in life during critical periods of brain growth.

In addition to age-related alterations in body composition, the neonatal period is characterized by certain physiologic alterations which are capable of reducing the plasma protein binding of drugs (Table 24-2).

Table 24-2. Plasma Protein Binding and Drug Distribution

	NEONATE	INFANTS	CHILDREN
Physiological Alteration			
Plasma Albumin	Reduced	Near normal	Near adult pattern
Fetal Albumin	Present	Absent	Absent
Total Proteins	Reduced	Decreased	Near adult pattern
Total Globulins	Reduced	Decreased	Near adult pattern
Serum Bilirubin	Increased	Normal	Normal adult pattern
Serum Free Fatty Acids	Increased	Normal	Normal adult pattern
Blood pH	7.1–7.3	7.4 (normal)	7.4 (normal)
Adipose Tissue	Scarce ($\uparrow$ CNS)	Reduced	Generally reduced
Total Body Water	Increased	Increased	Near adult pattern
Extracellular Water	Increased	Increased	Near adult pattern
Endogenous Maternal Substances (Ligands)	Present	Absent	Absent
Possible Pharmacokinetic Consequences			
Free Fraction	Increased	Increased	Slightly increased
Apparent Volume of Distribution			
Hydrophilic drugs	Increased	Increased	Slightly increased
Hydrophobic drugs	Reduced	Reduced	Slightly decreased
Tissue/Plasma Ratio	Increased	Increased	Slightly increased

Direction of alteration given relative to expected normal adult pattern
Adapted from Morselli, P. L. (1983)

In the neonate, the free fraction of drugs which are extensively (i.e., >60%) bound to circulating plasma proteins is markedly increased, largely due to lower concentrations of drug binding proteins (i.e., a lower number of binding sites), reduced binding affinity (e.g., lower binding affinity for weak acids to fetal albumin, presence of acidic plasma pH and endogenous competing substrates such as bilirubin, free fatty acids). This is exemplified by phenytoin, a weak acid which is 94 to 98% bound to albumin in adults (i.e., free fraction = 2 to 4%) but only 80 to 85% bound in the neonate (i.e., free fraction = 15 to 20%). Consequent to developmental immaturity in the activity of hepatic microsomal enzymes which are responsible for phenytoin biotransformation, compensatory clearance of the increased free fraction does not occur, thereby producing an increased amount of free phenytoin in the plasma and CNS. This particular age-dependent alteration in drug binding functionally reduces the total plasma phenytoin level associated with both efficacy and toxicity in the newborn, as compared to older infants and children where phenytoin protein binding is normal.

Reduced plasma protein binding associated with absolute and relative differences in the sizes of various body compartments (e.g., total body water, extracellular fluid, composition of body tissues) frequently influences the apparent volume of distribution for many drugs and also influences their localization (i.e., both uptake and residence) in tissue. As illustrated by the examples contained in Table 24-3, the apparent volume of distribution of small molecular weight compounds which are not extensively bound to plasma proteins (e.g., ampicillin, cefotaxime, gentamicin) corresponds to age-related alterations in the total body water space and extracellular fluid pool (Figure 24-1). In contrast, the apparent volume of distribution for digoxin, a drug extensively bound to muscle tissue, does not decrease during the first years of life but rather increases to values (i.e., 10–15 L/kg for infants) which exceed those reported for adults (e.g., 5 to 7 L/kg), alterations that reflect both age-related changes in body composition and the affinity of digoxin for its binding sites.

Drug Metabolism

In general, most of the enzymatic activities responsible for metabolic degradation of drugs are reduced in the neonate. Certain phase I biotransformation reactions (e.g., hydroxyla-

Table 24-3. Examples of Age-Related Differences in Pharmacokinetics

DRUG	$V_{d\,ss}$ (L/kg)			ELIMINATION $t_{1/2}$ (hr)		
	PT	T	INFANT	PT	T	INFANT
Ampicillin	0.7	0.65	0.6	4–6	2–3	0.8–1.5
Cefotaxime	0.7	0.6	0.5	5–6	2–3	1.1–1.5
Vancomycin	0.9	0.7	0.6	6–10	4–6	2.5–3
Gentamicin	0.5	0.45	0.35	4–12	3–4	2–3
Chloramphenicol	1.2	0.8	0.5–0.7	20–24	10–12	1.5–3.5
Digoxin	5–7	8–10	10–15	60–170	34–45	18–25

Abbreviations include: PT, preterm neonate; T, term neonate; $V_{d\,ss}$, apparent steady state volume of distribution; and $t_{1/2}$, half-life

tions) appear to be more compromised than others (e.g., dealkylation reactions). This is reflected by prolonged clearance of compounds such as phenytoin, phenobarbital, diazepam, lidocaine, meperidine, and indomethacin, during the first two months of life. Phase II reactions are also unevenly reduced with sulfate and glycine conjugation activities present at near adult levels during the first month of life as opposed to glucuronidation (i.e., the activity of specific UDP glucuronosyltransferase isoforms) which is reduced as reflected by prolonged elimination of chloramphenicol (Table 24-3) in the neonate.

It must be recognized that developmental differences in hepatic drug metabolism occur consequent to reductions in the activity of specific drug metabolizing enzymes and their respective isoforms. For most enzymes, the greatest reduction of activity is seen in premature infants where immature function may also accompany continued organogenesis. As reflected by an examination of the ontogeny of important drug metabolizing enzymes as summarized in Table 24-4, it is apparent that maturation of activity is enzyme, and in some cases, isoform-specific. It is also important to note that for enzymes which are polymorphic in their expression (i.e., more than one phenotype for activity), development per se may produce a discordance between the phenotype and genotype. This is exemplified by N-acetyltransferase-2 (NAT2) where reduced enzyme activity results in over 80% of infants being classified as the poor-metabolizer phenotype during the first two months of age.

As denoted in Table 24-4, the activity of selected phase I and phase II enzymes in young infants can exceed that for adults. The potential pharmacologic implications of this particular developmental alteration in drug metabolism is exemplified by examining the impact of age on the predicted steady state plasma concentrations of theophylline (a predominant CYP1A2 and xanthine oxidase substrate) from a fixed dose of the drug (Figure 24-2). In the first two weeks of life, the activity of all of the cytochromes P450 and other enzymes (e.g., xanthine oxidase) responsible for theophylline biotransformation is virtually absent, leaving renal excretion of unchanged drug and trans-methylation of theophylline to caffeine as the predominant clearance pathways. By 3 to 6 months of postnatal age, CYP1A2 ontogeny results in activity of the enzyme which can exceed adult levels, thus increasing the plasma clearance of theophylline to maximum values as reflected in Figure 24-2.

While there is considerable evidence for dynamic, developmental regulation of drug-metabolizing enzymes reflected by pharmacokinetic data in pediatric patients, it is not generally known what is responsible for these changes in activity. In the case of some enzymes (e.g., CYP1A2, CYP3A4), age-associated changes in activity appear to temporally correspond to periods of rapid somatic growth and/or sexual maturation, thus implying a role for neuroendocrine regulation (e.g., growth hormone, sex hormones). As discussed elsewhere (see Chapters 13 and 39), pharmacogenetics may modulate the "pattern" of developmental differences in drug metabolism, especially for enzymes and transporters that are polymorphically expressed. Finally, certain disease states that present in childhood (e.g., cystic fibrosis, sickle cell anemia, Down syndrome) may alter the developmental profile for activity of drug-metabolizing enzymes by virtue of disease modulation of activity as compared to normal infants and children.

As expected, age-related differences in the activity of drug metabolizing enzymes can have dramatic clinical implications for dose and dose interval selection. An understanding of the basic clinical pharmacology of a given drug (often available from studies conducted in older children or adults), the ontogeny of drug metabolizing enzymes (Table 24-4) and of the other physiological alterations which occur during development that potentially

Table 24-4. Developmental Patterns for the Ontogeny of Important Drug Metabolizing Enzymes in Man

ENZYME(S)	KNOWN DEVELOPMENTAL PATTERN
Phase I Enzymes	
CYP2D6	Low to absent in fetal liver but present at 1 week of age. Poor activity (i.e., 20% of adult) by 1 month. Adult competence by 3 to 5 years of age.
CYP2C19, CYP2C9	Apparently absent in fetal liver. Low activity in first 2 to 4 weeks of life with adult activity reached by approximately 6 months. Activity may exceed adult levels during childhood and declines to adult levels after conclusion of puberty.
CYP1A2	Not present in appreciable levels in human fetal liver. Adult levels reached by approximately 4 months and exceeded in children at 1 to 2 years of age. Adult activity reached after puberty.
CYP3A7	Fetal form of CYP3A which is functionally active (and inducible) during gestation. Virtually disappears by 1 to 4 weeks postnatal when CYP3A4 activity predominates, but remains present in approximately 5% of individuals.
CYP3A4	Extremely low activity at birth reaching approximately 30 to 40% of adult activity by 1 month and full adult activity by 6 months. May exceed adult activity between 1 and 4 years of age, decreasing to adult levels after puberty.
Phase II Enzymes	
NAT2	Some fetal activity by 16 weeks gestation. Poor activity between birth and 2 months of age. Adult phenotype distribution reached by 4 to 6 months with adult activity reached by 1 to 3 years.
TPMT	Fetal levels approximately 30% of adult values. In newborns, activity is approximately 50% higher than adults with phenotype distribution which approximates adults. Exception is Korean children where adult activity is seen by 7 to 9 years of age.
UGT	Ontogeny is isoform specific. In general, adult activity is reached by 6 to 24 months of age.
ST	Ontogeny is isoform specific and appears more rapid than that for UGT. Activity for some isoforms may exceed adult levels during infancy and early childhood.

Abbreviations include: CYP, cytochrome P450; NAT2, N-acetyltransferase-2; TPMT, thiopurine methyltransferase; UGT, glucuronosyltransferase; and ST, sulfotransferase
Adapted from Leeder, J. S. and Kearns, G. L. (1997)

impact hepatic drug metabolism (Table 24-5) can enable prediction of the possible pharmacokinetic consequences as summarized in Table 24-5. Determination of the developmental "breakpoints" for the activity of drug metabolizing enzymes can also enable effective guidance of drug dosing and/or the study of new drugs by eliminating arbitrary age-based categories (e.g., infant, child, and adolescent) which may or may not have anything to do with the competence of a specific drug metabolizing enzyme.

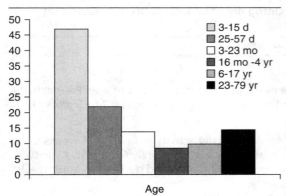

Figure 24-2. Impact of development on theophylline plasma concentrations. Predicted steady state mean serum theophylline concentrations from a dose of 20 mg/kg/day administered to patients of varying age. (Adapted from Aranda, 1983)

Renal Drug Excretion

At birth, the kidney is anatomically and functionally immature. This is illustrated by Figure 24-3, which summarizes the ontogeny of glomerular filtration in term and preterm infants. The acquisition of renal function depends, more than any other organ, on gestational age and postnatal adaptations. In the preterm infant, renal function is dramatically reduced, largely due to the continued development of functioning nephron units (i.e., nephrogenesis). In contrast, the acquisition of renal function in the term neonate represents, to a great degree, recruitment of fully developed nephron units. In both term neonates and preterm infants who have birth weights >1500 grams, glomerular filtration rates increase dramatically during the first two weeks of postnatal life (Figure 24-3). This particular dynamic change in function is a direct result of postnatal adaptations in the distribution of renal blood flow (i.e., medullary distribution to corticomedullary border), resulting in dramatic recruitment of functioning nephron units. In addition, there is a situation of glomerular/tubular imbalance due to a more advanced maturation of glomerular function. Such an imbalance may persist up to 6 months of age where both tubular and glomerular function approach normal values for adults.

Table 24-5. Drug Metabolism in the Neonate, Infant, and Child

	NEONATE	INFANTS	CHILDREN
Physiological Alteration			
Liver/Body Weight Ratio	Increased	Increased	Slightly increased
Cytochromes P450 Activity	Reduced	Increased	Slightly increased
Blood Esterase Activity	Reduced	Normal (by 12 mo)	Adult pattern
Hepatic Blood Flow	Reduced	Increased	Near adult pattern
Phase II Enzyme Activity	Reduced	Increased	Near adult pattern
Possible Pharmacokinetic Consequences			
Metabolic Rates	Reduced	Increased	Near adult pattern*
Presystemic Clearance	Reduced	Increased	Near adult pattern
Total Body Clearance	Reduced	Increased	Near adult pattern*
Inducibility of Enzymes	More evident	Slightly increased	Near adult pattern*

Direction of alteration given relative to expected normal adult patterns
*Denotes assumption of adult pattern of activity after the conclusion of puberty. The activity of all drug metabolizing enzymes is generally higher before vs. after puberty.
Adapted from Morselli, P. L. (1983)

The ontogeny of renal function and the potential pharmacokinetic consequences which occur during development are summarized in Table 24-6.

The fact that the ontogeny of renal function has been the most well characterized of any organ responsible for drug elimination makes it possible to accurately predict the potential impact of development on the elimination characteristics of drugs which are predominantly excreted by the kidney. This is well illustrated by a recent study of famotidine, an H_2 receptor antagonist which in older children and adults is approximately 80% excreted unchanged in the urine. A comparison of the pharmacokinetics of famotidine in neonates and older children is presented in Table 24-7. As illustrated by these data, the renal clearance of famotidine in children was approximately five-fold higher than that observed in neonates; populations where the average glomerular filtration rates would

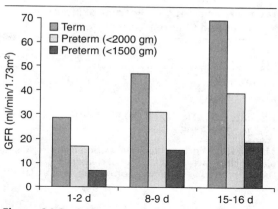

Figure 24-3. Ontogeny of glomerular filtration in the neonate.

Table 24-6. Renal Function in the Neonate, Infant, and Child

	NEONATE	INFANTS	CHILDREN
Physiological Alteration			
Kidney/Body Weight Ratio	Increased	Increased	Near adult values
Glomerular Filtration Rate	Reduced	Normal (by 12 mo)	Normal adult values
Active Tubular Secretion	Reduced	Near normal	Normal adult values*
Active Tubular Reabsorption	Reduced	Near normal	Normal adult values
Proteins Present in Urine	Present (30%)	Low to absent	Normally absent
Urinary Acidification Capacity	Low	Normal (by 1 mo)	Normal adult activity
Urine Output (ml/hr/kg)	3 to 6	2 to 4	1 to 3
Urine Concentrating Capacity	Reduced	Near normal	Normal adult values
Possible Pharmacokinetic Consequences			
Active Drug Excretion	Reduced	Near normal	Normal adult pattern
Passive Drug Excretion	Reduced to increased	Increased	Normal adult pattern
Excretion of Basic Drugs	Increased	Increased	Near normal

Direction of alteration given relative to expected normal adult patterns
*Denotes slight increase in excretion rate for basic compounds
Adapted from Morselli, P. L. (1983)

Table 24-7. Famotidine Pharmacokinetics in Neonates and Children

PATIENT GROUP	$t_{1/2}$ (hr)	Cl (L/hr/kg)	Cl_{renal} (L/hr/kg)
Children (n = 12, 1.1–12.9 yr)	3.2	0.70	0.45
Neonates (n = 10, 936–3495 g)	10.9	0.13	0.09

Abbreviations include: $t_{1/2}$, elimination half-life; Cl, total plasma clearance; and Cl_{renal}, renal clearance
Data expressed as mean values from James et al. (1998)

be expected to be approximately 100 and 20 ml/min/1.73 m^2, respectively. As well, correlations between post-natal age, renal function status (i.e., glomerular filtration rate and tubular secretory capacity), and drug clearance have been demonstrated for aminoglycoside antibiotics, vancomycin, beta-lactam antibiotics, and ranitidine, all of which are predominantly excreted via renal mechanisms.

Scaling of Clearance Based on Ontogeny

The pattern reflected by the ontogeny of a drug-metabolizing enzyme and/or physiologic indicator of renal function (e.g., glomerular filtration rate) now enables more refined approaches for scaling drug clearance as opposed to traditionally used allometric approaches based upon relative proportionality of body size and/or liver weight as compared to adults (Figure 24-4).

These newer approaches (described in detail by Alcorn and McNamara; see Reference 1) are based upon the determination of an "infant scaling factor" that is derived from information describing the metabolism of a given drug (e.g., V_{max}, K_m), physiologic data profiling the ontogeny of organ function (in the case of the kidneys), and, for drugs that are metabolized by one or more enzymes, the rate/pattern of acquisition of activity from birth through adulthood. Generally, these new approaches provide reasonable concordance between predicted and observed clearance values early in life (i.e., 0–3 months) when intersubject variability in the activity of a drug-metabolizing enzyme may be lower (as compared to older infants and children) consequent to ontogeny and also for drug-metabolizing enzymes with lower normal interindividual variability in activity and which are monomorphically expressed.

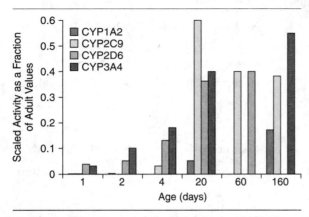

Figure 24-4. Ontogeny of Selected Cytochromes P450 Expressed as Activity Relative to Adult Values (adapted from Alcorn and McNamara 2002).

Pediatric Dose Selection

As illustrated by the aforementioned sections of this chapter, the physiological changes which occur consequent to the process of development are capable of altering the determinants of both dose size (i.e., apparent volume of distribution) and dose frequency (i.e., drug clearance). Ideally, pediatric dose selection for any drug should consider the potential impact of both normal and abnormal physiology (i.e., that induced by disease states) on the physiologic determinants of drug disposition at a given point in time. In a perfect clinical setting, this would be accomplished through individualization of the dose regimen based upon patient-derived pharmacokinetic parameters (e.g., half-life, apparent volume of distribution, total plasma clearance). The pediatric dose for a given drug could then be calculated to achieve either desired target plasma concentrations or alternatively, a drug "exposure" similar to adults as reflected by the dose-normalized AUC. While this may be possible for some drugs whose plasma concentrations are either routinely measured on a clinical basis (e.g., aminoglycoside antibiotics, anticonvulsants, chloramphenicol, cyclosporine, tacrolimus, methotrexate, theophylline, caffeine) or alternatively whose pharmacokinetic characteristics were defined in pediatric subjects during the drug development process, it is not possible for most drugs in many clinical environments. Accordingly, alternative methods must often be employed.

To date, over 20 different "approaches" for pediatric dose selection have been published over the last four decades. The majority of these utilize either body weight (BW) or body surface area (BSA) as an "index" which reflects the maturation/development of either body composition (e.g., body water spaces) or organ function required for drug clearance. Body weight based dosing approaches make the following basic assumptions: (1) that total body weight correlates with organ size and hence function and (2) that basal metabolism is proportional to the body weight potency $BW^{0.75}$, known as the Kleiber potency. A simple and infrequently used BW dosing approach is reflected by Clark's Rule, which is illustrated by Equation 24.1:

$$\text{Infant Dose} = (BW_{infant}/BW_{adult}) \cdot \text{Adult Dose} \tag{1}$$

This dosing method assumes that the infant dose represents a fraction of the adult dose determined solely upon developmental differences in body size and, presumably, organ function as reflected by age-dependent differences in body weight. In those instances where the weight normalized plasma clearance (e.g., L/hr/kg) of a drug in an infant may exceed that of an adult consequent to developmental increases in the activity of one or more drug metabolizing enzymes (see Tables 24-4 and 24-5), it is readily apparent that selection of a proper pediatric dose using Equation 24.1 (or any similar BW-based scaling approach) may not always be successful.

An alternate approach for pediatric dosing utilizes BSA, which can be readily determined for neonates or infants from established nomograms found in many pediatric textbooks or by using the following equations:

$$BSA_{neonate} = 0.0224265 \cdot BW^{0.5378} \cdot Ht^{0.3964} \tag{2}$$

$$BSA_{infant} = 0.007184 \cdot BW^{0.425} \cdot Ht^{0.725} \tag{3}$$

where BW is expressed in kilograms, Ht reflects height in cm, and BSA is body surface area per m^2. Dosing approaches based on BSA assume that body size (i.e., incorporating both height and weight) correlates with not only body composition but also organ size and function.

Generally speaking, pediatric dose selection based either upon BW or BSA will produce similar relationships between drug dose and resultant plasma concentration. There are subtle differences, however, which are illustrated by the following example contained in Table 24-8. Selection of a BSA- vs. BW-based dosing approach will result in drug concentrations

Table 24-8. Drug Concentrations in Body Fluids in Newborns and Adults

REFERENCE PARAMETER AND DOSE SIZE	PATIENT	DRUG CONCENTRATION RATIO IN:		
		ECF	ICF	TBW
Surface Area	Newborn	1	1	1
D = 100 mg/m²	Adult	1	0.35	0.5
Body Weight	Newborn	1	1	1
D = 100 mg/kg	Adult	2	0.8	1.1

Abbreviations include: D, dose; ECF, extracellular fluid; ICF, intracellular fluid; and TBW, total body water

which reach quite different percentages in extracellular, intracellular, and whole body fluid. Accordingly, for those drugs whose distribution space corresponds to the extracellular fluid pool (i.e., V_d < 0.3 L/kg), a BSA-based dosing approach (i.e., mg/m²) would appear to be preferable over the use of BW (i.e., mg/kg). This is especially true for infants and young children where the BSA correlates much better to both extracellular and intracellular fluid than does BW. In contrast, for those drugs where the apparent volume of distribution exceeds the extracellular fluid space (i.e., V_d > 0.3 L/kg), a BW-based approach to dose selection appears preferable and consequently is the most frequently used dosing approach used in pediatrics.

Finally, when the pediatric dose of a given drug is not established or known, the aforementioned principles can be used to best approximate a proper drug dose for the initiation of therapy. An approach to determine dose size in infants has been described by Ritschel and is illustrated by the following equations:

$$\text{Infant Dose (if } V_d < 0.3 \, \text{L/kg}) = (\text{BSA}/1.73) \cdot \text{Adult Dose} \tag{4}$$

$$\text{Infant Dose (if } V_d \geq 0.3 \, \text{L/kg}) = (\text{BW}/70) \cdot \text{Adult Dose} \tag{5}$$

where V_d is the apparent volume of distribution for a drug in normal adults, BSA reflects the body surface area of the infant in m², BW reflects the body weight of the infant, and Adult Dose is the usual adult dose of a drug in mg/m² (Eq. 24.4) or mg/kg (Eq. 24.5), as appropriate. *It must be emphasized that all of the aforementioned approaches (Equations 24.1 through 24.5) assume that the body height and weight of a given child are appropriate for age (i.e., the absence of obesity, malnourishment, or other conditions which could perturb the height:weight ratio).*

The dose frequency (i.e., dosing interval) for drugs with significant (i.e., >50%) excretion by glomerular filtration in neonates and young infants can be approximated by estimation of the apparent elimination half-life ($t_{1/2}$) of the drug at a given point in development. This can be accomplished through application of the following equations:

$$k_{\text{el infant}} = k_{\text{el adult}} \{[((\text{GFR}_{\text{infant}} - /\text{GFR}_{\text{adult}}) - 1) \cdot F_{\text{el}}] + 1\} \tag{6}$$

$$t_{1/2 \, \text{infant}} = 0.693/k_{\text{el infant}} \tag{7}$$

where k_{el} represents the average apparent terminal elimination rate constant, GFR is an estimate of the glomerular filtration rate (which can be obtained from a creatinine clearance determination or from average age-related normal values), and F_{el} is the fraction of drug excreted unchanged in the urine.

In conclusion, it is readily apparent that children are not miniature adults but rather human beings in a phase of somatic, neurologic, and metabolic development which is dynamic and can markedly influence the dose *versus* concentration *versus* effect relationship for a given drug. Failure to recognize developmental immaturity in organ function and resultant reductions in drug clearance can easily produce significant therapeutic misadventures if the pediatric dose (and dosing interval) is not selected based upon age-dependent alterations in pharmacokinetics. Alternatively, failure to recognize developmental periods which are associated with increased activity of specific drug metabolizing enzymes with resultant enhanced drug clearance can produce therapeutic failure if pediatric dose selection does not take into account these differences. Finally, the selection of an appropriate drug dose for an infant, child, or adolescent requires consideration of not only the developmental differences in drug disposition but also other concurrent factors/conditions (e.g., gender, disease, diet, environmental exposure, drug therapy) which may further influence either the pharmacokinetics or pharmacodynamics of a given drug.

Selected References

1. Alcorn, J. and McNamara, P. J.: Ontogeny of Hepatic and Renal Systemic Clearance Pathways in Infants: Part II. *Clin. Pharmacokinet.* 41:1077–1094 (2002).

2. Aranda, J. V.: Maturational Changes in Theophylline and Caffeine Metabolism and Disposition: Clinical Implications, In *Proceedings of the Second World Conference on Clinical Pharmacology and Therapeutics,* American Society for Pharmacology and Experimental Therapeutics, Bethesda, pp. 868–877, (1984).

3. Friis-Hansen, B.: Water Distribution in the Foetus and Newborn Infant, *Acta Paediatr. Scand.* 305:7–11 (1983).

4. Haycock, M. B., Schwartz, G. J. and Wistosky, D. H.: Geometric Method for Measuring Body Surface Area: A Height-Weight Formula Validated in Infants, Children and Adults, *J. Pediatr.* 93:62–68 (1978).

5. Hines, R. N. and McCarver, D. G.: The Ontogeny of Human Drug-Metabolizing Enzymes: Phase I Oxidative Enzymes. *J. Pharmacol. Exp. Ther.* 300:355–360 (2002).

6. James, L. P., Marotti, T., Stowe, C., Farrar, H. C., Taylor, B. J. and Kearns, G. L.: Pharmacokinetics and Pharmacodynamics of Famotidine in Infants, *J. Clin. Pharmacol.* 38:1089–1095 (1998).

7. Johnson, T. N., Tanner, M. S., Taylor, C. J. and Tucker, G. T.: Enterocytic CYP3A4 in a Paediatric Population: Developmental Changes and the Effect of Coeliac Disease and Cystic Fibrosis. *Br. J. Clin. Pharmacol.* 51:451–460 (2001).

8. Kauffman, R. E. and Kearns, G. L.: Pharmacokinetic Studies in Pediatric Patients: Clinical and Ethical Considerations, *Clin. Pharmacokinet.* 1:10–29 (1992).

9. Kearns, G. L., Abdel-Rahman, S. M., Alander, S. W., Blowey, D. L., Leeder, J. S. and Kauffman, R. E.: Developmental Pharmacology: The Impact of Ontogeny on Drug Disposition, Action and Therapy, *N. Engl. J. Med.,* in press, August (2003).

10. Kearns, G. L. and Reed, M. D.: Clinical Pharmacokinetics in Infants and Children: A Reappraisal, *Clin. Pharmacokinet.* 17(Suppl. 1):29–67 (1989).

11. Kearns, G. L.: Pharmacogenetics and Development: Are Infants and Children at Increased Risk for Adverse Outcomes?, *Curr. Opin. Pediatr.* 7:220–233 (1995).

12. Leeder, J. S.: Developmental and Pediatric Pharmacogenomics. *Pharmacogenomics* 4:331–341 (2003).

13. Leeder, J. S. and Kearns, G. L.: Pharmacogenetics in Pediatrics: Implications for Practice, *Pediatr. Clin. North Am.* 44:55–77 (1997).

14. McCarver, D. G. and Hines, R. N.: The Ontogeny of Human Drug-Metabolizing Enzymes: Phase II Conjugation Enzymes and Regulatory Mechanisms. *J. Pharmacol. Exp. Ther.* 300:361–366 (2002).

15. Morselli, P. L.: Development of Physiological Variables Important for Drug Kinetics, In *Antiepileptic Drug Therapy in Pediatrics,* P. L. Morselli, C. E. Pippenger and J. K. Penry (editors), Raven Press, New York, NY, pp. 1–12, (1983).

16. Morselli, P. L.: Clinical Pharmacology of the Perinatal Period and Early Infancy, *Clin. Pharmacokinet.* *17*(Suppl. 1): 13–28 (1989).

17. Radde, I. C. and MacLeod, S. M. (editors). Pediatric Pharmacology and Therapeutics, second edition, Mosby, St. Louis, (1993).

18. Taketomo, C. K., Hodding, J. H. and Kraus, D. M. (editors): Pediatric Dosage Handbook, Fourth Edition, American Pharmaceutical Association, Washington, D.C. (1997).

19. Wilson, J. T., Kearns, G. L., Murphy, D. and Yaffe, S. J.: Paediatric Labelling Requirements: Implications for Pharmacokinetic Studies, *Clin. Pharmacokinet. 26*:308–325 (1994).

20. Yaffe, S. J. and Aranda, J. V. (editors): Pediatric Pharmacology: Therapeutic Principles in Practice, Second Edition, W. B. Saunders Co., Philadelphia, PA, (1992).

25

Drug Dosage in Elderly Patients

With increasing age, physiologic and pathologic changes occur which may greatly influence drug concentration and availability of receptors. The change of drug concentration in the organism upon administration of a drug can be explained pharmacokinetically by the LADMER System.

Absorption

A decrease in gastric secretion, i.e., volume of gastric fluid and strength of hydrochloric acid, can change the rate of dissolution of a tablet or capsule and the drug and the degree of ionization. Thus, the rate of absorption can be decreased. Due to changes in the gastrointestinal mucosa, active transport may be delayed. In addition, changes in the gastric emptying rate and intestinal motility and decreased mesenteric blood flow can alter the rate of absorption. Usually we find a slower absorption rate in the aged, whereas the extent of absorption seems not to be reduced.

Distribution

The total systemic perfusion or flow rates decrease with age and, although there is no significant change in blood or plasma volume per unit of body weight with age, cardiac output decreases with age.

The total body fluid (TBF) decreases significantly with age. The extracellular fluid (ECF) remains unchanged but constitutes a larger portion of the TBF in the aged. Since the intracellular water concentration does not change with age, it is interpreted that the reduction in TBF reflects loss of viable tissue with increasing age, and, hence, the intracellular fluid (ICF) is also reduced. The reduction in TBF in males is 0.37 percent and in females 0.27 percent per year. This is verified by the fact that the cell mass (CM) decreases at approximately parallel slopes.

Since the drug receptors are usually found in the cell and since the cell mass and the total body fluid decrease at an apparently constant rate, it might be reasonable to assume that the volume of distribution decreases proportionally with increasing age. Furthermore, there is a small but significant reduction in albumin. Hence, when drugs are being largely bound to protein, the result is increased concentration of the free unbound drug with increasing age. Both decreased volume of distribution and decreased amount of albumin would therefore result in a higher drug concentration in the aged than in the young adult. Even if the body weight remains constant, the body composition changes, resulting in less lean body mass and more fat tissue with increasing age.

Metabolism

Although there are definite structural changes of the liver and its size decreases with increasing age, there seems to be no significant change in the liver function. However, rates of metabolism for some drugs are changed with advancing age.

Elimination

The glomerular filtration rate (GFR) and the transport maximum (T_m) for active secretion decrease at a rate of 0.66 percent and 0.62 percent per year after age 25, respectively. The larger the fraction of drug eliminated via the kidney (F_{el}), the slower the drug will be eliminated from the body with increasing age.

Often drugs are not only given occasionally, such as aspirin against acute headache, but may be administered for days, weeks, months, or years. Whenever the dosing interval is shorter than the time required to eliminate the drug, accumulation of the drug in the body occurs until steady state is reached. A decreased volume of distribution and decreased rate of elimination will, therefore, result in higher accumulation and higher steady state blood levels which in turn might be responsible for higher incidence of side effects and increased toxicity in the aged. Reduction in viable tissue with decreased numbers of receptors available could aggravate the situation. The reduced rate of absorption will not be enough to compensate for these changes.

Table 25-1 summarizes the pharmacokinetic and therapeutic consequences of physiologic and pathologic changes with increasing age. It should be emphasized that these changes and their consequences are valid for the "healthy" geriatric patient in the absence of severe liver, kidney, or heart failure. However, the implications become even more pronounced if one or more of these diseases are present.

Factors possibly affecting drug liberation and absorption in the aged patient are summarized in Tables 25-2 and 25-3.

Drugs for which changes in pharmacokinetic parameters have been found with increasing age are listed in Table 25-4.

Dosage Regimen

Dose sizes for "normal" geriatric patients, i.e., those who do not suffer from acute congestive heart failure or renal or hepatic impairment, can be calculated according to the C_{av}^{ss}-method (for drugs following the log-dose response curve) or the C_{min}^{ss}-method (for drugs when it is essential to maintain a minimum effective concentration throughout the dosing interval).

Table 25-1. Physiologic and Pathologic Changes and Their Pharmacokinetic and Therapeutic Consequences in the Geriatric Patient

PARAMETER	PHYSIOLOGIC OR PATHOLOGIC CHANGE	ORGAN CONSEQUENCES	PHARMACOKINETIC CONSEQUENCES	THERAPEUTIC CONSEQUENCES
Body weight	generally reduced, including vital organs	loss of fluid, reduction in heart, kidney and muscle tissue, atrophic tissue	normal adult dose results in higher blood levels, higher drug concentration-receptor ratio	overdosing, increased side effects and toxic effects
GI-secretion, GI-tract	reduced secretion reduced GI-motility	higher gastric pH, longer stomach emptying rate, less mixing of GI-contents	altered dissolution rate of tablets and capsules, delayed transition to small intestine; prolonged absorption rate	longer time for onset of effect, lower intensity of effect, prolonged duration of effect
Body fluid	TBF and ICF reduced	hypokalemia and hypernatremia	reduced volume of distribution, increased blood levels	overdosing, increased side effects and toxic effects, dehydration
Heart and blood flow	reduced cardiac output, reduced vascular elasticity and permeability, reduced blood flow	possible venous congestion and arterial hypovolemia	slower absorption rate from GI-tract, muscle, skin, rectum, delayed distribution; reduced volume of distribution, increased blood levels	longer time for onset, overdosing, increased side effects and toxic effects, hypoxia

(continued)

Table 25-1. Physiologic and Pathologic Changes and Their Pharmacokinetic and Therapeutic Consequences in the Geriatric Patient (*Continued*)

PARAMETER	PHYSIOLOGIC OR PATHOLOGIC CHANGE	ORGAN CONSEQUENCES	PHARMACOKINETIC CONSEQUENCES	THERAPEUTIC CONSEQUENCES
Body composition	reduced lean body mass, increased fat tissue	organ function changed	decrease in volume of distribution in general storage of drugs with high lipid solubility in fat depots, and slower elimination	overdosing, increased side effects; reduced response for drugs of high lipid solubility, hangover phenomenon, delayed onset followed by accumulation and overdosing in multiple dosing
Kidney	reduced renal blood flow, reduced glomerular filtration and active secretion	lower creatinine clearance, reduced renal function	increase in elimination half-life of drugs eliminated via kidney	overdosing, longer duration of effect, increased side effects and toxic effects
Plasma proteins	reduction in albumin	hypoalbuminemia	saturation of protein binding and increased concentration of free drug, shorter half-life if highly bound	increased intensity of effect, increased side effects and toxic effects, overdosing
Homeostasis	abnormal lability	restricted range of regulatory functions	possible change in volume of distribution	paradoxic drug reactions

Table 25-2. Factors Possibly Affecting Drug Liberation in the Aged

ROUTE OF ADMINISTRATION	FACTORS ALTERED	POSSIBLE CONSEQUENCES
PO	Gastric secretion ↓	Delayed dissolution
	Gastric pH ↑	Change in degree of ionization
	Gastric motility ↓	Delayed dissolution
IM	Tissue perfusion rate ↓	Delayed dissolution of solid particles
Topical	Skin hydration ↓	Delayed release

↓ = decrease; ↑ = increase

These methods are applicable for drugs of low lipid solubility (digoxin, antibiotics, sulfonamides, etc.) and if F_{el} is > 0.5.

The maintenance dose sizes for males and females for the two methods are given in Equations 25.1 through 25.4. The corresponding loading doses are the same for both patterns and are given in Equations 25.5 and 25.6 on page 249.

Geriatric dose sizes of drugs following the MIC pattern are as follows.

Dose Size for Males (maintenance dose):

$$DM_{Ger.M.} = \frac{\left\{ \Delta' \cdot \left[\dfrac{54.25 - 0.199 \cdot (Age-25)}{54.25} \right] \cdot BW \right\} \cdot MIC \cdot \left(1 - e^{-k_{el} \cdot \left(\left\{ \left[\frac{120.7 - 0.988 \cdot (Age-25)}{120.7} - 1 \right] \cdot F_{el} \right\} + 1 \right) \cdot \tau} \right)}{\left(-e^{-k_{el} \cdot \left(\left\{ \left[\frac{120.7 - 0.988 \cdot (Age-25)}{120.7} - 1 \right] \cdot F_{el} \right\} + 1 \right) \cdot \tau} \right) \cdot f \cdot 1000} \tag{1}$$

Table 25-3. Factors Possibly Affecting Absorption in the Aged

SITE OF ABSORPTION	FACTORS ALTERED	POSSIBLE CONSEQUENCES
PO	Gastric emptying time ↑	Delayed transfer to small intestine
	Peristalsis ↓	Reduced mixing of intestinal content
	Mesenteric blood flow rate ↓	Decreased concentration gradient
	Macro- and microvilli of mucosa ↓ (atrophy)	Reduced absorbing surface area
	Mucosal connective tissue ↑	Change in epithelial transfer
	Submucosal amyloid content ↑	Change in epithelial transfer
IM	Connective tissue in muscle ↑	Change in permeability
	Blood flow rate ↓	Decreased concentration gradient
Topical	Skin hydration ↓	Reduced permeability
	Keratinization ↑	Reduced permeability
	Blood flow rate ↓	Decreased concentration gradient

↑ = increase; ↓ = decrease

Table 25-4. Survey of Drugs with Altered Pharmacokinetic Parameters in the Aged

DRUG	ELIMINATION HALF-LIFE	VOLUME OF DISTRIBUTION	TOTAL CLEARANCE
Acetaminophen	↑	U	↓
Acetanilid	↑	↓	U
Aminopyrine	↑	NI	NI
Amitriptyline	↑	NI	↓
Amobarbital	↑	U	↓
Ampicillin	↑	↓?	↓
Antipyrine	↑	↓	↓
Aspirin	↑	↑	↓
Atenolol	U	U	U
Carbenicillin	↑	↑	NI
Carbenoxolone	↑	↓	↓
Cefamandole	↑	↑	U
Cefazolin	↑	U	↓
Cefoxitin	↑	↑	↑
Cephradine	↑	U	↓
Clomethiazole	↑	↑	↓
Chlordiazepoxide	↑	↑	↓
Chlorthalidone	↑	U	↓
Cimetidine	↑	↓	↓
Clobazam	↑	↑	U
Cyclophosphamide	↑	↑	NI
Desipramine	↑	NI	NI
Desmethyldiazepam	↑	↑	↓
Diazepam	↑	↑	U or ↓
Digitoxin	U	U	U
Digoxin	↑	↓	↓
Dihydrostreptomycin	↑	NI	NI
Doxycycline	↑	U	↓
Gentamicin	↑	↓	↓
Heparin	U	U	U
Imipramine	↑	NI	U
Indomethacin	↑	NI	NI

(*continued*)

Table 25-4. Survey of Drugs with Altered Pharmacokinetic Parameters in the Aged (*Continued*)

DRUG	ELIMINATION HALF-LIFE	VOLUME OF DISTRIBUTION	TOTAL CLEARANCE
Kanamycin	↑	NI	NI
Levopromazine	↑	U	↓
Lidocaine	↑	↑	U
Lithium	NI	NI	↓
Lorazepam	U or ↑	NI	U or ↓
Methotrexate	↑	↓	↓
Metoprolol	↑	U	U
Morphine	↑	↑	U
Netilmicin	↑	U	↓
Nitrazepam	↑	↑	U
Nortriptyline	↑	U	↓
Oxazepam	U	U	U
Pancuronium	↑	U	↓
Penicillin G	↑	NI	NI
Penicillin G Procaine	↑	NI	NI
Phenobarbital	↑	NI	NI
Phenylbutazone	↑	U	↓
Phenytoin	NI	NI	↑
Practolol	↑	↓	NI
Prazosin	U	↑	U
Propicillin	↑	↓	NI
Propranolol	↑	↓	↓
Propylthiouracil	NI	U	U
Protriptyline	↑	↓	↓
Quinidine	↑	↓	↓
Quinine	U	↓	↓
Spironolactone	↑	NI	NI
Sulbenicillin	↑	↑	NI
Sulfamethizole	↑	U or ↓	↓
Sulfisomidine	↑	↑	↓
Tetracycline	↑	NI	NI
Theophylline	↑	U or ↓	↓

(*continued*)

Table 25-4. Survey of Drugs with Altered Pharmacokinetic Parameters in the Aged (*Continued*)

DRUG	ELIMINATION HALF-LIFE	VOLUME OF DISTRIBUTION	TOTAL CLEARANCE
Thiopental	↑	↑	↑
Thioridazine	↑	NI	NI
Tobramycin	↑	↓	↓
Tolbutamide	↑	↓	↓
Warfarin	↑ or U	U	↓ or U

↑ = increase; ↓ = decrease; U = unchanged; NI = no information

Dose Size for Females (maintenance dose):

$$DM_{Ger.F.} = \frac{\left\{ \Delta' \cdot \left[\dfrac{49.25 - 0.130 \cdot (Age - 25)}{49.25} \right] \cdot BW \right\} \cdot MIC \cdot \left(1 - e^{-k_{el} \cdot \left(\left\{ \left[\frac{105.9 - 0.988 \cdot (Age-25)}{105.9} - 1 \right] \cdot F_{el} \right\} + 1 \right) \cdot \tau} \right)}{\left(-e^{-k_{el} \cdot \left(\left\{ \left[\frac{105.9 - 0.988 \cdot (Age-25)}{105.9} - 1 \right] \cdot F_{el} \right\} + 1 \right) \cdot \tau} \right) \cdot f \cdot 1000} \quad (2)$$

Geriatric dose sizes of drugs following the log dose-response patterns are as follows. Dose Size for Males (maintenance dose):

$$DM_{Ger.M.} = \frac{C_{av}^{ss} \cdot \left\{ \Delta' \cdot \left[\dfrac{54.25 - 0.199 \cdot (Age-25)}{54.25} \right] \cdot BW \right\} \cdot \tau}{1.44 \cdot \left\{ \dfrac{t_{1/2}}{F_{el} \cdot \left[\dfrac{120.7 - 0.988 \cdot (Age-25)}{120.7} - 1 \right] + 1} \right\} \cdot f \cdot 1000} \; [mg] \quad (3)$$

Dose Size for Females (maintenance dose):

$$DM_{Ger.F.} = \frac{C_{av}^{ss} \cdot \left\{ \Delta' \cdot \left[\dfrac{49.25 - 0.130 \cdot (Age-25)}{49.25} \right] \cdot BW \right\} \cdot \tau}{1.44 \cdot \left\{ \dfrac{t_{1/2}}{F_{el} \cdot \left[\dfrac{105.9 - 0.988 \cdot (Age-25)}{105.9} - 1 \right] + 1} \right\} \cdot f \cdot 1000} \; [mg] \quad (4)$$

Corresponding geriatric loading doses are:

$$DL_{Ger.M.} = \frac{DM_{Ger.M.}}{1 - e^{-k_{el} \cdot \left(\left\{ \left[\frac{120.7 - 0.988 \cdot (Age-25)}{120.7} - 1 \right] \cdot F_{el} \right\} + 1 \right) \cdot \tau}} [mg] \qquad (5)$$

$$DL_{Ger.F.} = \frac{DM_{Ger.F.}}{1 - e^{-k_{el} \cdot \left(\left\{ \left[\frac{105.9 - 0.988 \cdot (Age-25)}{105.9} - 1 \right] \cdot F_{el} \right\} + 1 \right) \cdot \tau}} [mg] \qquad (6)$$

Selected References

1. Ritschel, W. A.: Pharmacokinetic Approach to Drug Dosing in the Aged, *J. Am. Geriat. Soc. 24*:344 (1976).

2. Ritschel, W. A.: Drug Action and Interaction in the Geriatric Patient, *Sci. Pharm. 45*:304 (1977).

3. Ritschel, W. A.: The Effect of Aging on Pharmacokinetics: A Scientist's View of the Future, *Contemp. Pharm. Pract. 5*:209 (1982).

4. Ritschel, W. A. and Eldon, M. A.: Prediction of Biological Half-Life and Volume of Distribution in Geriatric Patients: Limitations of a Recently Developed Pharmacokinetic Dosing Method, *Sci. Pharm. 47*:142 (1979).

5. Ritschel, W. A.: Disposition of Drugs in Geriatric Patients, *Pharm. Internat. 1*:226 (1980).

6. Ritschel, W. A.: Pharmacokinetics in the Aged. In *Pharmacologic Aspects of Aging*, Pagliaro, L. A. and Pagliaro, A. M., editors, The C. V. Mosby Co., St. Louis, 1983, p. 219.

7. Ritschel, W. A. In: *Gerontokinetics*. The Telford Press, Caldwell, NJ, 1988, pp. 23–48.

8. Ritschel, W. A.: Drug Disposition in the Elderly: Gerontokinetics, *Meth. Find. Exp. Clin. Pharmacol. 14*:555–572 (1992).

9. Ritschel, W. A.: Identification of Populations at Risk in Drug Testing and Therapy: Application to Elderly Patients, *Eur. J. Drug Metab. Pharmacokinet. 18*:101–111 (1993).

10. Ritschel, W. A.: Drug Disposition and Bioavailability in Elderly Patients, *Proceedings of Pharmaceutical Product Development Symposium*, Gifu, Japan, 13–14 September 1993, pp. 65–73.

11. Vestal, R. E.: Clinical Pharmacology, In *Principles of Geriatric Medicine*, Andres, R., Bierman, E. L. and Hazzard, W. R., editors, McGraw-Hill, New York, 1985, p. 424.

26

Drug Dosage in Obese Patients

The "normal" body weight (BW) is usually up to 10 percent above the "ideal" body weight (IBW). A BW of 10 to 20 percent above the IBW is considered as overweight, and 20 percent above IBW is considered as obesity. Twenty to 45 percent of the population of industrialized, western countries is suffering from obesity.

Obesity represents a therapeutic challenge in that both excess body weight and the concomitant medical conditions often associated with this problem (e.g., hypertension, diabetes, congestive heart failure, fatty infiltration of the liver) can profoundly impact upon the pharmacokinetics and/or pharmacodynamics of a given drug. Examples of factors affecting drug disposition in obesity are given in Table 26-1.

Drug dosing in obese patients may cause problems which are often due to the large deviation of body composition from that of the normal adult and the lipid solubility or the distribution of the drug between fat tissue and body water. For drugs of low lipid solubility (digoxin, gentamicin, kanamycin, streptomycin, etc.), it is recommended to base the dose size for obese patients on the lean body mass. For drugs of high lipid solubility (thiopental), the dose size should be based on the actual body weight.

The problem arises then with those drugs of intermediate lipid solubility for which the dose size should be somewhere between the two extremes. For practical reasons, a test dose may be given and dosage regimen adjustment made according to monitored drug concentrations in the patient.

Lean body weight (LBW), lean body mass (LBM), or ideal body weight (IBW) can be estimated as follows or taken from height/weight tables.

IBW for males:

$$\text{If } H > 152.5 \text{ cm} = 50 + [(H - 152.4) \cdot 0.89] \tag{1}$$

$$\text{If } H < 152.5 \text{ cm} = 50 - [(152.4 - H) \cdot 0.89] \tag{2}$$

IBW for females:

$$\text{If } H > 152.4 \text{ cm} = 45.4 + [(H - 152.4) \cdot 0.89] \tag{3}$$

Table 26-1. Factors Influencing Drug Disposition in Obesity

VARIABLE	PHYSIOLOGIC ALTERATION	PHARMACOKINETIC CONSEQUENCES
Absorption	No major alterations	

Distribution	Altered body composition
	   increased lean body mass
	   increased adipose tissue
	   increased organ size
	   increased blood volume
	   increased cardiac output
		Lipid-soluble drugs tend to have higher volume of distribution

	Protein binding alterations
	   increased AAG
	   increased plasma lipids
	   increased free fatty acids
		Decreased free fraction of basic drugs
		Potential displacement of highly bound acidic drugs

Metabolism	Altered hepatic function
	   increased splanchnic flow
	   increased number of hepatocytes
	   increased parencymal cell
	     degeneration
	   increased fatty infiltration
	   increased cholestasis
	   increased periportal fibrosis and
	     infiltration
		Generally reduced clearance of drugs with high hepatic extraction ratios
		
		Specific phase I enzymes may demonstrate reduced activity
		
		Glucuronidation and sulfation may be increased

Excretion	Altered renal function/structure
	   increased kidney size
	   increased glomerular filtration
	   increased tubular secretion
		General increase in the renal clearance of both filtered and actively secreted drugs

Abbreviations: AAG, alpha-1-acid glycoprotein
Adapted from Blouin, R. A., et al. (1987)

$$\text{If } H < 152.4 \text{ cm} = 45.4 - [(152.4 - H) \cdot 0.89] \tag{4}$$

where H is height in cm and IBW is in kg.

For an individual patient the IBW can also be calculated from skinfold measurements and corrected for age-dependent changes in muscle mass and bone mineral:

$$D_B = 1.02415 - 0.00169 \cdot SFB + 0.00444 \cdot H - 0.00130 \cdot SFA \, [g/ml] \tag{5}$$

D_B = body density [g/ml]
SFB = skinfold thickness on back (subscapular) [mm]
SFA = skinfold thickness of abdomen [mm]
H = height in decimeters [1 dm = 10 cm]

$$\% \, Fat = \left(\frac{4.57}{D_B} - 4.142 \right) \cdot 100 \tag{6}$$

Finally, the lean or ideal body weight is calculated following:

$$IBW = BW_{actual} - \left(\frac{BW_{actual} \cdot \% \, Fat}{100}\right) [kg] \qquad (7)$$

Percent overweight is:

$$\% \, Overweight = \frac{BW_{actual} - IBW}{IBW} \cdot 100 \qquad (8)$$

Recently, some equations were suggested to predict the apparent volume of distribution of drugs based on physicochemical properties of drugs as listed in Table 26-2.

Some drugs with altered pharmacokinetic parameters in obesity are given in Table 26-3.

Examples of drugs whose V_d in obesity can be predicted include: aminoglycosides (Equation 26.9); acetaminophen (Equation 26.10); antipyrine, digoxin, fentanyl, procainamide, theophylline (Equation 26.11); benzodiazepines (Equation 26.12).

To estimate age-dependent creatinine clearance, $Cl_{creat.}$, in obese subjects, the lean or ideal body weight, IBW, is used in the Cockcroft-Gault equation:

$$Cl_{creat. \, obese} = \frac{(140 - Age) \cdot IBW \cdot S}{72 \cdot S_{creat.}} \qquad (9)$$

where Age is in years, IBW is in kg, S = 1 for males and 0.9 for females, and $S_{creat.}$ is the serum creatinine in mg/100 ml.

To normalize $Cl_{creat. \, obese}$ to 1.73 m², one needs to calculate the patient's body surface area (see Equation 32.1), SA. In obese subjects, the IBW should be used instead of the total BW.

In obese elderly subjects, the maintenance dose (DM) of a drug can be calculated based upon knowledge of the glomerular filtration rate (GFR), the fraction of the drug eliminated unchanged in the urine (F_{el}), the normal elimination rate constant which correlates with GFR (β), the APC, the extent of protein binding (EPB), the pK_a, and the fraction of drug absorbed (F). This technique is illustrated in the following equations.

Step 1: If $F_{el} > 0.5$, determine β for geriatric patient as follows:

$$\beta_{ger} = \beta_{norm} \cdot \left\{\left[\left(\frac{GFRs_{normal} - 0.988 \cdot (Age - 25)}{GFRs_{normal}} - 1\right)F_{el}\right] + 1\right\} \qquad (10)$$

GFRs for males = 120 ml/min/1.73 m²
for females = 105 ml/min/1.73 m²

Step 2: Look up APC, EPB, and pK_a, and make a decision of the type of $V_{d \, obese}$ equation listed in Table 26-2.

Step 3: Estimate total plasma clearance for obese geriatric subject as follows:

$$Cl_{tot \, obese \, ger} = V_{d \, obese} \cdot \beta_{ger} \qquad (11)$$

Table 26-2. Physicochemical Properties of Drugs and Equations of Choice for Predicting Apparent Volume of Distribution in Obesity

	PHYSICOCHEMICAL PROPERTIES			
APC	Low <0.2	Medium <5.0	Medium <5.0	High >5.0
EPB	Low <10	Medium <70	Medium <70	High >70
Ionization	$pH-pK_a>1$ or <1	$pK_a-pH>1$	$pH-pK_a>1$ or <1	$pH-pK_a>1$
Equation	$V_0 = V_N + 1.111$ • APC • ATW • $(1 - EPB)$	$V_0 = (0.1302$ • APC $+ 0.9314)$ • $(1 - EBP)$ • ABW_0	$V_0 = V_N$ • $(IBW_0 + 0.15$ • ATW$)$	$V_0 = \dfrac{(ATW/TBW)_0}{(ATW/TBW)_N} \cdot V_N$
No.	Eq. 26.9	Eq. 26.10	Eq. 26.11	Eq. 26.12

APC = n-octanol/buffer pH 7.4 apparent partition coefficient; EPB = extent of protein binding to 4% human albumin (fraction of 1); V = apparent V_d; ATW = adipose tissue weight; ABW = actual body weight; TBW = total body water; IBW = ideal body weight; the indices 0 and N refer to obese and normal (lean) condition; V_N = normal apparent volume of distribution ($V_{d\ area}$ or $V_{d\beta}$) in liters.
ATW = ABW − IBW
TBW = $58.3 • e^{-0.0043059 • \% \text{ overweight}}$

$(ATW/TBW)_N$ males: 0.353548
females: 0.67329

Table 26-3. Survey of Drugs with Altered Pharmacokinetic Parameters in Obesity

DRUG	ELIMINATION HALF-LIFE	VOLUME OF DISTRIBUTION	TOTAL CLEARANCE
Acetaminophen	↓	↓	↓*
Acetyl Procainamide	↓	?	↓
Amikacin	↓	↓	↓*
Antipyrine	↑	↓	↓
Caffeine	↑	↑	U
Diazepam	↑	↑	?
Digoxin	↓	↓	↓*
Fentanyl	↑	↑	U
Gentamicin	↓	↓	↓*
Procainamide	↓	↓	U
Theophylline	↑	↓	↓*
Thiopental	↑	↑	↓*
Tobramycin	↓	↓	↓*
Vancomycin	↓	↑	↑*

↑ = increase; ↓ = decrease; U = unchanged; *might be of significant importance.

Step 4: Calculate DM as follows:

$$DM_{obese\ ger} = (Cl_{tot\ obese\ ger} \cdot Desired\ C_{av}^{ss} \cdot \tau)/f \tag{12}$$

where τ is the selected dosing interval and f is the absolute bioavailability (fraction of 1).

Selected References

1. Abernethy, D. R. and Greenblatt, D. J.: Pharmacokinetics of Drugs in Obesity, *Clin. Pharmacokinet.* 7:108–124 (1982).

2. Blouin, R. A., Kolpek, J. H. and Mann, H. J.: Influence of Obesity on Drug Disposition, *Clin. Pharm.* 6:706–714 (1987).

3. Forsyth, H. L. and Sinning, W. E.: The Anthropometric Estimation of Body Density and Lean Body Weight of Male Athletes, *Med. Sci. Sports* 5:174 (1973).

4. Groves, B. M., Ewy, G. A., Ball, M. F., Jackson, B. E., Nimmo, L. E. and Marcus, F. I.: Digoxin Metabolism in Obesity, *Clin. Res.* 19:114 (1971).

5. Mitzkat, H. J.: Übergewicht und Folgeerkrankungen für den Stoffwechsel, *Österr. Apoth. Ztg.* 31:1010 (1977).

6. Norris, A. H., Lundy, T. and Shock, N. W.: Trends in Selected Indices of Body Composition in Men Between Ages 30 and 80 Years, *Ann. N.Y. Acad. Sci. 110*:623 (1963).

7. Ritschel, W. A. and Kaul, S.: Prediction of Apparent Volume of Distribution in Obesity, *Methods Find. Exp. Clin. Pharmacol. 8*:239–247 (1986).

27

Drug Disposition in Pregnancy

The course of a blood concentration-time profile depends on the physicochemical properties of the drug and the physiologic/pathologic properties of the body. Because a number of physiologic functions are altered during pregnancy, and at least two further compartments (at least during the later part of pregnancy), namely, the fetus and the amniotic fluid, have to be added to the system, it becomes plausible that pharmacokinetics may be different in the pregnant woman from that in the nonpregnant one. The situation is complicated by the fact that pregnancy is not just one single physiologically altered entity, but rather a complex and constantly changing phenomenon.

Consideration of drug exposure during pregnancy must encompass the aspects of not only the physiologic changes associated with pregnancy but also the fact that these changes in both the mother and developing fetus are dynamic. During pregnancy, there are two predominant factors which are most often of clinical concern: (1) maternal alterations in drug pharmacokinetics and pharmacodynamics and (2) the extent of fetal drug exposure. These can be conceptualized by considering drug transfer between the maternal and fetal circulation via the diaplacental and paraplacental routes. As schematically illustrated in Figure 27-1, fetal localization and accumulation of drug is directly related to maternal dose, maternal drug clearance, the extent of fetal transfer (via the placenta and fetal membranes), incorporation of the drug in the fluids and tissues of the fetus, metabolism and excretion of the drug by the fetus, and fetal re-exposure via recirculation of drug through amniotic fluid (e.g., fetal drinking and recycling of amniotic fluid in the fetal lung). In addition to the physicochemical conditions required for the translocation of a drug (see Chapters 4 and 6), it must be recognized that the physiological characteristics of each component of the maternal—placental—fetal unit undergo dynamic change during parturition. This is best exemplified by specific routes of fetal drug metabolism (e.g., hydrolysis, sulfotransferase activity, activity of the fetal form of cytochrome P450 3A or CYP3A7) which are relatively absent for the first trimester of pregnancy but increase in activity over the second and third trimesters. These are of consideration not only for the localization of drugs in the fetal compartment and their attendant effects (e.g., teratogenicity, fetal toxicity), but also the potential for fetal pharmacotherapy (e.g., treatment

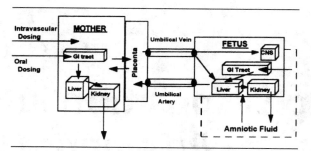

Figure 27-1. Relationships between maternal, placental, and fetal compartments and the distribution of drugs between them.

of fetal toxoplasmosis, masculinization secondary to 21-hydroxylase deficiency, and fetal tachyarrhythmias).

Recent evidence from human studies indicates that the activity of specific drug-metabolizing enzymes is altered by pregnancy. For example, the activity of CYP1A2 progressively declines during pregnancy (by approximately 50%) while those for xanthine oxidase (XO) and NAT2 appear to increase slightly. Also, CYP2D6 activity may increase during pregnancy. These changes are likely the result of alterations in either estrogen or progesterone that occur during the course of a normal pregnancy.

Although more research is needed regarding pharmacokinetic drug characterization in pregnancy and in the fetus, some generalizations which can now be made are summarized in Table 27-1.

Table 27-2 gives a survey of drug concentration ratios between maternal and fetal blood in humans.

Table 27-1. General Pharmacokinetic Aspects in Pregnancy

COMPARTMENT	PARAMETER	PHYSIOLOGIC CHANGES
Maternal organismus (Pregnancy)	Absorption:	P.O.-delayed due to delayed motility and decreased gastric secretion. I.M.-delayed from upper thigh due to decreased tissue perfusion. S.C.-delayed due to increase in subcutaneous fat.
	Distribution:	Increased volume of distribution due to increase in total body fluid by 5 to 8 liters, and formation of edema. Blood volume increases by 30–40%, plasma volume increases by 50%. Erythrocytes increase in number by 18%, yet the total hemoglobin level decreases. Body fat increases by 3–10 kg, hence increased V_d for highly lipid soluble drugs. Albumin concentration decreases by 15 to 30%, hence total conc. may decrease and unbound conc. may increase.
	Metabolism:	Enzyme specific up or down regulation.
	Elimination:	Drugs predominantly eliminated via the kidney are eliminated faster due to increase in total clearance (increase in renal blood flow). Renal plasma flow increases by up to 100%, glomerular filtration rate increases by about 70%. The elimination half-life of drugs that are largely or completely eliminated by the kidney in unchanged form should therefore be shorter in pregnancy.

(continued)

Table 27-1. General Pharmacokinetic Aspects in Pregnancy (*Continued*)

COMPARTMENT	PARAMETER	PHYSIOLOGIC CHANGES
	Blood levels:	Delayed peak time and decreased peak concentration. The concentration-time profile of free drug during a dosing interval may change with increased peak and decreased trough levels. To reduce these increased steady state fluctuations between C_{max}^{ss} and C_{min}^{ss} it may be appropriate to decrease the dosing interval.
Mother (During Labor)	Absorption:	P.O.-delayed due to decreased motility and decreased gastric secretion in maternal organism. I.M.-delayed from upper thigh due to decreased tissue perfusion. S.C.-delayed due to increase in subcutaneous fat.
	Distribution:	Increased volume of distribution due to increase in total body fluid and formation of edema.
	Metabolism:	Enzyme specific up or down regulation.
	Elimination:	Slower elimination of drugs excreted via kidney due to decreased total clearance.
	Blood levels:	Probably increased.
Fetus	Absorption:	In principle, all drugs may reach fetal circulation, depending on physicochemical characteristics of drug (lipid solubility, pK_a, molecular size) and transport mechanism. Amniotic fluid may act as absorption reservoir.
	Distribution:	Larger aqueous compartment per unit of body weight, reduced blood-barrier function, and less plasma protein probably result in extensive volume of distribution for most drugs.
	Metabolism:	Primarily depends on maternal and placental metabolic capacity.
	Elimination:	Depends on placental exchange, paraplacental recycling after micturition into amniotic fluid.
	Blood levels:	Acidic drugs may reach fetal blood levels up to maternal concentrations, whereas basic drugs may exceed maternal concentration. Possible accumulation due to additional drug depot in amniotic fluid.

Table 27-2. Ratios of Maternal/Fetal Drug Concentrations

DRUG	COMPARTMENT STUDIED	RATIO OF MATERNAL/FETAL BLOOD
Amikacin		<2
Amoxicillin		>2
Ampicillin		<2
	MB,FB,AF	1.5
	MB,FB,AF	2
		1.3
Antipyrine		1
Azidocillin	MB,FB,AF	3.8
Barbiturates	MB,FB	1.4
Bishydroxycoumarin		1.7
Bupivacaine	MB,FB	2.3–3.3
Carbenicillin		>2
Cefazolin	MB,FB,AF,P,M,E,D,C,PL,FM	1.3
Cephacetrile	MB,FB,AF	1.7
Cephalosporins		<2
Chloralhydrate	MB,FB	1
Chloramphenicol		>2
		1.3
Chlorothiazide		0.9
Chlorpromazine	MB,FB	<2
Clindamycin		<2
Clorazepate	MB,FB,AF	1.3
Colistimethate		<2
Cyclopropane		1.3
Diazepam	MB,FB	1.2
	MB,FB,AF	1
Dicloxacillin		<2
Diethyl ether		1
Erythromycin		<2
Ethanol		1.3
Gentamicin	MB,FB,AF	2
		1.3
Histidine	MB,FB	1
Imipramine		0.5
INH		1.1
Insulin		4
Kanamycin		2
Lidocaine	MB,FB	1.8
Meperidine	MB,FB	0.8–1.3
Mepivacaine	MB,FB	1.5
Methicillin		>2
Nafcillin		<2
Nitrofurantoin		>2
Nitrous oxide		1.7

Table 27-2. Ratios of Maternal/Fetal Drug Concentrations (*Continued*)

DRUG	COMPARTMENT STUDIED	RATIO OF MATERNAL/FETAL BLOOD
Oxacillin		<2
		1
Paraldehyde		1
Penicillin		1.4–5
Penicillin G		>2
	MB,FB,AF	3
Pentazocine	MB,FB	1.4–2.5
Pentobarbital		1.3
Procaine		1.7
Promethazine	MB,FB	1.4
Secobarbital		1.4
Streptomycin		2
Sulfonamides		>2
Sulphasalazine	MB,FB,AF	1.7
Tetracycline		1.4
		>2
Thiopental		1
Thiouracil		1
Ticarcillin	MB,FB,AF	1.7
Tobramycin		<2
Trichloroethylene		1
Trimethoprim		>2

MB = maternal blood
FB = fetal blood (venous or arterial or capillary blood)
AF = amniotic fluid
P = perimetrium
M = myometrium
E = endometrium
D = decidua
C = chorion
PL = placenta
FM = fetal membrane

Selected References

1. Farrar, H. C. and Blumer, J. L.: Fetal Effects of Maternal Drug Exposure, *Ann. Rev. Pharmacol. Toxicol.* 31:525–547 (1991).

2. Lobstein, R., Lalkin, A. and Koren, G.: Pharmacokinetic Changes During Pregnancy and Their Clinical Relevance, *Clin. Pharmacokinet.* 33:328–343 (1997).

3. Pacifici, G. M. and Nottoli, R.: Placental Transfer of Drugs Administered to the Mother, *Clin. Pharmacokinet.* 28:235–269 (1995).

4. Parker, W. A.: Effects of Pregnancy on Pharmacokinetics, in *Pharmacokinetic Basis for Drug Treatment,* Benet, L. Z., Massoud, N., Gambertoglio, J. G., (eds.), Raven Press, New York, 1984, pp. 249–268.

5. Ritschel, W. A.: Pharmacokinetic Characterization of Drugs, In *Clinical Pharmacology in Pregnancy,* Kuemmerle, H. P. and Brendel, K., Editors, Thieme-Stratton, New York, 1984, p. 59.

6. Ritschel, W. A.: Kinetic Model and Dosage Regimen, In *Clinical Pharmacology in Pregnancy,* Kuemmerle, H. P. and Brendel, K., Editors, Thieme-Stratton, New York, 1984, p. 217.

7. Tsutsumi, K., Kotegawa, T., Matsuki, S., Tanaka, Y., Ishii, Y., Kodama, Y., et al.: The Effect of Pregnancy on Cytochrome P4501A2, Xanthine Oxidase, and N-Acetyltransferase Activities in Humans. *Clin. Pharmacol. Ther.* 70:121–125 (2001).

28

Dosage Regimen Design

One of the practical applications of pharmacokinetics is the calculation of dose size and dosing intervals for drugs in patients with and without renal failure.

The purpose of a dosage regimen design is, for the drug-naive patient, to initiate therapy for multiple dosing. Since there is no drug in the body, mean literature pharmacokinetic parameters are used. The mean pharmacokinetic parameters should result at steady state in blood levels close to the desired ones but may result in greatly increased blood levels in case of renal and/or hepatic failure, myocardial or coronary infarction, other pathological conditions, or genetically different drug disposition. Edema and obesity may change the volume of distribution and consequently the blood level. In case of stabilized renal impairment, correction can be made based on the actual creatinine clearance or serum creatinine concentration.

In case of suspected alteration of normal pharmacokinetic parameters, the Repeated One-Point Method is recommended. This permits design of dosage regimen to be based on the pharmacokinetic parameters obtained from two blood samples after administration of two test doses.

This chapter deals with the determination of desired dose sizes and/or desired dosing intervals for multiple doses in patients with or without renal failure being treated with a particular drug. The objective is to maintain a minimum therapeutic concentration (MTC), a minimum inhibitory concentration (MIC), or a minimum effective concentration (MEC) or to obtain a desired peak or mean steady state concentration. Calculations are based on the equations on drug accumulation for multiple dosing with fixed dose sizes and fixed dosing intervals as discussed in Chapter 22, "Pharmacokinetics of Multiple Dosing."

The equations for determination of dose sizes and dosing intervals are based on the open one-compartment model. Therefore, one must recognize the implications, assumptions, and limitations. The following considerations especially must be kept in mind:

- It is assumed that all pharmacokinetic parameters remain constant during the course of therapy once a dosage regimen has been determined. In case one or more of the factors change, the once established dosage regimen is no longer valid.

- Change in urinary pH can cause deviation of actual blood levels from calculated ones.
- Change (decrease) in renal function will prolong elimination of those drugs which are at least partly excreted from the body in unchanged form via the kidneys. By determining the creatinine clearance or the serum creatinine a correction can easily be made.
- Change in hepatic clearance due to liver disease or saturation of metabolic pathways, enzyme induction, or enzyme inhibition can cause deviation of actual blood levels from calculated ones for those drugs which are at least partly metabolized and/or excreted via the liver. Unfortunately, we do not yet have any liver function test which permits us to determine a correction factor. The only way is to obtain information of changed pharmacokinetic parameters from blood level or urinary excretion studies in the particular patient.
- Congestive heart failure and myocardial infarction may cause reduction in blood flow, resulting in reduced volume of distribution and prolonged elimination of drugs. A reduction in V_d by 30 percent may be indicated for preliminary design of dosage regimen.
- Since the equations are based on the open one-compartment model they can be applied to the open two-compartment model if instead of k_{el}, the terminal rate constant β, and instead of V_d either $V_{d\beta}$ or V_{dss} are used. An exception is in the case of calculating the loading dose for IV infusions where the volume of the central compartment V_c is used.

A dosage regimen is characterized by the dose size and the dosing interval. In order to maintain a certain therapeutic blood level either the dose size can be varied keeping the dosing interval constant or both dose size and dosing interval are changed.

At a given minimum effective concentration, the longer the dosing interval the higher will be the required dose size and hence, the larger will be the fluctuations between the maximum and minimum blood levels C_{max}^{ss} and C_{min}^{ss}. This is of great clinical importance in dosage regimen calculation of toxic drugs and dosage regimen adjustment in renal failure. In the latter case it is safer to reduce the dose size and maintain the normal dosing interval than vice versa. Of the many different approaches for adjustment of dosage regimen five will be discussed:

- Calculation of dose size and dosing interval in patients without renal failure based on the steady state average blood level C_{av}^{ss} equation, and in patients with renal failure considering additionally the creatinine clearance (C_{av}^{ss} Method).
- Calculation of dose size and dosing interval in patients without renal failure based on the equation for minimum blood level concentration at steady state C_{min}^{ss}, and in patients with renal failure considering additionally the creatinine clearance (C_{min}^{ss} Method).
- Calculation of dose size and dosing interval in patients without renal failure based on the equation for maximum blood level concentration at steady state C_{max}^{ss}, and in patients with renal failure considering additionally the creatinine clearance (C_{max}^{ss} Method).
- Calculation of dose size and dosing interval in patients without renal failure based on the equations for maximum and minimum blood level concentration at steady state C_{max}^{ss} and C_{min}^{ss}, and in patients with renal failure considering additionally the creatinine clearance ($C_{max}^{ss} - C_{min}^{ss}$ Method).
- Calculation of dosage regimen for any of the above listed methods in patients where a change in volume of distribution is suspected and/or in patients with renal and/or liver impairment (Repeated One-Point-Method).

If one has determined the required maintenance dose size DM and the loading dose DL, calculation is identical regardless of whether or not renal failure is present, except that $k_{el\,r.f.}$ (elimination rate constant in renal failure) is used instead of k_{el}.

Loading Dose and Maintenance Dose

A particular dose size given repeatedly in constant dosing intervals results, after a few applications, usually 5–10—depending on the elimination half-life of the drug and the dosing interval—in a plateau where the drug concentration fluctuates between a maximum and minimum blood level. In order to obtain this plateau with the first dose, a larger dose has to be given as a loading dose.

If the dosing interval is equal to or similar to the elimination half-life, the loading dose is determined according to Table 28-1 (Equations 28.1–28.3). If the dosing interval differs from the elimination half-life, the loading dose is determined according to Table 28-2 (Equations 28.4–28.8).

This procedure (Table 28-1) is applicable if it is known either that the loading dose is already therapeutically effective, or that a sequence of maintenance doses will result in therapeutic effectiveness in a chosen dosage interval.

Intravenous Infusion

The infusion rate is the product of the effective blood level and the total clearance of the drug from the body:

$$R° = C_{av}^{ss} \cdot (V_d \cdot k_{el}) [\mu g/ml] \tag{9}$$

Since an IV infusion can be considered as multiple dose administration with an infinitely small dosing interval τ, no fluctuations between a minimum and maximum blood level concentration exist. Therefore $C_{max}^{ss} = C_{min}^{ss} = C_{av}^{ss}$. Equation 28.9 can be rewritten sub-

Table 28-1. General Rules for Loading Dose–Maintenance Dose Ratio if the Dosing Interval is Equal to or Shorter than the Elimination Half-Life

LOADING DOSE DL—MAINTENANCE DOSE DM—RATIO R

Rule of Thumb:
If the dosing interval τ is equal to or somewhat shorter than the elimination half-life $t_{1/2}$, then the dose Ratio R should be 2:1:

$$R = \frac{DL}{DM} = \frac{2}{1} (\text{if } \tau \lesssim t_{1/2}) \qquad \text{Eq. 28.1}$$

If a known dose of a drug yields satisfactory therapeutic effectiveness, then the maintenance dose DM should be ½ of the loading dose DL:

$$DM = \frac{DL}{2} [mg] (\text{if } \tau \lesssim t_{1/2}) \qquad \text{Eq. 28.2}$$

If a known maintenance dose DM yields satisfactory therapeutic effectiveness, then the loading dose DL should be twice the maintenance dose DM:

$$DL = 2 \cdot DM [mg] (\text{if } \tau \lesssim t_{1/2}) \qquad \text{Eq. 28.3}$$

Table 28-2. Calculation of Loading Dose and Maintenance Dose if the Dosage Interval Is Not Equal to the Elimination Half-Life

LOADING DOSE DL AND MAINTENANCE DOSE DM CALCULATION IF $\tau \neq t_{1/2}$	
Intravenous Infusion (§)	
$$DL = \frac{D_t}{t_t \cdot \ln 2} \cdot t_{1/2} \, [mg]$$	(Eq. 28.4)
Intravascular Administration	
$$DL = \frac{DM}{(1 - e^{-k_{el} \cdot \tau})} \, [mg]$$	(Eq. 28.5)
$$DM = DL \cdot (1 - e^{-k_{el} \cdot \tau}) \, [mg]$$	(Eq. 28.6)
Extravascular Administration	
$$DL = \frac{DM}{(1 - e^{-k_a \cdot \tau}) \cdot (1 - e^{-k_{el} \cdot \tau})} \, [mg]$$	(Eq. 28.7)
$$DM = DL \cdot (1 - e^{-k_{el} \cdot \tau}) \cdot (1 - e^{-k_a \cdot \tau}) \, [mg]$$	(Eq. 28.8)

(§) = a different approach is necessary if the I.V. curve follows the open two-compartment model. See under the paragraph on "Intravenous Infusion."
t = dosing interval [h]
D_t = dose which is infused over time period t_t [µg] or [mg]
t_t = time period of infusion [h]
k_a = absorption rate constant [h^{-1}]
k_{el} = elimination rate constant [h^{-1}]

stituting C_{min}^{ss}, or the minimum inhibitory concentration MIC (in the case of antibiotics and chemotherapeutics), or the minimum effective concentration MEC, or the minimum therapeutic concentration, MTC for C_{av}^{ss}:

$$R° = MEC \cdot \Delta' \cdot BW \cdot k_{el} \, [\mu g/ml] \tag{10}$$

$R°$ = infusion rate [µg/h]
C_{av}^{ss} = average blood level concentration at steady state [µg/ml]
V_d = volume of distribution [ml]
k_{el} = elimination rate constant [h^{-1}]
MEC = minimum effective concentration = MIC = MTC [µg/ml]
Δ' = distribution coefficient [ml/g]
BW = body weight [g]

If an IV infusion is started without giving a loading dose, several half-lives would pass before a therapeutic concentration could be reached. In the case in which the IV curve of a drug can be described by an open one-compartment model, either Equation 28.4 can be used to calculate the IV loading dose or:

$$DL = V_d \cdot C_{av}^{ss} = \Delta' \cdot BW \cdot C_{av}^{ss} \, [\mu g] \tag{11}$$

However, if the IV curve of a drug follows the open two-compartment model where distribution is slower, and one would use $V_{d\,ss}$ instead of V_d, too high a loading dose results.

In the case where the open two-compartment model applies, the volume of the central compartment V_c, or its distribution coefficient Δ' have to be used:

$$DL = V_c \cdot C_{av}^{ss} = \Delta'_c \cdot BW \cdot C_{av}^{ss} \ [\mu g] \tag{12}$$

DL = loading dose of IV infusion [μg]
V_d = volume of distribution [ml]
V_c = volume of central compartment [ml]
Δ'_c = distribution coefficient of central compartment [ml/g]

Dosage Regimen Design Based on C_{av}^{ss}

The C_{av}^{ss} or *log Dose-Response* or *Therapeutic Window Method* (see Figures 28-1 and 28-2) is used for those drugs whose clinical effect follows a log dose-response curve and an average concentration is desired within a therapeutic range. The lower level of the therapeutic range lies somewhat above the dose size at which the log dose-response curve starts. In most cases, drug doses are selected to be in the lower-half portion of the log dose-response curve, so that the desired mean steady state concentration is about in the lower third of the log dose-response curve. The log dose-toxicity curve may start already in the upper region of the log dose-response curve. For drugs following the log dose-response the intensity of effect (and of toxicity) increases with increasing peak height (Figure 28-1). Drugs that are often based on this pattern are digoxin, lidocaine, procainamide, theophylline, quinidine, bactericidal antibiotics, analgesics, antipyretics, and hypoglycemic agents.

For some drugs, such as antidepressants and antipsychotics, the clinical effect increases with dose size only up to a certain point and then actually diminishes as the dose size is further increased. Instead of a therapeutic range, there exists a therapeutic window, showing a more or less bell-shaped log dose-response curve (Figure 28-2). A desired C_{av}^{ss} concentration is selected which is about in the middle of the therapeutic window.

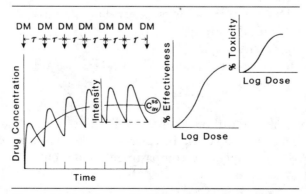

Figure 28-1. Schematic diagram of a drug accumulation blood level-time curve and selection of desired mean steady state concentration C_{av}^{ss} according to the drug's log dose-response and log dose-toxicity curves.

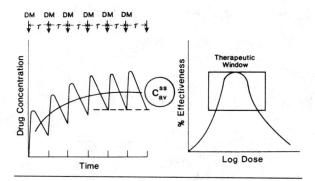

Figure 28-2. Schematic diagram of a drug accumulation blood level-time curve and selection of desired mean steady state concentration C_{av}^{ss}, to be about in the middle of the height of the therapeutic window of the log dose-response curve.

This approach is based on the average blood level equation at steady state C_{av}^{ss}:

$$C_{av}^{ss} = \frac{f \cdot DM}{k_{el} \cdot V_d \cdot \tau} \tag{13}$$

which can be expressed in different forms as are given in Equation 28.14:

$$C_{av}^{ss} = \left(\frac{1}{V_d \cdot k_{el}}\right) \cdot \frac{f \cdot DM}{\tau} = \left(\frac{1}{V_d \cdot \dfrac{0693}{t_{1/2}}}\right) \cdot \frac{f \cdot DM}{\tau} = \left(\frac{1.44 \cdot t_{1/2}}{V_d}\right) \cdot \frac{f \cdot DM}{\tau} \tag{14}$$

Since the amount of drug in the body (A) at equilibrium state can be expressed by Equation 28.15:

$$A = C_{av}^{ss} \cdot V_d \tag{15}$$

and the reciprocal of the overall elimination rate constant can be expressed according to Equation 28.16:

$$\frac{1}{k_{el}} = 1.44 \cdot t_{1/2} \tag{16}$$

A can be expressed as given in Equation 28.17:

$$A = \frac{1.44 \cdot t_{1/2} \cdot f \cdot DM}{\tau} \tag{17}$$

DOSE SIZE DESIGN IN PATIENTS WITHOUT RENAL FAILURE (C_{av}^{ss} METHOD)

$$DM = \frac{C_{av}^{ss} \cdot V_d \cdot \tau}{1.44 \cdot t_{1/2} \cdot f} \tag{18}$$

DOSING INTERVAL DESIGN WITHOUT RENAL FAILURE (C_{av}^{ss} METHOD)

$$\tau = \frac{f \cdot DM \cdot 1.44 \cdot t_{1/2}}{C_{av}^{ss} \cdot V_d} [h] \tag{19}$$

DOSE SIZE DESIGN IN PATIENTS WITH RENAL FAILURE (C_{av}^{ss} METHOD)

$$t_{1/2 \, r.f.} = \frac{t_{1/2}}{\left[\left(\dfrac{Cl_{creat.\,obs.}}{Cl_{creat.\,norm.}} - 1 \right) \cdot F_{el} \right] + 1} [h] \tag{20}$$

The patient's observed creatinine clearance, $Cl_{creat.obs.}$, must be corrected for 1.73 m². The $Cl_{creat.norm.}$ is 120 for males and 105.9 for females and:

$$DM_{r.f.} = \frac{C_{av}^{ss} \cdot V_d \cdot \tau}{1.44 \cdot t_{1/2 \, r.f.} \cdot f} \tag{21}$$

Knowing the half-life in renal failure $t_{1/2 \, r.f.}$, one can also use one of the following equations:

$$DM_{r.f.} = DM \cdot \left(\frac{t_{1/2}}{t_{1/2 \, r.f.}} \right) = \frac{DM}{t_{1/2 \, r.f.}/t_{1/2}} \tag{22}$$

$$DM_{r.f.} = DM \cdot \left(\frac{k_{el \, r.f.}}{k_{el}} \right) = \frac{DM}{k_{el}/k_{el \, r.f.}} \tag{23}$$

DOSING INTERVAL DESIGN IN PATIENTS WITH RENAL FAILURE (C_{av}^{ss} METHOD)

$$\tau_{r.f.} = \frac{f \cdot D \cdot 1.44 \cdot t_{1/2 \, r.f.}}{C_{av}^{ss} \cdot V_d} [h] \tag{24}$$

Knowing the half-life in renal failure $t_{1/2 \, r.f.}$ one can also use one of the following methods:

$$\tau_{r.f.} = \tau \cdot \left(\frac{t_{1/2 \, r.f.}}{t_{1/2}} \right) = \frac{\tau}{t_{1/2}/t_{1/2 \, r.f.}} [h] \tag{25}$$

$$\tau_{r.f.} = \tau \cdot \left(\frac{k_{el}}{k_{el \, r.f.}} \right) = \frac{\tau}{k_{el \, r.f.}/k_{el}} [h] \tag{26}$$

C_{av}^{ss} = average blood level during dosing interval after steady state is reached [mg/l]
f = fraction of drug absorbed [fraction of 1]
DM = dose size [mg]
k_{el} = elimination rate constant [h⁻¹]
V_d = volume of distribution [l/kg]
τ = dosing interval [h]

A $\quad$ = amount of drug in the body at steady state [mg/kg]

$t_{1/2}$ $\quad$ = elimination half-life [h]

$DM_{r.f.}$ = dose size in renal failure [mg]

$k_{el\,r.f.}$ = elimination rate constant in renal failure [h⁻¹]

$t_{1/2\,r.f.}$ = elimination half-life in renal failure [h]

$\tau_{r.f.}$ $\quad$ = dosing interval in renal failure [h]

F_{el} $\quad$ = fraction of drug excreted via kidney [fraction of 1]

Dosage Regimen Design Based on C_{min}^{ss}

The C_{min}^{ss} or *Trough* or *MIC* or *MEC* or *MTC* Method (see Figure 28-3) is used for those drugs where it is necessary to maintain a minimum inhibitory, effective, or therapeutic concentration throughout the entire dosing interval. Above the MIC or MEC the drug will be effective regardless of how high a peak level is reached as long as the entire steady state blood level-time curve is above the required minimum concentration. If the blood level-time curve falls below the MIC or MEC level, the drug will be ineffective as long as the concentration stays below this level. Drugs that are often based on this method are bacteriostatic antibiotics and other antimicrobial agents (sulfonamides) that have a relatively large therapeutic index.

However, one has to realize that each drug has a different MIC for each type of microorganism, and even then there are sometimes wide ranges for different strains of the same microorganism, e.g., the MIC of erythromycin against *S. aureus* is 0.01 to 2.5 µg/ml. For the proper selection of the MIC a microbiological sensitivity test is indicated.

This approach is based on the minimum blood level concentration at equilibrium C_{min}^{ss} which can be set equal to the required minimum effective, minimum inhibitory, or minimum therapeutic concentration:

$$C_{min}^{ss} = \frac{C(0) \cdot e^{-k_{el} \cdot \tau}}{1 - e^{-k_{el} \cdot \tau}} \tag{27}$$

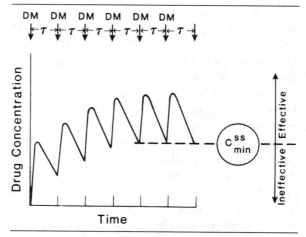

Figure 28-3. Schematic diagram of a drug accumulation blood level-time curve and selection of desired trough C_{min}^{ss} to be maintained.

The advantage of the C_{min}^{ss} method is that the actual blood level will remain above the minimum required therapeutic concentration during the entire dosing interval (as seen in Figure 28-3), whereas using the C_{av}^{ss} method the actual blood level falls for part of the dosing interval below the MEC.

DOSE SIZE DESIGN IN PATIENTS WITHOUT RENAL FAILURE (C_{min}^{ss} METHOD)

$$DM = \frac{\Delta' \cdot BW \cdot MTC \cdot (1 - e^{-k_{el} \cdot \tau})}{(e^{-k_{el} \cdot \tau}) \cdot f \cdot 1000} [mg] \tag{28}$$

DOSING INTERVAL DESIGN IN PATIENTS WITHOUT RENAL FAILURE (C_{min}^{ss} METHOD)

$$\tau = \frac{1}{k_{el}} \cdot \ln\left(1 + \frac{DM \cdot f}{\Delta' \cdot BW \cdot MTC}\right)[h] \tag{29}$$

DOSE SIZE DESIGN IN PATIENTS WITH RENAL FAILURE (C_{min}^{ss} METHOD)

$$DM_{r.f.} = \frac{\Delta' \cdot BW \cdot MTC \cdot \left(1 - e^{-k_{el} \cdot \left\{\left[\left(\frac{Cl_{creat.\ obs.}}{Cl_{creat.\ norm.}} - 1\right) \cdot F_{el}\right] + 1\right\} \cdot \tau}\right)}{e^{-k_{el} \cdot \left\{\left[\left(\frac{Cl_{creat.\ obs.}}{Cl_{creat.\ norm.}} - 1\right) \cdot F_{el}\right] + 1\right\} \cdot \tau} \cdot f \cdot 1000}[mg] \tag{30}$$

DOSING INTERVAL DESIGN IN PATIENTS WITH RENAL FAILURE (C_{min}^{ss} METHOD)

$$\tau_{r.f.} = \frac{1}{k_{el} \cdot \left\{\left[\left(\frac{Cl_{creat.\ obs.}}{Cl_{creat.\ norm.}} - 1\right) \cdot F_{el}\right] + 1\right\}} \cdot \ln\left(1 + \frac{DM \cdot f}{\Delta' \cdot BW \cdot MTC}\right)[h] \tag{31}$$

DM = maintenance dose [mg]

τ = dosing interval [h]

$DM_{r.f.}$ = maintenance dose in renal failure [mg]

$\tau_{r.f.}$ = dosing interval in renal failure [h]

Δ = distribution coefficient [ml/g]

BW = body weight of patient [g]

MTC = minimum therapeutic concentration of drug or minimum inhibitory concentration of drug against a specific microorganism, determined in vitro by serial dilution, agar plate, or filter disk methods in media containing serum [µg/ml], or MEC = minimum effective concentration of drug in blood, plasma, or serum [µg/ml]

k_{el} = overall elimination rate constant of the drug [h^{-1}], i.e., rate of loss of unchanged drug from the systemic circulation by renal and extrarenal excretion and metabolism, in the open two-compartment model termed β.

$Cl_{creat.obs.}$ = creatinine clearance observed in a particular patient corrected for 1.73 m^2 surface area [ml/min] or,

$$Cl_{creat.\,obs.} = \frac{(140 - Age) \cdot BW}{72 \cdot S_{cr}} \tag{32}$$

where $Cl_{creat.obs.}$ is the creatinine clearance in ml/min, age is in years, BW in kg, and S_{cr} in mg/100 ml. The patient's clearance must be corrected for 1.73 m² (see Chapter 17, "Excretion and Clearance of Drugs").

$Cl_{creat.norm.}$ = normal creatinine clearance = 120.7 for males and 105.9 for females [ml/min]
f = fraction of dose absorbed [fraction of 1]
F_{el} = fraction of unchanged drug which is eliminated by renal excretion [fraction of 1]

Dosage Regimen Design Based on C^{ss}_{max}

The C^{ss}_{max} or *Peak Method* (see Figure 28-4) is used for those drugs for which it is desired to reach a certain peak concentration within each dosing interval. However, for the remainder of the dosing interval it is not required that the drug concentration remains above a minimum level. On the contrary, sometimes it is believed to be desirable that the drug blood level drops below a MIC or MEC value. This is particularly the case with bactericidal drugs which act only on the proliferating microorganisms. In these cases one does not wish to inhibit the growth of those microorganisms that have not been killed by the previous dose. Drugs often based on the C^{ss}_{max} method are penicillins, cephalosporins, gentamicin, kanamycin, etc.

The maintenance dose size DM for the C^{ss}_{max} method is given in Equation 28.33:

$$DM = \frac{\Delta' \cdot BW \cdot C^{ss}_{max} \cdot (1 - e^{-k_{el} \cdot \tau})}{(e^{-k_{el} \cdot t_{max}}) \cdot f \cdot 1000} \tag{33}$$

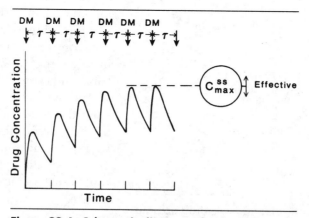

Figure 28-4. Schematic diagram of a drug accumulation blood level-time curve and selection of desired peak concentration C^{ss}_{max} to be reached within each dosing interval.

where t_{max} is the time in h to reach the peak after dosing. The other parameters were defined above for the C_{min}^{ss} method.

In the case of renal failure k_{el} has to be corrected as outlined above for the C_{min}^{ss} method.

Dosage Regimen Design Based on Fixed $C_{max}^{ss} - C_{min}^{ss}$

The fixed $C_{max}^{ss} - C_{min}^{ss}$ or *Limited Fluctuation Method* (see Figure 28-5) may be used for drugs to be dosed according to a pattern where within a dosing interval the steady state blood levels shall not exceed a maximum level C_{max}^{ss} and not undercut a desired minimum level C_{min}^{ss}. Drugs often based on this method are the aminoglycosides, INH, and theophylline. Having the range of fluctuations set, first the necessary dosing interval τ' is calculated:

$$\tau' = \left(\frac{1}{k_{el}} \cdot \ln \frac{C_{max}^{ss}}{C_{min}^{ss}} \right) + t_{max} \, [h] \tag{34}$$

The dose size is then calculated according to Equation 28.35:

$$DM = \frac{\Delta' \cdot BW \cdot C_{min}^{ss} \cdot (1 - e^{-k_{el} \cdot \tau'})}{(e^{-k_{el} \cdot \tau'}) \cdot f \cdot 1000} \tag{35}$$

The parameters have been defined above for the C_{min}^{ss} method. In the case of renal failure k_{el} has to be corrected as outlined above for the C_{min}^{ss} method.

Dosage Regimen Design According to the Repeated One-Point Method

(Use if pharmacokinetic data are not available or if changes in renal and/or hepatic function and/or in volume of distribution are expected.)

In some clinical situations such as acute heart failure, liver failure, renal failure, hypoalbuminemia, displacement from protein binding, obesity, severe edema, etc., both the volume of distribution and the elimination rate may change. The determination of the creatinine clearance may be too time consuming, and the serum creatinine concentration may be an unreliable indicator in some situations, such as in renal failure, uremia, muscular diseases, and old age. Besides, neither creatinine clearance nor serum creatinine data indicate changes in elimination by extrarenal routes, such as metabolism in hepatic failure. For these instances the *Repeated One-Point Method* has been proposed which is based on the determination of one drug blood level concentration each taken after the first

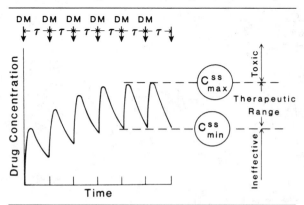

Figure 28-5. Schematic diagram of a drug accumulation blood level-time curve and selection of extent of fluctuation between a maximum C_{max}^{ss} and minimum C_{min}^{ss} steady state concentration within each dosing interval.

and second dose size towards the end of the dosing interval. The procedure is shown in Figure 28-6. A smaller than usual maintenance dose is administered as test dose (D_t) at the normal dosing interval (τ) as the first and second dose. The two blood samples taken must be exactly one dosing interval apart. The individual patient's elimination rate constant is then predicted according to Equation 28.36:

$$k_{el\,pred.} = \frac{\ln \dfrac{C_1}{C_2 - C_1}}{\tau}\,[h^{-1}]$$

(36)

where $k_{el\,pred.}$ is the individual patient's overall elimination rate constant in h^{-1}, C_1 and C_2 are the blood level concentrations in $\mu g/ml$ during the first and second dosing interval, respectively, and τ is the dosing interval in h.

Next, the minimum steady state concentration $C^{ss}_{min\,test\,dose}$ is calculated which would be obtained if the test doses were continued:

$$C^{ss}_{min\,test\,dose} = \frac{\dfrac{C_1}{e^{-k_{el\,pred.}\cdot t_1}} \cdot e^{-k_{el\,pred.}\cdot \tau}}{1 - e^{-k_{el\,pred.}\cdot \tau}}$$

(37)

where t_1 is the time when C_1 was sampled.

In Equation 28.37 the first term (fraction) of the denominator represents the extrapolated intercept B of the first test dose with the ordinate at time zero:

$$B = \frac{C_1}{e^{-k_{el\,pred.}\cdot t_1}}$$

(38)

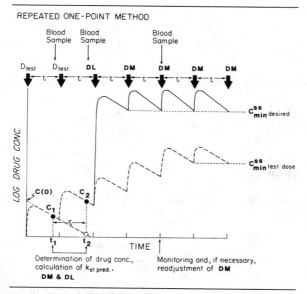

Figure 28-6. Schematic presentation of the use of the repeated one-point method for dosage regimen design.

This information can now be used to calculate the dosage regimen by the four methods discussed below.

Since the test dose was given to the same patient for whom the dosage regimen is determined the volume of distribution is not required in any calculation.

C_{av}^{ss} Method

If the test dose would be continued the following steady state would result:

$$C_{av \text{ test dose}}^{ss} = \frac{B}{k_{el \text{ pred.}} \cdot \tau} \tag{39}$$

The desired maintenance dose size $DM_{desired}$ for the patient is then:

$$DM_{desired} = \frac{C_{av \text{ desired}}^{ss}}{C_{av \text{ test dose}}^{ss}} \cdot D_{test} \tag{40}$$

C_{min}^{ss} Method

The desired maintenance dose is given by Equation 28.41:

$$DM_{desired} = \frac{C_{min \text{ desired}}^{ss}}{C_{min \text{ test dose}}^{ss}} \cdot D_{test} \tag{41}$$

C_{max}^{ss} Method

If the test dose would be continued the following maximum steady state concentration would result:

$$C_{max \text{ test dose}}^{ss} = \frac{B}{1 - e^{-k_{el \text{ pred.}} \cdot \tau}} \tag{42}$$

and the desired maintenance dose is then calculated according to Equation 28.43:

$$DM_{desired} = \frac{C_{max \text{ desired}}^{ss}}{C_{max \text{ test dose}}^{ss}} \cdot D_{test} \tag{43}$$

Fixed C_{max}^{ss} — C_{min}^{ss} Method

The required dosing interval τ for this fixed steady state concentration method is obtained by using Equation 28.44:

$$\tau' = \left(\frac{1}{k_{el \text{ pred.}}} \cdot \ln \frac{C_{max \text{ desired}}^{ss}}{C_{min \text{ desired}}^{ss}} \right) \cdot t_{max} \tag{44}$$

The desired maintenance dose size is then calculated by applying Equations 28.37 and 28.41.

Note: In Equation 28.37 τ' is used instead of τ.

Loading Dose

The two test doses may not result in the desired steady state concentration. The loading dose will build up the blood level from the concentration maintained from the test doses to the desired level:

$$DL = \frac{DM_{desired}}{1 - e^{-k_{el\,pred.} \cdot \tau'}} - D_{test} \cdot \left(\sum_{n=1}^{n=n} e^{-n \cdot k_{el\,pred.} \cdot \tau} \right) \tag{45}$$

where n is the number of test doses given before the new loading dose will be administered.

Note: To calculate DL for the Repeated One-Point Method based on C_{av}^{ss}, C_{min}^{ss}, or C_{max}^{ss}, τ' is τ. Only if based on $C_{max}^{ss} - C_{min}^{ss}$ has τ' to be used for calculating the amount of the loading dose with $DM_{desired}$, and τ for the amount of the test doses persisting in the body.

Application of Pharmacokinetic Methods to Optimize Antibiotic Effect

Any method that enables the prediction of the excursion between C_{max}^{ss} and C_{min}^{ss} for a given drug dose and dosing interval can be used to optimize antimicrobial therapy. By integrating the pharmacokinetic parameters of an antibiotic with measures of microorganism susceptibility (e.g., the MIC), it is possible to optimize bacterial eradication and thereby accomplish a more rapid clinical cure.

The most simple approach used to optimize antimicrobial effect entails prediction of the time during a fixed dosing interval where the plasma concentrations of a given antimicrobial agent are greater than the MIC (or minimum bactericidal concentration, MBC). This parameter can be estimated from Equation 28.46 as follows:

$$T > MIC = (\ln C_{max}^{ss} - \ln MIC)/k_{el} \tag{46}$$

where T > MIC is the time above the MIC during a dosing interval.

Alternatively, the area under the inhibitory curve (AUIC), the quotient of AUC and MIC, has been proposed to be an "index" of antibacterial action for the cephalosporins, quinolones, and aminoglycosides. More recent studies (see *Amsden, G. W., et al. 1993*) have shown that a 24-hour steady state AUIC of at least 125 is necessary for the adequate eradication of bacterial pathogens.

Application of the AUIC first involves calculation or estimation of the total plasma clearance for a given drug using plasma drug concentration data (see Equations 17.51 through 17.55) or through determination of the patient's creatinine clearance (e.g., correction of the "normal" Cl_{tot} for a given value of Cl_{cr}). The 24-hour steady state AUC can then be estimated according to Equation 28.47:

$$AUC_{0-24h}^{ss} = \frac{\text{Total daily dose (mg/24 h)}}{Cl_{tot}} \tag{47}$$

The AUIC is then determined as follows according to Equation 28.48:

$$AUIC = AUC_{0-24h}^{ss}/MIC \tag{48}$$

where MIC represents the minimum inhibitory concentration of the infecting pathogen.

Generally, AUIC "target values" of between 250 and 350 are utilized for dose selection. If the calculated AUIC is too low (i.e., risk of potential loss of efficacy) or too high (i.e., risk of potential concentration and time dependent drug toxicity), the maintenance dose and/or dosing interval can be easily readjusted to obtain a desired AUIC value by application of the Fixed $C_{max}^{ss} - C_{min}^{ss}$ or Limited Fluctuation Method (see Figure 28-5 and Equations 28.34, 28.35, 28.44, 28.49) or the Repeated One-Point Method (Equations 28.36–28.38).

Both the T > MIC (Eq. 28.46) and AUIC methods are based upon *in vivo* determination (or estimation) of plasma drug concentrations and *in vitro* determinations of antimicrobial susceptibility (i.e., MIC or MBC). Implicit assumptions in both of these methods entail a predictable relationship between the pharmacokinetics of the drug in plasma and at the site(s) of infection, and that *in vitro* microbial susceptibility reflects pharmacodynamic characteristics of microbial killing/eradication (e.g., the potential for an inoculum effect, postantibiotic effect) *in vivo*. Additionally, it should also be noted that the AUIC provides a rapid method for estimating doses necessary to target the desired amount of antimicrobial action and technically provides an assessment of the area above the inhibitory curve for a given pathogen.

Assumptions and Limitations

The assumption must be made that the pharmacokinetic parameters do not change during the time period of administration of the first test dose through the time the loading dose is given. After that time, an observed steady state concentration $C_{observed}$ (either C_{av}^{ss}, C_{max}^{ss}, or C_{min}^{ss}) different from the desired one $C_{desired}$ can be used to readjust the dosage regimen:

$$\text{DM}_{\text{readjusted}} = \frac{C_{\text{desired}}^{ss}}{C_{\text{observed}}^{ss}} \cdot \text{DM}_{\text{used}} \tag{49}$$

The limitations are that the two blood samples taken during the first and second dosing interval are exactly one dosing interval apart and that the drug assay is reliable.

There are advantages of the Repeated One-Point Method over taking only two blood samples after one dose. Accumulation of two doses results in higher drug concentrations, thus probably increasing assay accuracy. Also fluctuations in V_d, creatinine clearance, circadian rhythm, etc., will approach a mean value. The longer the dosing interval the less will be the impact of small fluctuations on the predicted dose.

New Approaches in Pharmacokinetics

Population Pharmacokinetics

Population Pharmacokinetic analysis is a relatively new approach which can be used to obtain important pharmacokinetic and pharmacodynamic information. Specifically, it enables the prediction of patient-specific pharmacokinetic (or pharmacodynamic) parameters for a given drug from data obtained in a group of patients having similar characteristics (i.e., age, disease state, concomitant therapy, etc.) and thus enables the projection of dosing regimens from patient-specific data. As well, these techniques enable the assessment of factors which impact drug disposition and/or effects such as the physiological changes which occur during development/aging, pathophysiologic effects, interindividual variability, residual or intraindividual variability and variability in data introduced by measurement errors in quantitating drug concentration or response and random changes in a given patient's parameter values over time. Knowledge about the quantitative aspects of interindividual variation is important in that it can provide information to assess how well an individual value can be predicted from patient characteristics and other factors which, in turn, makes the prediction of pharmacokinetic parameters more accurate or precise.

Typically, utilization of specific population approaches (e.g., nonlinear mixed-effects modeling or NONMEM) enables prediction of important parameters from studies involving many patients but with few observations (e.g., sparse blood levels, intermittent assessments of biologic markers of drug action) per patient. The precision of population pharmacokinetic approaches to either predict a given pharmacokinetic parameter or an appropriate initial dosing regimen rests completely on the quality (i.e., the confidence in) of the prior mean parameter estimates from a given patient population which are incorporated in the model. However, if a feedback technique (e.g., Bayesian estimation) is used wherein measurements of drug concentration and/or response are obtained during an initial trial regimen, then patient-specific information can be combined with prior information about the mean values, their variances, and the variance of the intrasubject errors. This enables the prediction of the most probable parameter value(s) for an individual patient from *observed* concentrations or responses. However, population pharmacokinetic approaches can be limited in their accuracy (and hence, clinical utility) if a given patient for whom parameter estimates are being generated is not represented by the population from which prior estimates of mean parameters or variance were derived.

Presently, the U.S. Food and Drug Administration is advocating the use of population pharmacokinetic approaches to gather pharmacokinetic information during the development of new drugs. In Phase II studies (i.e., those which define the disposition profile of a drug in patients who would be likely to receive it therapeutically), population-based approaches have been successfully used to characterize the pharmacokinetics and pharmacodynamics of drugs with multiple dosing. This particular application holds promise for the study of new drugs in infants and children where logistical constraints often prohibit excessive blood sampling required to support more traditional approaches to data analysis. In Phase III studies (i.e., investigations of efficacy, safety, and tolerance of a new drug used to treat a disease for which it is intended), population-based approaches enable the collection of pharmacokinetic data in relatively large numbers of patients from sparse numbers of blood samples during therapy. Thus, pharmacokinetic data sufficient to examine the impact of disease state, age, and/or concomitant therapy can be generated with sufficient accuracy so as to enable a more complete characterization of a drug's disposition profile. Presently, applications of population pharmacokinetic methods to medical practice are limited consequent to technological constraints (e.g., the general availability of software and professionals skilled in its use). However, when appropriately applied, these techniques can be valuable in that they enable the prediction of steady state dose vs. concentration and/or effect relationships from limited amounts of non-steady state data in patients. In addition, they can be used to model exposure-response relationships and to derive drug doses for patients of a specific age with a given disease state.

Increasingly, pharmacokinetic/pharmacodynamic modeling is being used in drug research and development. The attribute of population-based approaches that resides with sparse sampling ostensibly permits examination of both pharmacokinetics and pharmacodynamics during phase III of drug development (i.e., the conduct of pivotal safety and efficacy trials). This approach not only enables evaluation in larger numbers of subjects (i.e., hundreds to thousands in phase III development versus tens to hundreds in phase II) but, most importantly, in the context of a disease under treatment for which the test article is intended. Consequently, the true variability in drug disposition and action is better reflected by incorporating population-based pharmacokinetics and pharmacodynamics into treatment trials. As well, this approach may also reduce the time for drug development by enabling greater adaptive control over dose selection and attainment of target levels of drug exposure than traditional phase III approaches where multiple fixed doses of a drug were evaluated.

Finally, an important caveat to be considered in the application of population-based approaches is that of model appropriateness. The nature of the application of a population-based model must be taken into account during the entire modeling process. The intended use of a model should influence both the attitude of the pharmacokineticist and also the modeling approaches used during the analyses. An a priori determination of covariates considered physiologically/pharmacologically relevant should be made, along with a determination of which parameters are of primary concern (i.e., are clinically relevant). Also, the extent and method of model evaluation and validation must be considered to ensure the appropriateness of the model for a given drug and the set of experimental conditions (e.g., sampling times relative to expected disposition/action profile of the drug).

Projection of Human Pharmacokinetics from Animal Data

The prediction of pharmacokinetic parameters and dosing regimens in man from data obtained in laboratory animals is referred to as *interspecies scaling*. Interspecies scaling is most commonly achieved through the allometric approach which establishes quantitative relationships between the pharmacokinetic parameters of interest and a physiological characteristic of the animal. Simply, allometry is a method used for interpolation and extrapolation based on physiologic, anatomic, and biochemical similarities between species. These techniques assume that physiologic variables which govern drug disposition (e.g., organ weight, organ clearance, heart rate, and biochemical processes) are related to the weight or body surface area of the animal species (including human).

To facilitate the process of interspecies scaling, artificial *neural networks* have been developed. These computer-based techniques are used in the prediction of response variables from a set of input and target parameters. The most commonly used network in the area of pattern recognition is the feed forward/back propagation (BPN) network. BPN with a combination of physicochemical properties and pharmacokinetic parameters derived from animals has been used to predict important pharmacokinetic parameters (e.g., V_d, Cl_{tot}) with reasonable accuracy. In the drug development process, data available from preclinical testing can be applied using interspecies scaling to project both drug disposition characteristics in man and also dosing regimens for consideration of use during Phase I of drug development (i.e., the first-dose in man to evaluate pharmacokinetics and tolerance).

Selected References

1. Amsden, G. W., Ballow, C. H. and Schentag, J. J.: Population Pharmacokinetic Methods to Optimise Antibiotic Effects, *Drug Invest.* 5:256–268 (1993).

2. Derendorf, H., Lesko, L. J., Chaikin, P., Colburn, W. A., Lee, P., Miller, R., Powell, R., et al.: Pharmaco-kinetic/Pharmacodynamic Modeling in Drug Research and Development. *J. Clin. Pharmacol. 40*: 1399–1418 (2000).

3. Dettli, L.: *Elimination Kinetics and Dosage Adjustment of Drugs in Patients with Kidney Disease,* Progress in Pharmacology, Vol. 1, No. 4. Gustav Fischer Verlag Stuttgart, 1977.

4. Ette, E. I., Williams, P. J., Kim, Y. H., Lane, J. R., Liu, M-J. and Capparelli, E. W.: Model Appropriateness and Population Pharmacokinetic Modeling. *J. Clin. Pharmacol. 43*:610–623 (2003).

5. Hussain, A. S., Johnson, R. D., Vachharajani, N. N. and Ritschel, W. A.: Feasibility of Developing a Neural Network for Prediction of Human Pharmacokinetic Parameters from Animal Data, *Pharm. Res. 10*:466–469 (1993).

6. Ludden, T. M.: Population Pharmacokinetics, *J. Clin. Pharmacol. 28*:1059–1063 (1988).

7. Ritschel, W. A.: Dose Size and Dosing Interval Determination. *Arzneim. Forsch. 25*:1442 (1975).

8. Ritschel, W. A. and Thompson, G. A.: The One-Point Method in Predicting Dosage Regimen in Case of Hepatic and/or Renal Failure in Presence or Absence of Change in Volume of Distribution. *J. Clin. Pharmacol. 19*:350 (1979).

9. Ritschel, W. A., Vachharajani, N. N., Johnson, R. D. and Hussain, A. S.: Allometric Approach for Interspecies Scaling of Pharmacokinetic Parameters. *Comp. Biochem. Physiol. 103*:249–253 (1992).

10. Ritschel, W. A., Akileswaran, R. and Hussain, A. S.: Application of Neural Networks for the Prediction of Human Pharmacokinetic Parameters, *Meth. Find. Exp. Clin. Pharmacol. 17*:629–643 (1995).

11. Samara, E. and Granneman, R.: Role of Population Pharmacokinetics in Drug Development: A Pharmaceutical Industry Perspective. *Clin. Pharmacokinet. 32*:294–312 (1997).

12. Sheiner, L. B. and Ludden, T. M.: Population Pharmacokinetics/Dynamics. *Ann. Rev. Pharmacol. Toxicol. 32*:185–209 (1992).

29

Drug Monitoring and Dose Adjustment

A patient receiving drug therapy, regardless of whether the dosage regimen designed is based on literature mean pharmacokinetic parameters as discussed in Chapter 28 or on implementation of an empirical dosage regimen, should be clinically evaluated for response. If the clinical response is satisfactory, there is no reason for change of the dosage regimen. If the response does not reach the expected effect or side effects or toxicity is observed, the dosage regimen may have to be adjusted or a different drug or therapy used.

One aspect of total monitoring is the therapeutic drug monitoring via blood level determination. Another reason for drug monitoring via blood levels is *noncompliance* with a prescribed dosage regimen. It is believed that about 60 percent of the patients fail to take their medications as directed.

However, drug monitoring for all drugs and in all patients is neither possible nor feasible because of problems with logistics, manpower, time, and for economic reasons. Furthermore, total drug monitoring, at least at present, is not relevant for all drugs. For the so-called *hit-and-run drugs,* i.e., those drugs for which, at this time, there is no known correlation between pharmacologic response and pharmacokinetic disposition (antidepressants during the first 2 to 3 weeks, antihypertensives such as bethanidine, debrisoquin, and guanethidine, azathioprine, monoamine oxidase inhibitors, nitroglycerin, reserpine, nonmercurial diuretics), therapeutic drug monitoring via blood levels is not feasible.

For those drugs for which a pharmacological response is easily, quickly, and accurately measured (blood pressure, blood glucose, electrolyte excretion, urinary output, etc.), it is clinically more relevant to directly monitor the response.

Therapeutic drug monitoring via blood levels is indicated for a number of drugs or drug groups that either show normally large interindividual variation or have a narrow therapeutic range. These include the antiepileptics (phenytoin, carbamazepine, phenobarbital), antiarrhythmics (digoxin, lidocaine, procainamide, acetylprocainamide), theophylline, tricyclic antidepressants, lithium, and the aminoglycosides.

Blood level adjustment, wherever possible, should be done for a dosage regimen when steady state has been reached. As a rule of thumb, steady state is assumed if dosing has been done for at least $5 \cdot t_{1/2}$ of the drug.

Whenever possible, the trough concentration at steady state C_{min}^{ss} should be used for dosage adjustment. However, in some cases (aminoglycosides), one may use the peak level C_{max}^{ss}, particularly at the end of short-term infusions. For adjustment of sustained release preparations (theophylline) a C_{av}^{ss} about 2/3 in the dosing interval may be used.

One has to be aware of pitfalls and errors, such as time of sampling relative to the dose administration, exact recording of dose, route of administration, and sampling time.

Adjustment of Dose at Steady State

If a present dosage regimen results in a steady state concentration C_{found}^{ss} that deviates from the desired target concentration $C_{desired}^{ss}$, adjustment can be made as follows:

$$DM_{adjusted} = \frac{C_{av\ desired}^{ss}}{C_{av\ found}^{ss}} \cdot DM_{used} \tag{1}$$

$$DM_{adjusted} = \frac{C_{max\ desired}^{ss}}{C_{max\ found}^{ss}} \cdot DM_{used} \tag{2}$$

$$DM_{adjusted} = \frac{C_{min\ desired}^{ss}}{C_{min\ found}^{ss}} \cdot DM_{used} \tag{3}$$

where $DM_{adjusted}$ and DM_{used} are in mg and C_{index}^{ss} (C_{av}^{ss} or C_{max}^{ss} or C_{min}^{ss} for desired and found concentration) in μg/ml.

If the found blood level is much higher than the desired therapeutic concentration, $C_{found}^{ss} \gg C_{desired}^{ss}$, dosing should be interrupted until the actual blood level has returned to the desired one. The time required to discontinue dosing, $t_{discontinue}$, is calculated by:

$$t_{discontinue} = \frac{\ln C_{min\ found}^{ss} - \ln C_{min\ desired}^{ss}}{0.693/t_{1/2}} [h] \tag{4}$$

where $t_{1/2}$ is the terminal half-life in hours. For correction of $t_{1/2}$ in renal failure, see Equation 28.20.

After $t_{discontinue}$ has passed, the $DM_{adjusted}$ is implemented, maintaining the dosing interval as used before adjustment.

Adjustment of Dose for Drugs with Saturation Kinetics

For drugs exhibiting saturation or Michaelis-Menten kinetics at steady state, such as in case of phenytoin, the steady state concentration C_1^{ss} and C_2^{ss} in mg/l after two different dose rates R_1 and R_2 in mg/day must be known. Then the clearance (Cl) in 1/day, Michaelis-Menten constant K_m in mg/l, and the maximum rate of metabolism V_{max} in mg/day are calculated which are used to determine the adjusted dose rate $R_{adjusted}$ in mg/day:

$$Cl_1 = \frac{R_1}{C_1^{ss}}; \quad Cl_2 = \frac{R_2}{C_2^{ss}} \tag{5}$$

$$K_m = \frac{R_1 - R_2}{C_1 - C_2} \tag{6}$$

$$V_{max} = \frac{C_1^{ss} - C_2^{ss}}{1/Cl_1 - 1/Cl_2} \tag{7}$$

$$R_{adjusted} = \frac{V_{max} \cdot C_{desired}^{ss}}{K_m + C_{desired}^{ss}} [mg/day] \tag{8}$$

If the found steady state concentration is higher than the desired therapeutic concentration, $C_{found}^{ss} \gg C_{desired}^{ss}$, dosing should be halted for some time, $t_{discontinue}$, before the $R_{adjusted}$ is implemented:

$$t_{discontinue} = \frac{K_m \cdot \ln(C_{found}^{ss}/C_{desired}^{ss}) + (C_{found}^{ss} - C_{desired}^{ss})}{V_{max}/V_d} [h] \tag{9}$$

Drugs which usually follow Michaelis-Menten kinetics in the therapeutic dose range are listed at the end of Chapter 13, "Drug Metabolism."

Conversion from IV Constant Rate Infusion to IV or EV Multiple Dosing

Often an acutely ill patient may be on IV constant rate infusion until clinically improved. It may then be desirable to switch therapy to either IV push injection or EV administration. Knowing the last, effective rate of infusion R° in mg/h, the new dosage regimen for IV or EV administration is calculated after having selected an appropriate dosing interval τ in h:

$$DM_{for\ I.V.\ or\ E.V.} = \frac{R^\circ}{f} \cdot \tau \tag{10}$$

where f is the absolute bioavailability.

Selected References

1. Ritschel, W. A.: Pitfalls and Errors in Drug Monitoring: Pharmacokinetic Aspects, *Methods Find. Exp. Pharmacol.* 5:559 (1983).

2. Ritschel, W. A.: Therapeutic Drug Monitoring, In: *Clinical Chemistry: Theory, Analysis, and Correlation,* Kaplan, L. A. and Pesce, A. J., editors, The C. V. Mosby Co., St. Louis, 1984, p. 962 ff.

3. Witmer, D. R. and Ritschel, W. A.: Phenytoin-Isoniazid Interaction: A Kinetic Approach to Management, *Drug Intell. Clin. Pharm.* 18:483–486 (1984).

30

Physiological and Pathological Factors Influencing Drug Response

Whereas *classical* pharmacokinetics is concerned with establishing models to describe the drug's LADMER system and to elaborate on the "normal" pharmacokinetic parameters in healthy man, *clinical* pharmacokinetics is concerned with the adaptation of the drug concentration-time pattern in the body to one or more altered physiological and/or pathological conditions in the individual patient to optimize drug therapy.

There are so many factors involved which are often interwoven and overlapping that the entire aspect of physiologically and pathologically altered drug disposition is extremely complex. The purpose of this basic handbook and the space available do not permit adequate coverage of this area. Therefore, only the most important factors are listed with a brief description of their impact on pharmacokinetics.

Body Weight

Normal dose sizes are designed for the average adult body weight of 70 kg. Hence, such a dose size will result in lower drug concentrations in patients of high body weight and in higher drug concentrations in those of lower body weight. Dose size adjustment, if necessary, can simply be made on a mg/kg basis:

$$D_{desired} = \frac{BW_{patient}}{70} \cdot D_{normal} \tag{1}$$

However, this adjustment is not applicable for obese (i.e., if the actual BW is more than 20 percent of the BW_{ideal}; see Chapter 26) and edematous (>5 liters of edema fluid) patients.

Newborns and Children

The newborn has a different body composition than the adult with respect to amount and distribution of body fluids and fat and has immature hepatic and renal functions. Both hepatic and renal function, although not fully developed, are, at the age of 6 months in term infants, similar to that of the adult. The maturation process may take longer in premature infants. For dosing in children see Chapter 24. Beyond the age of two years, dosing adjustment can usually be made on a mg/kg basis. Special care in dosing is warranted in newborns.

Aged

With increasing age the fraction of lean body mass decreases and that of fat tissue increases, even if the body weight remains unchanged throughout adulthood. The various organ and tissue blood flow rates and the renal function decrease. Also, the rate of metabolism may change. Literature reports on more than 70 drugs indicate that, in general, the elimination half-life increases with advancing age. However, it would be erroneous to adjust the dosage regimen based solely on the half-life, because the volume of distribution may also change by either an increase or decrease. If V_d increases it may compensate for a prolonged $t_{1/2}$ resulting in unchanged drug clearance. In this case the dosage regimen should not be changed, but it will take longer to achieve steady state which depends on $t_{1/2}$ and τ. This aspect should be kept in mind for the monitoring of drug concentrations. If the V_d decreases, smaller dose sizes are required. For dosing in geriatric patients see Chapter 25.

Temperature

Decreased body temperature (hypothermia) may influence all phases of the LADMER-system. Exposure to heat (hyperthermia) and high relative humidity may result in depletion of body water and salt (decrease in ECF) and, hence, change the V_d.

Gastric Emptying Time

The transit time of a drug through the stomach may profoundly influence the rate and extent of absorption. Factors influencing the gastric emptying time are: amount and type of solid food, amount of fluid, viscosity of GI-content, pH, position of patient (slowest emptying when lying in the left supine position), stress, drugs given concomitantly, and temperature. Enteric coated preparations and those inactivated by gastric fluid should be given with 250 ml of ice-water ($\simeq 5°C$) to ensure rapid stomach emptying ($\simeq 15$ min), whereas warm fluid significantly delays stomach emptying time (see also Chapter 10).

Blood Flow Rates

Drugs are distributed within the body leaving the systemic circulation in the capillary bed and entering interstitial fluid and tissue cells. The total length of capillaries in man is approximately 95,000 km. In the perfused tissue no cell is further apart from a capillary than approximately 0.125 mm. A decrease in perfusion results in a temporary closing of the capillaries and, hence, a reduced rate and extent of distribution.

The tissue perfusion depends on the blood flow rates in the various tissues, which in turn depend on the cardiac output. Bed rest, hypothermia, shock, and heart failure reduce blood flow rates, and physical exercise increases them. The blood flow rates may influence all phases of the LADMER system.

Environment

Environmental factors such as smoking, living in a city or an industrial area, and exposure to various insecticides may play an important role in regulating the activity of metabolic enzyme systems, resulting in enzyme induction of various drugs. In contrast, some industrial chemicals such as the halogenated hydrocarbons may produce renal and hepatic damage, thus prolonging the $t_{1/2}$ of some drugs.

High altitude reduces the cardiac output and may delay all phases of the LADMER system.

Nutrition

The nutritional status influences the activities of the hepatic enzyme systems. Undernutrition and vitamin deficiencies exist not only in developing countries but are also frequent in highly industrialized countries. The lack of adequate protein synthesis may cause hypoalbuminemia and reduced rate of metabolism. Thus, the V_d may be changed, resulting in a higher fraction of free drug in plasma (increased intensity of effect, increased toxicity) and higher accumulation of drug due to reduced metabolic capacity.

Pregnancy

During pregnancy the fraction of fat tissue increases, the change in hormonal secretion may cause changes in drug metabolism, and the increase in renal blood flow may enhance renal elimination of drugs. Additionally, during pregnancy another pharmacokinetic compartment, the fetus, must be added to which the drug distributes (see Chapter 27).

Genetics

Genetically based variations in drug response are primarily caused by mutations of DNA, which result in structural changes of proteins involved in the different pharmacokinetic phases of absorption, distribution, metabolism, and elimination and in drug-receptor interactions. Drugs for which differences in response and/or disposition have been found to be due to genetic control are: antipyrine, bishydroxycoumarin (dicumarol), ethanol, halothane, hydralazine, INH, nortriptyline, phenylbutazone, succinylcholine, and warfarin.

Circadian Rhythm—Diurnal Rhythm

The biological clock controlling rhythms of life processes in the body may influence all phases of the LADMER system. The circadian rhythm is caused by endogenous rhythms (hormones) whereas the diurnal rhythm is caused by external synchronizers or "zeitgeber" (dark-light, sleep-awake, etc.).

Differences in blood concentration-time curves were found for acetaminophen, aminopyrine, amphetamine, antipyrine, carbamazepine, cortisol, ethanol, ethosuximide, glucose, guanethidine, iron, lithium, meperidine, methylene blue, minocycline, nortriptyline, phenacetin, phenytoin, prednisolone, potassium, prostaglandins, salicylate, sulfisomidine, tetracycline, tolbutamide, thyroxine, valproic acid, and others.

The pharmacologic response to various drugs has been found to follow a circadian or diurnal rhythm. It is not yet established whether or not there are differences in the blood concentration-time curves; it might be that these variations are caused by variations in the receptor sensitivity. Examples include antihistamines, local anesthetics, and chlorpromazine.

Cardiovascular Diseases

The increased filling pressure resulting in increased stroke volume may congest vital organs, which in association with sodium retention leads to formation of edema. The reduced cardiac output results in reduced perfusion of liver, kidney, splanchnic area, muscle tissue, and skin. Pulmonary edema and reduced perfusion may result in hypoxia and systemic acidosis.

Decreased absorption rates in congestive heart failure have been found for a number of drugs: aprindine, digoxin, hydrochlorothiazide, metolazone, procainamide, and quinidine. A prolonged hepatic clearance in congestive heart failure was found for lidocaine and theophylline. A reduced volume of distribution in congestive heart failure was documented for digoxin and other drugs (see next section under Renal Diseases).

Renal Diseases

Drugs which are predominantly cleared via the kidney will accumulate to higher drug concentrations in the plasma of patients with poor renal perfusion (congestive heart failure, shock, trauma) or with intrinsic renal diseases (acute renal failure, chronic renal failure) than in normal subjects.

In the presence of renal diseases some metabolic functions seem to be impaired. These have been documented for: reduction (hydrocortisone), acetylation (INH, hydralazine, sulfisoxazole, PAS), and ester hydrolysis (clindamycin phosphate, erythromycin estolate, indanyl carbenicillin, prednisolone hemisuccinate). Recent studies have demonstrated that the activity of specific drug-metabolizing enzymes is altered in patients with renal disease. As reflected by the erythromycin breath test, the activity of CYP3A4 is approximately 30% lower in adults with end-stage renal disease. Similar reductions have been reported for both CYP2D6 and CYP2C9 (50% reduction). Currently, the reasons for these disease-associated changes are not readily apparent. Possibilities include increased carbon dioxide production rates in patients with chronic renal failure and exposure to environmental contaminants (e.g., polyvinyl chloride plastics) associated with dialysis treatment.

A reduced volume of distribution in renal failure has been documented for ampicillin, cephacetrile, cephalexin, digoxin, insulin, lincomycin, methicillin, metolazone, quinidine, and propranolol.

Liver Diseases

Liver disease is not a single well defined status but comprises a number of various structural and functional conditions, ranging from inflammatory and degenerative to neoplastic insults to the hepatic parenchyma and biliary tree, often associated with reduced blood flow to the organ.

Table 30-1 lists the most important pharmacologic consequences due to pathophysiologic abnormalities in patients with various liver impairments.

Table 30-1. Pharmacological Consequences Due to Pathophysiological Abnormalities in Liver Diseases

PATHOPHYSIOLOGIC CONDITION	PHARMACOLOGICAL CONSEQUENCES
Impaired hepatic blood flow (heart failure, cirrhosis, portal vein thrombosis)	↓ systemic clearance for drugs with high hepatic extraction (E > 0.7)
Reduced hepatic cell mass (cirrhosis, acute and chronic active hepatitis, acute alcohol intoxication)	↓ FPE for drugs with high hepatic extraction (E > 0.7) ↓ systemic clearance for drugs with low hepatic extraction (E < 0.3)
Decreased protein binding (hepatitis, cholestasis, cirrhosis)	Increased distribution of drugs into liver (increased elimination) and other tissues
Cholestasis (primary biliary cirrhosis, common duct obstruction, drug induced)	Impaired metabolism
Portal-systemic shunt (cirrhosis, portal vein thrombosis, shunt operation)	Increased systemic bioavailability for drugs with high hepatic extraction (E > 0.7)

At present there is no single liver function test available which would permit generation of a correction factor for dosage regimen design. However, some general guidelines have been suggested as listed in Table 30-2.

In cirrhosis, a chronic condition, the total clearance of all but one of the drugs tested decreased (amobarbital, ampicillin, antipyrine, chloramphenicol, diazepam, INH, lidocaine, meperidine, phenobarbital, and phenylbutazone). Only tolbutamide clearance was not changed. In acute viral hepatitis a decreased clearance was found for antipyrine, diazepam, hexobarbital, and meperidine. No change in clearance was found for lidocaine, phenobarbital, phenylbutazone, phenytoin, and warfarin. For tolbutamide an increased clearance was observed. In chronic active hepatitis and obstructive jaundice the total clearance seems to be decreased.

In liver disease, particularly in cirrhosis, the ability for synthesis of serum albumin and other macromolecules is impaired, resulting in hypoalbuminemia which, as a consequence, may change the drug's volume of distribution, rate of metabolism and renal elimination. The distribution of the drug is a complicating factor in drug disposition in the case of hypoalbuminemia caused by liver disease. With decreasing binding it can be expected that the volume of distribution will increase. An increase in V_d in liver disease was observed in cirrhotic patients for amobarbital, ampicillin, diazepam, lidocaine, propranolol, and thiopental. However, these increases in V_d sometimes cannot be explained on a basis of reduced binding alone. A change in body composition, such as ascites, may also be responsible (e.g., for diazepam, lidocaine, and propranolol).

The rate of metabolism is primarily a function of the activity of the hepatic microsomal drug metabolizing enzyme system, the LBF, and, in some cases, the ratio of free to bound drug and the normal extent of metabolism. In acute hepatitis the plasma concentration of methyldigoxin is increased, whereas that of digoxin remains unchanged, because the first drug (methyldigoxin) is predominantly eliminated by metabolism, and the latter (digoxin) by

Table 30-2. Pharmacokinetic Classification of Drugs in Risk Groups for PO Use in Patients with Liver Impairment

RISK GROUP	HEPATIC ELIMINATION	EXAMPLES	CONSEQUENCES FOR DOSAGE DESIGN
High	high extraction (E > 0.7), flow limited	clomethiazole, ergotamine tartrate, labetolol, lorcainide, meperidine, niridazol, nitroglycerin, pentazocine, propoxyphene, propranolol, salicylamide, verapamil	Reduce DL and DM
Limited	low extraction (E < 0.3), capacity limited	aminopyrine, antipyrine, azapropazone, caffeine, cefoperazone, chloramphenicol, chlordiazepoxide, clindamycin, diazepam, hexobarbital, methyldigoxin, paracetamol, pentobarbital, phenobarbital, rifampicin, theophylline, zomepirac	Reduce DM only
Low	Little or no change	ampicillin, carbenicillin, cimetidine, clofibrate, colchicine, digoxin, furosemide, isoniazid, lorazepam, methadone, morphine, naproxen, oxazepam, PAS, phenylbutazone, prednisone, prednisolone, spironolactone, thiamphenicol, tolbutamide, valproic acid	No change in dosage regime

renal excretion. The rate of metabolism of diazepam and meperidine is reduced in acute viral hepatitis, and that of barbiturates and phenytoin was found to be decreased in patients with hepatic necrosis.

Liver disease may also alter extrahepatic drug metabolism. The pseudocholinesterase activity in blood may be reduced in liver impairment, resulting in prolongation of the effect of succinylcholine.

It should also be noted that in liver disease some portion of portal blood may be deviated from the liver to the systemic circulation. Hence, in such cases the first-pass effect may be diminished and an increased systemic availability results which may increase the pharmacologic response or lead to toxicity.

Selected References

1. Benet, L. Z., editor: *The Effect of Disease States on Drug Pharmacokinetics*—American Pharmaceutical Association, Washington, D.C., 1976.
2. Bircher, J.: Altered Drug Metabolism in Liver Disease—Therapeutic Implications. In: *Recent Advances in Hepatology*, Thomas, H. C. and MacSween, R. N. M., editors, Churchill Livingstone, Edinburgh, 1983, p. 101.
3. Bonate, P. L.: Gender-Related Differences in Xenobiotic Metabolism, *J. Clin. Pharmacol.* 31:684–690 (1991).
4. Creasey, W. A.: *Drug Disposition in Humans*, Oxford University Press, New York—Oxford, 1979.
5. Curry, S. H.: *Drug Disposition and Pharmacokinetics*, Blackwell, Oxford-London-Edinburgh-Melbourne, 1974.
6. Dowling, T. C., Briglia, A. E., Fink, J. C., Hanes, D. S., Light, P. D., Stackiewicz, L., Karyekar, C. S., et al.: Characterization of Hepatic Cytochrome P4503A Activity in Patients with End-Stage Renal Disease. *Clin. Pharmacol. Ther.* 73:427–434 (2003).

7. Dreisbach, A. W., Japa, S., Gebrekal, A. B., Mowry, S. E., Lertora, J. J. L., Kamath, B. L., Rettie, A. E.: Cytochrome P4502C9 Activity in End-Stage Renal Disease (letter). *Clin. Pharmacol. Ther. 73*:475–477 (2003).

8. Gibaldi, M. *Biopharmaceutics and Clinical Pharmacokinetics,* 2nd Ed., Lea and Febiger, Philadelphia, 1977.

9. Guttendorf, R. J. and Wedlund, P. J.: Genetic Aspects of Drug Disposition and Therapeutics, *J. Clin. Pharmacol. 32*:107–117 (1992).

10. Houghton, I. T., Chan, K., Wong, Y. C., Aun, C. S. T., Lau, O. W. and Lowe, D. M.: Pethidine Pharmacokinetics After Intramuscular Dose: A Comparison in Caucasian, Chinese and Nepalese Patients, *Meth. Find. Exp. Clin. Pharmacol. 14*:451–458 (1992).

11. Levy, G., editor: *Clinical Pharmacokinetics—A Symposium,* American Pharmaceutical Association, Washington, D.C., 1974.

12. Mauro, V. P., Mauro, L. S. and Hageman, J. H.: Comparison of Pentoxifylline Pharmacokinetics Between Smokers and Nonsmokers, *J. Clin. Pharmacol. 32*:1054–1058 (1992).

13. Niazi, S.: *Textbook of Biopharmaceutics and Clinical Pharmacokinetics,* Appleton-Century-Crofts, New York, 1979.

14. Ritschel, W. A., Editor: *Clinical Pharmacokinetics—Proceeding of an International Symposium at Saltzgitter—Ringelheim,* Gustav Fischer Verlag, Stuttgart—New York, 1977.

15. Ritschel, W. A.: Clinical Pharmacokinetics. In: *Remington's Pharmaceutical Sciences,* 16th Ed. Osol, P., editor 1980, p. 702.

16. Ritschel, W. A. and Forusz, H.: Chronopharmacology: A Review of Drugs Studied, *Meth. Find. Exp. Clin. Pharmacol. 16*:57–75 (1994).

17. Smith, S. E. and Rawlings, M. D.: *Variability in Human Drug Response,* Butterworth, London, 1973.

18. Zhou, H. H., Sheller, J. R., Nu, H., Wood, M. and Wood, A. J. J.: Ethnic Differences in Response to Morphine, *Clin. Pharmacol. Ther. 54*:507–513 (1993).

31

First Dose Size in Man

The question of the magnitude of the first dose size to be administered to man in Phase I drug study poses a problem which should be considered from three different points of view: safety, analytical sensitivity, and pharmacokinetics.

Safety. The dose should be as low as possible in order not to expose the subject to undue risk.

Analytical sensitivity. The dose must be high enough to obtain measurable drug concentrations in blood which can reproducibly be followed up for a length of time as dictated by the drug's disposition.

Pharmacokinetics. In order to obtain relevant pharmacokinetic information, the drug concentration-time profile in blood should be followed up for at least $3 \cdot t_{1/2}$, or 10 percent of the peak concentration.

However, since the drug has not been given to man, no information on the volume of distribution is available. Before the first dose is given to man, one should know what drug concentration can be expected, and consequently have an analytical method available to accurately determine the drug concentration for pharmacokinetic evaluation. The following procedure is suggested.

Dose Size Estimate

An estimate on the first dose to be used in man is usually obtained from LD_{50} values from acute toxicity studies in various animal species. The first dose in man with reasonable safety is:

$$\text{1st Dose in man} < \frac{LD_{50}}{200} \tag{1}$$

where LD_{50} is the lowest LD_{50} found in any of the tested animal species. (For toxic compounds, 600 is used in the denominator of Equation 31.1.)

Let us assume the LD_{50} was 200 mg/kg. One two-hundredth of this dose is 1 mg/kg. Since the first dose shall be $<LD_{50}/200$, a dose of 50 mg might be considered for a man of 70 kg body weight.

Estimate on Volume of Distribution in Man

The volumes of distribution for the one-compartment model V_d, and the two-compartment model V_c, V_{dss}, and $V_{d\beta}$ can be estimated from in vitro data, namely the apparent lipid/water (*n*-octanol/buffer pH 7.4) partition coefficient APC, and the extent of protein binding (fraction) p (to 4 percent human albumin).

One-Compartment Model:

$$V_d = (0.0955 \cdot APC + 1.2232) \cdot (1-p) \cdot BW \, [ml] \qquad (2)$$

Two-Compartment Model:

$$V_c = (0.0397 \cdot APC + 0.0273) \cdot (1-p) \cdot BW \, [ml] \qquad (3)$$

$$V_{dss} = (0.1141 \cdot APC + 0.6611) \cdot (1-p) \cdot BW \, [ml] \qquad (4)$$

$$V_{d\beta} = (0.1302 \cdot APC + 0.9314) \cdot (1-p) \cdot BW \, [ml] \qquad (5)$$

Let us assume the drug has an APC of 5.4 and is 85 percent bound to protein. For a 70 kg person the volumes of distribution are:

$$V_d = 18,258 \, ml$$
$$V_c = 2538 \, ml$$
$$V_{dss} = 13,411 \, ml$$
$$V_{d\beta} = 17,162 \, ml$$

However, we do not know whether the drug would follow a one- or two-compartment model. An APC of 5.4 and high protein binding suggest that a two-compartment model might apply after IV dosing.

Estimate on Initial Concentration

The fictitious zero-time concentration after IV administration is:

$$C(0) = \frac{Dose}{V_d} \, (\text{one-compartment model}) \qquad (6)$$

$$C(0) = \frac{Dose}{V_c} \, (\text{two-compartment model}) \qquad (7)$$

If the one-compartment model applies, the $C(0)$ would be 2.7 µg/ml, and if the two-compartment model applies, $C(0)$ would be 19.7 µg/ml.

Required Analytical Sensitivity

Since the drug concentration-time profile has to be followed up to 10 percent of the peak concentration, the lowest concentration would be 10 percent of the $C(0)$ value for the one-compartment model.

The lowest expected concentration would be 0.27 µg/ml, and the highest could be about 19.7 µg/ml in our example. Hence, the assay range for the first dose size should be between 20 and 0.25 µg/ml.

Selected References

1. Ritschel, W. A.: Planning, Executing and Evaluating the Pharmacokinetics in Phase I Studies, In *Problems of Clinical Pharmacology in Therapeutic Research: Phase I,* Kuemmerle, H. P., Shibuya, T. K. and Kimura, E., editors, Urban and Schwarzenberg, Munich, 1977, p. 212.

2. Ritschel, W. A. and Hammer, G. V.: Prediction of the Volume of Distribution from In Vitro Data and Use for Estimating the Absolute Extent of Absorption, *Int. J. Clin. Pharmacol. Ther. Toxicol. 18*:298 (1980).

32

Forensic Pharmacokinetics

In forensic medicine it is often required to estimate the dose size administered or ingested by the deceased, based on either a postmortem blood level or urine drug concentration. Ideally, creatinine clearance should be known, or serum creatinine should be determined in the blood sample, and converted to creatinine clearance, which is corrected for age and sex and normalized for body surface area:

$$SA = \frac{167.2 \cdot \sqrt{BW} \cdot \sqrt{H}}{10000} [m^2] \tag{1}$$

$$Cl_{\text{creat. observed}} = \frac{(140 - A) \cdot BW \cdot S}{72 \cdot Cr_{\text{ser found}}} [ml/min] \tag{2}$$

$$Cl_{\text{creat. observed corrected}} = \frac{Cl_{\text{creat. observed}} \cdot 1.73}{SA} [ml/min/1.73\,m^2] \tag{3}$$

SA   = body surface area $[m^2]$
BW   = body weight [kg]
H   = body height [cm]
A   = age [years]
S   = correction factor for sex: males $S = 1$
        females $S = 0.9$
$Cr_{\text{serum found}}$ = serum creatinine in deceased [mg/100 ml]
$Cl_{\text{creat. observed}}$ = observed creatinine clearance in deceased [ml/min]
$Cl_{\text{creat. observed corrected}}$ = corrected creatinine clearance in deceased [ml/min/1.73 m²]

Estimate on Ingested or Administered Dose Size from Postmortem Blood Sample

$$D_{\text{estimated}} = \frac{C_{\text{found}} \cdot \Delta' \cdot BW}{f \cdot e^{-k_{el}} \cdot \left\{ \left[\left(\frac{Cl_{\text{creat. observed corrected}}}{120 \cdot S} - 1 \right) \cdot F_{el} \right] + 1 \right\} \cdot (t_d - t_{int})} [mg] \tag{4}$$

291

$D_{estimated}$ = estimated dose size of drug taken before death [mg]
C_{found} = drug concentration in postmortem blood sample [µg/ml]
Δ' = apparent volume of distribution of drug [l/kg]
BW = body weight [kg]
f = absolute bioavailability (fraction of drug absorbed)
k_{el} = elimination rate constant [h⁻¹]
F_{el} = fraction of unchanged drug eliminated in urine (fraction of 1)
S = correction factor for Sex:
males S = 1
females S = 0.9
t_d = decimal clock time of death [h]
t_{int} = decimal clock time of assumed drug intake [h]

Notes:

1. If t_d and t_{int} are not known, it is assumed that death occurs at or shortly after peak concentration. Hence, carry out calculations twice: once, substituting t_{max} for ($t_d - t_{int}$), and once substituting $2 \cdot t_{max}$ for ($t_d - t_{int}$). This will give the probable range for $D_{estimated}$. The peak time t_{max} in hours can be obtained from literature mean data.
2. If $Cr_{serum\ found}$ is not available, Equations 32.1, 32.2, and 32.3 are not relevant and not to be used. In Equation 32.4 substitute $120 \cdot S$ for $Cl_{creat\ observed\ corrected}$.
3. For compilation of pharmacokinetic parameters see Appendix.

Estimate on Ingested or Administered Dose Size from Postmortem Urine Sample

$$D_{estimated} = \frac{Ae_{found}}{(1 - e^{-k_{el}} \cdot \left\{ \left[\left(\frac{Cl_{creat.\ observed\ corrected}}{120 \cdot S} - 1 \right) \cdot F_{el} \right] + 1 \right\} \cdot (t_d - t_{int}) \cdot f \cdot F_{el})} [mg] \quad (5)$$

Ae_{found} = amount of drug found in postmortem urine sample [mg] (the amount is calculated from the drug concentration in urine Ae_u [mg/ml] and the volume of urine recovered from the bladder V [ml]; $Ae_{found} = Ae_u \cdot V$)

For definitions of other parameters see those listed for Eq. 32.4, including the Note.

Lethal Concentrations of Some Important Drugs

The lethal concentrations listed in Table 32-1 are not absolute values. Certain disease states and concomitant intake of alcohol and/or of other drugs may have increased toxicity; hence, lower than listed concentrations may be lethal. A comprehensive list of therapeutic, toxic, and lethal concentrations can be found by consulting the primary literature (*Meyer, 1994*).

Postmortem Changes in Pharmacokinetics

Postmortem changes begin at a cellular level with the onset of ischemia. As the duration of ischemia increases and death ensues, both the structure and function of organs and tissues

Table 32-1. Lethal Blood Concentrations of Drugs

DRUG	LETHAL CONCENTRATION [µg/ml]	DRUG	LETHAL CONCENTRATION [µg/ml]
Acetaminophen	1500	Imipramine	2
Alcohol	3500	Lidocaine	25
Allobarbital	20	Lithium	35
Amitriptyline	10–20	Meperidine	30
Amobarbital	10	Meprobamate	140–350
Amphetamine	2	Methadone	4
Aprobarbital	50	Methamphetamine	10–40
Aspirin	500	Methanol	900
Barbital	100	Methapyrilene	50
Brallobarbital	15	Methaqualone	30
Bromide	2000	Methylphenidate	2–3
Butabarbital	30	Methyprylone	50
Butalbital	25	Morphine	0.05–4
Caffeine	100	Nicotine	50–500
Carbamazepine	15	Nitrazepam	9
Carbromal	40	Nortriptyline	13
Chloral Hydrate	250	Orphenadrine	4–8
Chlordiazepoxide	20	Oxazepam	3
Chlorpromazine	3–12	Paraldehyde	500
Cocaine	1–20	Pentazocine	10–20
Codeine	0.2–0.6	Pentobarbital	15
Cyclobarbital	20	Phenobarbital	69
Desipramine	10–20	Phenytoin	100
Diazepam	20	Primidone	100
Diethylallylacetamide	45	Propallylonal	10
Digitoxin	0.3	Propoxyphene	0.8–2
Digoxin	0.015	Propranolol	8–12
Diphenhydramine	10	Propylhexedrine	2–3
Disopyramide	26	Quinidine	30–50
Doxepin	10	Quinine	12
Ethchlorvynol	150	Secobarbital	10
Flurazepam	0.5	Theophylline	210–250
Glutethimide	20–100	Thiopental	10–400
Halothane	200	Thioridazine	20–80
Heptabarbital	20	Trifluoperazine	3–8
Hexobarbital	50	Vinylbital	8
Hydromorphone	0.1–0.3		

progressively deteriorate. These changes may influence the distribution of drugs in body fluids and tissues, particularly those whose distribution is dependent upon molecular size, lipophilicity, pH, energy-dependent transport, and tissue binding (e.g., tricyclic antidepressants, digoxin, cimetidine, procainamide).

When evaluating drug concentrations after death, it is important to consider the phenomenon of **postmortem redistribution.** Specifically, it should be noted that postmortem drug concentrations may not reflect those at the time of death. Accordingly, it is possible that wrong conclusions can be drawn from postmortem blood level data if they cannot be reliably used to simulate the dose versus concentration versus effect (toxicity) relationship.

Selected References

1. Kulpmann, W. R.: *Internist 25*:60 (1984).
2. Meyer, F. P.: Indicative Therapeutic and Toxic Drug Concentrations in Plasma: A Tabulation: *Int. J. Clin. Pharmacol. Ther. 32*:71–81 (1994).
3. Shepherd, M. F., Lake, K. D. and Kamps, M. A.: Postmortem Changes and Pharmacokinetics: Review of the Literature and Case Report, *Ann. Pharmacother. 26*:510–514 (1992).
4. Winek, C. L.: *Drug and Chemical Blood Level Data 1980*, Fisher Scientific Co., Pittsburgh, 1980.

33

Nonlinear Pharmacokinetics

Detection of Nonlinearity

The classical pharmacokinetics as discussed thus far implies that with increased dose size peak height and amount of drug transferred to tissue will be directly proportional to the dose. However, it is evident that there are many deviations from linear pharmacokinetics with respect to one or more processes in absorption, distribution, binding to biological material in tissue, plasma protein binding, metabolism, and elimination of a drug.

Deviations from linearity with respect to absorption may be due to low solubility of the drug, low dissolution and/or release rate of the drug from the dosage form, changes in intestinal flow rate, change in pH of the intestinal content during intestinal transit, and, in the case of active absorption processes, due to saturation of the carriers.

Deviation from linearity with respect to tissue distribution may occur when tissues or active transport systems in the tissue compartment(s) become saturated. In this case one would find that the slope of the hybrid rate constant α in the open two-compartment model becomes smaller, hence the distribution phase becomes prolonged as seen from Figure 33-1.

The tissue concentration after IV administration is:

$$A_2 = \frac{k_{12} \cdot D}{\alpha - \beta} \cdot (e^{\beta \cdot t} - e^{\alpha \cdot t}) \, [\text{mg/kg}] \tag{1}$$

And after extravascular administration, it is:

$$A_2 = D \cdot f \cdot k_a \cdot k_{12} \cdot \left[\frac{e^{-\alpha \cdot t}}{(k_a - \alpha) \cdot (\beta - \alpha)} + \frac{e^{-\beta \cdot t}}{(k_a - \beta) \cdot (\alpha - \beta)} \right.$$
$$\left. + \frac{e^{-k_a \cdot t}}{(\alpha - k_a) \cdot (\beta - k_a)} \right] [\text{mg/kg}] \tag{2}$$

If one calculates the amount of drug in tissue A_2 at a given time t according to Equation 33.1 or 33.2 for intravascular and extravascular administration, respectively, for different dose

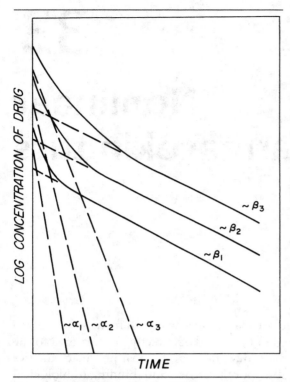

Figure 33-1. Schematic plot of log concentration versus time curves following the open two-compartment model of a hypothetical drug in three different dose sizes. Due to nonlinear pharmacokinetics with respect to distribution the slopes of α become more shallow, hence the distribution phase becomes prolonged with increasing dose size.

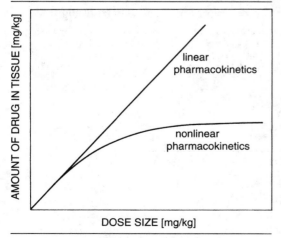

Figure 33-2. Schematic plot of amount of drug in tissue versus dose size.

sizes and plots the data on numeric graph paper, a straight line will be obtained in the case of linear pharmacokinetics, whereas in nonlinear pharmacokinetics a curve becoming asymptotic to the abscissa will be obtained (Figure 33-2).

To detect nonlinearity for one or more of the pharmacokinetic parameters, one can construct similar plots using $AUC^{0\rightarrow\infty}$, $t_{1/2}$, α, β, Δ'_c, Δ'_β, k_{13}, or Cl_{tot} versus dose size. (See also Chapter 20, Section on AUC as Test for Dose Dependency.)

Deviation from linearity with respect to protein binding can occur if increasing dose sizes approach saturation of binding sites, or if only a limited number of binding sites is available in plasma.

Nonlinearity with respect to excretion can be caused by changes of urinary pH for weak electrolytes undergoing urinary recycling, by saturation of reabsorptive processes, or by diurnal variation in the elimination of drugs. Also in the case of enterohepatic recycling, nonlinearity can be found due to saturation of active transport into bile.

In order to detect nonlinear pharmacokinetics it is recommended that one studies distinctly different dose sizes in individual subjects, or animals, upon IV administration of the drug and begins blood sampling as early as possible. Changing of pharmacokinetic parameters in a uniform manner with dose size indicates some type of nonlinear pharmacokinetics.

Consequences of nonlinear pharmacokinetics are that a given blood level curve, or given pharmacokinetic parameters, do not necessarily allow "translation" or prediction of blood levels for dose sizes differing widely from those for which the pharmacokinetic parameters have been determined. Furthermore, in case of poisoning where unusually large doses have been taken, predictions might be erroneous due to largely increased elimination half-lives and/or nonlinearities.

Michaelis-Menten Kinetics

In all biological processes where enzymes, carriers, or active processes are involved, as in biotransformation, renal tubular secretion, and active transport, saturation may occur. These processes may be relatively specific with respect to the substrate and may have finite or limited capacities. For these specialized processes often the use of Michaelis-Menten kinetics is applicable.

If we look at first-order and capacity-limited (saturation) kinetics (Table 33-1), the following picture is obtained on semi-log plot (Figure 33-3). The curves I and II in A and III in B of Figure 33-3 are described by the differential equation for loss of drug:

$$\frac{dc}{dt} = -k_1 \cdot C \tag{3}$$

which upon solution to the differential equation can be rewritten as Equation 33.4:

$$C = C_o \cdot e^{-k_1 \cdot t} \tag{4}$$

In A of Figure 33-3, both the small (a) and large (b) dose follow first-order kinetics. So does the small (a) dose in B of Figure 33-3. However, the large dose (b) in B of Figure 33-3

Table 33-1. Examples of Capacity-Limited Behavior for Various Pharmacokinetic Processes

PHARMACOKINETIC PROCESS/ PARAMETER	MECHANISM	EXAMPLES
Absorption	saturable transport intestinal metabolism	penicillins, riboflavin prodrugs, salicylamide
Distribution	plasma protein binding CSF transport tissue binding cellular uptake hepatic uptake	aftriaxone, prednisolone benzylpenicillins prednisolone methicillin indocyanine green
Metabolism	saturable metabolism product inhibition co-substrate depletion plasma protein binding	phenytoin phenytoin acetaminophen prednisolone
Elimination	glomerular filtration tubular secretion tubular reabsorption biliary secretion biliary recycling	naproxen mezlocillin, PAH cephapirin, riboflavin BSP, iodipamide cimetidine, isotretinoin
Response	saturable receptor binding	phenytoin

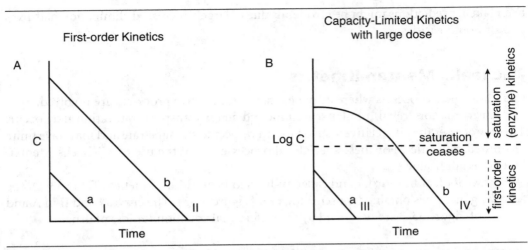

Figure 33-3. Schematic presentation of first-order and Michaelis-Menten kinetics for different dose sizes. a = small dose size; b = large dose size. (For explanation see text.)

shows saturation in the upper portion of the curve. In this case the Michaelis-Menten equation is applicable:

$$\frac{dc}{dt} = \frac{V_{max} \cdot C}{K_m + C} \tag{5}$$

where dc/dt is the rate of decline of drug concentration at time t, V_{max} is the theoretical maximum rate of the process, and K_m is the Michaelis-Menten constant. Upon integration of Equation 33.5 between the limits $C = C_o$ at $t = t_o$ and $C = C$ at $t = t$, Equation 33.6 is obtained:

$$V_{max} \cdot (t - t_o) = C_o - C + K_m \cdot \ln \frac{C_o}{C} \tag{6}$$

A zero-order rate constant k_o in the postdistributive phase can be calculated. In this range of saturation, drug concentration can be assumed to be much higher than K_m; hence, k_o would represent V_{max} in the limiting case of the Michaelis-Menten equation.

Since K_m often cannot be calculated directly from the blood level data, arbitrary values between 60 and 99 may be selected for percent saturation to generate possible K_m data. The percent saturation is given in Equation 33.7:

$$\% \text{ saturation} = \frac{C_o}{K_m + C_o} \cdot 100 \tag{7}$$

Equation 33.7 represents the concentration-time course of the drug that is eliminated only by a single capacity-limited process. Since Equation 33.6 cannot be solved explicitly for C, a series of data points can be generated by reiteration using V_{max}, determined from the postdistributive phase, and C_o, the starting concentration in the postdistributive phase.

The parameters V_{max} and K_m can also be estimated from a Michaelis-Menten drug concentration-time curve by the following procedure as shown in Figure 33-4.

From the terminal slope of the plot the global rate constant K is determined. The rate constants for parallel first-order processes have to be determined from separate plots, such as a dAe/dt versus midpoint time plot for the first-order rate constant for renal elimination k_u (see Chapter 19).

From the graph (Figure 33-4) the actual intercept of the blood concentration-time curve with the ordinate is marked "A," and the intercept of the back-extrapolated mono-exponential K-slope with the ordinate is marked "A*."

Since:

$$\ln A^* = \ln A + \frac{A}{K_m} \tag{8}$$

K_m can be calculated:

$$K_m = \frac{A}{\ln\left(\dfrac{A^*}{A}\right)}[\mu g/ml] \tag{9}$$

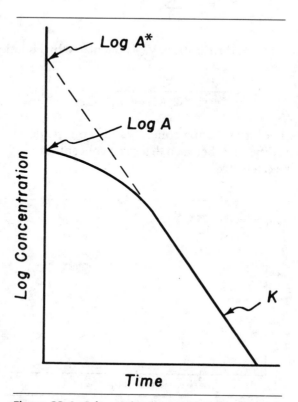

Figure 33-4. Schematic presentation for determination of V_{max} and K_m. (For explanation see text.)

Since:

$$\frac{V_{max}}{K_m} = K - (k_u + k_{er}) \tag{10}$$

$$V_{max} = [K - (k_u + k_{er})] \cdot K_m [\mu g/h] \tag{11}$$

Usually, pharmacokinetic parameters for drugs following Michaelis-Menten kinetics are determined from two steady state concentrations, C_1^{ss} and C_2^{ss}, obtained with two dose rates, R_1 and R_2. Each of the dose rates results in a dose-dependent clearance, Cl_1 or Cl_2:

$$Cl_1 = \frac{R_1}{C_1^{ss}}; \quad Cl_2 = \frac{R_2}{C_2^{ss}} [1/d] \tag{12}$$

From a direct linear plot of dose rate in mg/d on the ordinate versus clearance in l/d on the abscissa (see Figure 33-5), the intercept with the ordinate is V_{max} in mg/d, and the slope is K_m in mg/l.

$$V_{max} = R_1 - K_m \cdot Cl_1 [mg/d] \tag{13}$$

$$K_m = \frac{R_1 - R_2}{Cl_1 - Cl_2} [mg/l] \tag{14}$$

The apparent volume of distribution, V_d, is calculated by Equation 33.15:

$$V_d = \frac{V_{max} \cdot t}{K_m \cdot \ln(C_1/C_2) + (C_1 - C_2)} [1/kg] \tag{15}$$

where C_1 and C_2 are two drug plasma concentrations on the decaying blood level-time curve, and t is the time difference between these two concentrations. Knowing V_d, the area under the curve can be calculated.

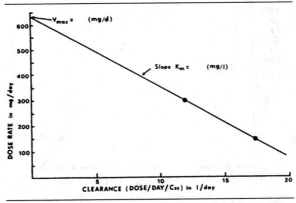

Figure 33-5. Direct linear plot for dose rate versus clearance.

Whereas with linear drugs there is a direct proportion between the total area under the curve $AUC^{0 \to \infty}$, and the clearance, nonlinear drugs exhibit a parabolic behavior with the AUC of higher doses disproportionate to those of lower doses. The AUC is calculated according to Equation 33.16:

$$AUC^{0 \to \infty} = \frac{D}{V_{max}} \cdot \left(\frac{D}{2 \cdot V_d} + K_m \right) [(mg/l) \cdot d] \qquad (16)$$

For nonlinear drugs, the usual, noncompartmental calculation of clearance as the ratio of dose to area under the curve results in a concentration-average clearance, $\overline{Cl}$, which decreases with dose:

$$\overline{Cl} = \frac{D}{AUC^{0 \to \infty}} = \frac{V_{max}}{K_m + \dfrac{C(0)}{2}} = \frac{V_{max}}{K_m + \dfrac{D}{2V_d}} [1/d] \qquad (17)$$

The mean residence time, MRT, can be obtained as follows:

$$MRT = \frac{V_d}{Cl} \cdot \frac{V_d \cdot AUC^{0 \to \infty}}{D} = \frac{V_d}{V_{max}} \cdot \left(\frac{D}{2V_d} + K_m \right) [h] \qquad (18)$$

Capacity-limited behavior may occur in practically all pharmacokinetic phases and processes. Some examples are given in Table 33-1.

Selected References

1. DiSanto, A. R. and Wagner, J. G.: Potential Erroneous Assignment of Nonlinear Data to the Classical Linear Two-Compartment Model, *J. Pharm. Sci. 61*:552 (1972).

2. Ginneken, van, C. A. M., Rossum, van, J. M. and Fleuren, H. L. J. M.: Linear and Nonlinear Kinetics of Drug Elimination. I. Kinetics on the Basis of a Single Capacity-Limited Pathway of Elimination With or Without Simultaneous Supply-Limited Elimination, *J. Pharmacokinet. Biopharm. 2*:395 (1974).

3. Hofstee, B. H. J.: On the Evaluation of the Constants V_{max} and K_m in Enzyme Reactions, *Science 116*:329 (1952).

4. Jusko, W. J.: Pharmacokinetics of Capacity-Limited Systems, *J. Clin. Pharmacol. 29*:488–493 (1989).

5. Jusko, W. J.: Guidelines for Collection and Analysis of Pharmacokinetic Data. In: *Applied Pharmacokinetics*, 2nd Ed., W. E. Evans, J. J. Schentag and W. J. Jusko, Eds., Applied Therapeutics Inc., San Francisco, CA, 1986, pp. 9–54.

6. Levy, G.: Pharmacokinetics of Salicylate Elimination in Man. *J. Pharm. Sci. 54*:959 (1965).

7. Michaelis, L. and Menten, M. L.: Die Kinetik der Invertinwirkung, *Biochem. Z. 49*:333 (1913).

8. Tozer, T. N. and Rubin, G. M.: Saturable Kinetics and Bioavailability Determination, In *Pharmacokinetics*, P. G. Welling and F. L. S. Tse, Eds., Marcel Dekker, Basel, 1988, pp. 473–513.

9. Wagner, J. G.: Theophylline: Pooled Michaelis-Menten Parameters (V_{max} and K_m) and Implications, *Clin. Pharmacokin. 10*:432–442 (1985).

10. Wagner, J. G.: Properties of the Michaelis-Menten Equation and Its Integrated Form Which are Useful in Pharmacokinetics. *J. Pharmacokinet. Biopharm. 1*:103 (1973).

11. Wagner, J. G.: A Modern View of Pharmacokinetics, *J. Pharmacokinet. Biopharm. 1*:363 (1973).

12. Wagner, J. G.: *Fundamentals of Clinical Pharmacokinetics*, Drug Intelligence Publications, Hamilton, Ill. 1975, p. 247.

13. Witmer, D. R. and Ritschel, W. A.: Phenytoin-Isoniazid Interaction: A Kinetic Approach to Management, *Drug Intell. Clin. Pharm. 18*:483–486 (1984).

34

Curve Fitting

When experimental points—such as drug concentrations in blood, plasma, or serum at given times—are plotted on graph paper, one often finds it difficult to draw a line through the points in order to find an equation describing the relationship between x and y within the range of the observed values. The difficulty in fitting a line to the data points is due to the random scatter among points. This is caused by experimental errors, such as inaccuracy of measuring blood volumes for analysis (usually between 1 and 5 ml of blood is measured with the syringe used for blood sampling), low sensitivity of analytical method etc., and assuming that the x data (usually time) are valid. Among the many types of relations between variables, the straight-line relationship is the one used most often in pharmacokinetics. For zero-order kinetics a straight line is obtained on a numeric plot, for first-order kinetics on a semilog plot.

Eye Fitting

Often it will be possible and even practical to fit the data points by eye to a straight line. If one uses "eye-balling" to fit data points to a straight line on a semilog plot care must be taken not to draw a line which lies visually best between scattered points. One has to be aware that the data points above the straight line will be further distant than those below the straight line due to the logarithmic scale.

Least Square Fitting

A commonly preferred method for obtaining estimates of parameters used in curve fitting is the method of least squares. The least square method is based on the equation which minimizes the sum of the squares of the deviations of the observed values from the line. In other words the line of best fit is obtained when the sum of the squares of the vertical distances from the points to the line is a minimum (Figure 34-1).

The functional relationships are such that the y value (drug concentration) is the dependent variable which is to be predicted in terms of the independent variable, x (time).

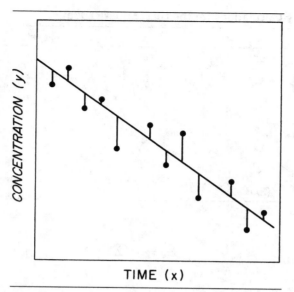

Figure 34-1. Schematic plot of curve fitting by the least square method.

Let us assume we have n pairs of data (x_1, y_2), (x_2, y_2), ... (x_n, y_n) which represent the times of sampling and the drug concentrations in blood of n samples. The predicting or estimating equation used to represent the experimental data is:

$$y' = a + b \cdot x \tag{1}$$

Thus for each observed value of x we have both an observed and a calculated value for y. The calculated or predicted value y' is determined by substituting the appropriate x value into Equation 34.1 once values of a and b are known. The least square criterion requires one to find the numerical values of the constants a and b in Equation 34.1, for which the sum of the squares $\Sigma (y - y')^2$ is as small as possible. Estimates of a and b can be made by solving Equations 34.2 and 34.3:

$$\Sigma y = n \cdot a + b \cdot (\Sigma x) \tag{2}$$

$$\Sigma(x \cdot y) = a \cdot (\Sigma x) + b \cdot (\Sigma x^2) \tag{3}$$

The data points are best compiled in a table and the necessary calculations are carried out as given in Table 34-1.

Using the values obtained as per Table 34-1, the constants a and b are then calculated using Equations 34.4 and 34.5, which are the solutions to Equations 34.2 and 34.3. Although there are different equations available it is easiest first to solve the equation for b and then for a:

$$b = \frac{n \cdot (\Sigma x \cdot y) - (\Sigma x) \cdot (\Sigma y)}{n \cdot (\Sigma x^2) - (\Sigma x)^2} \tag{4}$$

Table 34-1. Necessary Calculations for the Least Square Equation

NUMBER	x	y	x^2	$x \cdot y$
1	x_1	y^1	x_1^2	$x_1 \cdot y_1$
2	x_2	y^2	x_2^2	$x_2 \cdot y_2$
3	x_3	y^3	x_3^2	$x_3 \cdot y_3$
↓	↓	↓	↓	↓
n	Σx	Σy	Σx^2	$\Sigma(x \cdot y)$
	↓			
	$(\Sigma x)^2$			

$$a = \frac{\Sigma y - b \cdot (\Sigma x)}{n} \tag{5}$$

The constants a and b are then submitted into Equation 34.1 in order to obtain the calculated value of y′ for any given time x. Also, a is the intercept of the least square line with the ordinate, and b is the slope of the line.

Equations 34.1 through 34.5 are applicable for a least square fit of a straight line on a numeric plot. If a semilog plot is used, one has to use the logarithm for all y values, and consequently the two normal equations become:

$$\Sigma \log y = n \cdot (\log a) + b \cdot (\Sigma x) \tag{6}$$

$$\Sigma(x \cdot \log y) = (\log a) \cdot (\Sigma x) + b \cdot (\Sigma x^2) \tag{7}$$

which can be solved for log a and b and, hence, for a and b.

The equation for the exponential curve is:

$$y = a \cdot 10^{bx} \tag{8}$$

or in logarithmic form:

$$\log y = \log a + x \cdot b \tag{9}$$

Often it is simpler to proceed as per Table 34-1 but substituting log y for y. The predicting or estimating equation then becomes:

$$y' = \text{antilog}\,(a + b \cdot x) \tag{10}$$

The least square method as outlined above is applicable to any straight line, such as the monoexponential k_{el} slope in the open one-compartment model upon intravascular route of administration, the monoexponential slopes of k_{el} and k_a in the open one-compartment model upon extravascular route of administration, the monoexponential slopes of β and α in the open two-compartment model upon intravascular route of administration, and the monoexponential slopes of β, α, and k_a in the open two-compartment model upon extravascular administration.

In any bi- or triexponential equation the least square method should be applied to each exponential segment of the blood level versus time curve. Often it is not easy to find the "starting" point for a least square line. In this case one should try to start the least square line at different points (see Figure 34-2) and select the equation which results in a correlation coefficient closest to 1.0.

Correlation Coefficient

The correlation coefficient r is calculated using Equation 34.11:

$$r = \frac{n \cdot (\sum x \cdot y) - (\sum x) \cdot (\sum y)}{\sqrt{n \cdot (\sum x^2) - (\sum x)^2} \cdot \sqrt{n \cdot (\sum y^2) - (\sum y)^2}} \tag{11}$$

A minus in front of r indicates a negative correlation, or descending slope, and a plus indicates a positive correlation, or ascending slope.

However, one has to be aware that a correlation coefficient r closer to 1.0 with fewer points included may not be a better fit of curve than a lower r for more data points on the curve. In order to find out the statistical significance of the correlation coefficient depending on the number of pairs of x and y, Table 34-2 should be consulted.

Tilt of a Line

The tilt of a line method is a robust procedure of drawing a line through a series of experimental points. The term robust implies that a procedure is relatively insensitive to any one value. In this robust method, one point should not have large influence even as one point does not largely influence a median while it may largely influence a mean value. The tilt of line is based on the median. The x and y points are considered separately, not as pairs. If the number of x and of y points can be divided by 3, then 3 groups of upper, middle, and lower x and y points are formed. If there is a remainder, the extra point is added to the middle group; if there are two remainders, one each is added to the upper and lower

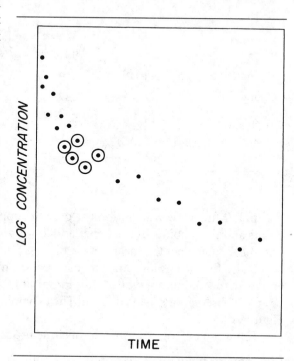

Figure 34-2. Schematic plot of an intravascular blood level versus time curve. The ○ indicate possible "starting" points for the least square calculations of the monoexponential β phase.

Table 34-2. Values of r at the 5 Percent and 1 Percent Levels of Significance

DEGREES OF FREEDOM (DF)	5 PERCENT	1 PERCENT	DEGREES OF FREEDOM (DF)	5 PERCENT	1 PERCENT
1	.997	1.000	24	.388	.496
2	.950	.990	25	.381	.487
3	.878	.959	26	.374	.478
4	.811	.917	27	.367	.470
5	.754	.874	28	.361	.463
6	.707	.834	29	.355	.456
7	.666	.798	30	.349	.449
8	.632	.765	35	.325	.418
9	.602	.735	40	.304	.393
10	.576	.708	48	.288	.372
11	.553	.684	50	.273	.354
12	.532	.661	60	.250	.325
13	.514	.641	70	.232	.302
14	.497	.623	80	.217	.283
15	.482	.606	90	.205	.267
16	.468	.590	100	.195	.254
17	.456	.575	125	.174	.228
18	.444	.561	150	.159	.208
19	.433	.549	200	.138	.181
20	.423	.537	300	.113	.148
21	.413	.526	400	.098	.128
22	.404	.515	500	.088	.115
23	.396	.505	1000	.062	.081

group. For further consideration use only the upper and lower groups. List separately the x points and the y points of the upper and lower group in increasing or decreasing order and find the median (not the mean!). One obtains for the upper group a median x and a median y, and also for the lower group a median x and a median y. These upper and lower median x and median y points are plotted. It is important to note that these two points do not have to be actual observations in the data set! The two points are then connected by a straight line (see Figure 34-3).

One can derive from this tilt of a line procedure the following equations:

upper point: median x_1; median y_1
lower point: median x_2; median y_2

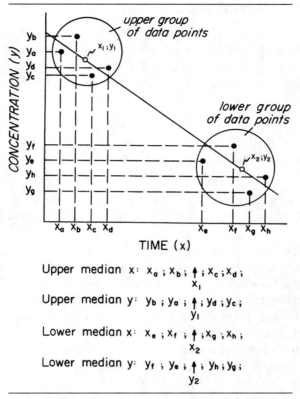

Figure 34-3. Schematic diagram for curve fitting by tilt of a line method.

$$slope = \frac{y_1 - y_2}{x_1 - x_2} \qquad (12)$$

$$y_1 = b + slope \cdot x_1 \qquad (13)$$

$$y_2 = b + slope \cdot x_2 \qquad (14)$$

$$b = y_{1\,or\,2} - slope \cdot x_{1\,or\,2} \qquad (15)$$

The equation for the line of best fit y' by the tilt of line method is given in Equation 34.16:

$$y' = b + slope \cdot x \qquad (16)$$

The tilt of a line method is a statistically robust procedure relatively insensitive to deviant points, but useful for practical purposes since the line can be drawn without preceding calculations in a matter of seconds.

Problems in Fitting of Rate Constants

Experimental data or published graphs are often not easy to evaluate. Usually preliminary estimates on rate constants are made from graphs which are later used for computer analysis. A problem frequently encountered is that the differences in values obtained by the residual method do not result in a straight line when connected with each other. Among the reasons for this problem are:

- Analytical error in drug concentration determination;
- Insensitive analytical method, particularly at low concentrations;
- Wrongly recorded or unreliable sampling times; and
- Poor estimate of the monoexponential line of the succeeding phase.

In Figure 34-4 examples of frequently observed evaluation problems are given along with suggestions for solution. Without question these solutions can be applied for preliminary evaluation only.

The residuals for the α-line in plot "a" of Figure 34-4 show a perfect fit to a straight monoexponential line. If one would combine the residuals (difference values) for the α-line in plot "b" of Figure 34-4, a concave curve would result indicating that a higher than a two-compartment model is applicable where the drug apparently distributes into a "shallow" and a "deep" peripheral compartment. There are two possible solutions, either to treat it as a three-compartment open model or to collapse it to a two-compartment model. For treatment as a three-compartment open model (plot b), a straight line is drawn through the last few points of the residuals resulting in the α-line. Then again the differences are taken between the first residuals and the corresponding concentrations on the α-line which, when connected by a straight line, result in the γ-line.

To collapse the apparent three-compartment open model to a two-compartment open model the α-line should be forced through all residuals (plot "c" in Figure 34-4).

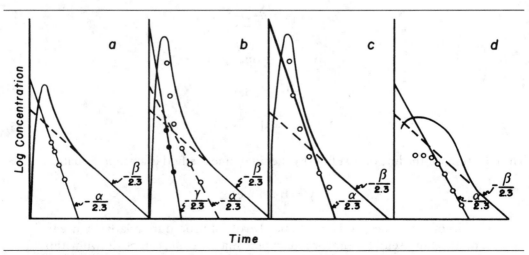

Figure 34-4. Schematic diagram for evaluation of residuals for estimating α-phase. (For explanation see text.)

In plot "d" of Figure 34-4 connecting of the residuals for the α-line would result in a convex curve, indicating either still ongoing absorption for same period after the peak, or presence of a lag-time. In order to obtain a good estimate on the α-slope the last residuals must be considered for the monoexponential line, neglecting all early residuals. Before the residual method is used again to "peel off" the k_a-line, correction should be tried for possible presence of a lag-time.

Determination of Lag-Time

The lag-time (t_{lag}) is the time interval between administration of a drug product (dosage form) and first appearance of drug in systemic circulation. It can only be observed upon extravascular (EV) route of administration.

In the EV one-compartment open model a lag-time is present if the semilog plot of the blood level *vs.* time curve shows an intercept of A larger than B as shown in Figure 34-5A. Graphically t_{lag} can be read off where the back-extrapolated elimination and the absorption slopes intercept. The lag-time can also be calculated from the intercepts A and B and the rate constants k_a and k_{el}:

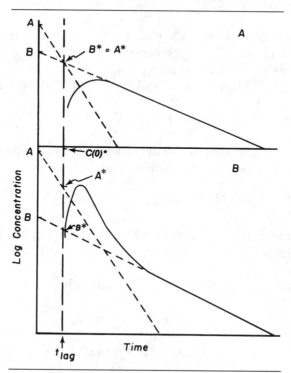

Figure 34-5. Schematic diagram for determination of lag-time. (For explanation see text.)
A = one-compartment open model.
B = two-compartment open model.

$$t_{tag} = \frac{\ln \dfrac{A}{B}}{k_a - k_{el}} [h] \tag{17}$$

Another approach is to increase the time t from t = 0 in small increments of about 0.01 h in the corresponding equations for the monoexponential slopes of the absorption and elimination phase. Since t_{lag} is where these lines intercept, the equations must at this point be equal:

$$B \cdot e^{-k_{el} \cdot t_{lag}} = A \cdot e^{-k_a \cdot t_{lag}} \tag{18}$$

Once t_{lag} has been determined, new intercepts A* and B* have to be calculated because A = B = C(0) in the one-compartment model:

$$B^* = B \cdot e^{-k_{el} \cdot t_{lag}} [\mu g/ml] \tag{19}$$

$$A^* = A \cdot e^{-k_a \cdot t_{lag}} [\mu g/ml] \tag{20}$$

Hence, the new general blood level equation in presence of a lag-time is:

$$C(t) = B^* \cdot e^{-k_{el} \cdot (t - t_{lag})} - A^* \cdot e^{-k_a \cdot (t - t_{lag})} [\mu g/ml] \tag{21}$$

If an EV blood level-time curve following the two-compartment model is plotted on semilog paper one would find that in presence of a lag-time C(0) > A + B as shown in Figure 34-5B. From the graph an estimate on t_{lag} can be obtained by reading the concentrations on the k_a-slope C(0)′, the α-slope A′, and the β-slope B′ at small time intervals until:

$$C(0)' = A' + B' \tag{22}$$

Since Equation 34.22 must be met in the two-compartment open model, the following Equation 34.23 can be used to accurately calculate t_{lag}:

$$C(0) \cdot e^{-k_a \cdot t_{lag}} = -A \cdot e^{-\alpha \cdot t_{lag}} + B \cdot e^{-\beta \cdot t_{lag}} \tag{23}$$

by using small increments for t_{lag} of about 0.01 h until Equation 34.23 is fulfilled. The t_{lag} now permits one to calculate the new intercepts C(0)*, A*, and B*:

$$C(0)^* = C(0) \cdot e^{-k_a \cdot t_{lag}} [\mu g/ml] \tag{24}$$

$$B^* = B \cdot e^{-\beta \cdot t_{lag}} [\mu g/ml] \tag{25}$$

$$A^* = A \cdot e^{-\alpha \cdot t_{lag}} [\mu g/ml] \tag{26}$$

Finally, the new general blood level equation in presence of a lag-time is obtained:

$$C(t) = B^* \cdot e^{-\beta \cdot (t - t_{lag})} + A^* \cdot e^{-\alpha \cdot (t - t_{lag})} - C(0)^* \cdot e^{-k_a \cdot (t - t_{lag})} [\mu g/ml] \tag{27}$$

35

Correlation of Clinical Response with Drug Disposition

Various models have been described to correlate the pharmacological or clinical response to drugs with their disposition in the body or one or more pharmacokinetic parameters. The classical model is the relationship between the log dose-response curve and the blood concentration-time curve. Such a relationship can be established for drugs showing reversible action and for which some type of log dose or log concentration-response can be established and for drugs which do not show nonlinear kinetics, dose-dependency, development of tolerance, etc. For these drugs we assume that the free plasma concentration is in equilibrium with the free drug concentration in the biophase, i.e., at the receptor site.

Having response data at hand, such as intensity of pain relief upon administration of an analgesic measured at various times after dosing, one can construct a numeric plot of intensity (response) versus time as shown in Figure 35-1A. The intercept with the ordinate gives the maximum intensity of effect E°.

Then the response is plotted versus log concentration of drug in plasma as determined from blood samples collected after dosing. From this plot (see Figure 35-1B) the slope m is determined. Note that usually a log dose-response plot shows a linear segment between approximately 20 and 80 percent response.

Finally, the drug concentration is plotted versus time (see Figure 35-1C), and the overall elimination rate constant k_{el} is determined.

The relationship between pharmacological or clinical response and time can be expressed by Equation 35.1:

$$E = E° = \frac{k_{el} \cdot m \cdot t}{2.303} \text{ [intensity of effect]} \tag{1}$$

$E° =$ maximum intensity of effect
E = intensity of effect at time t
k_{el} = overall elimination rate constant $[h^{-1}]$
m = slope of the log concentration-response curve
t = time after administration

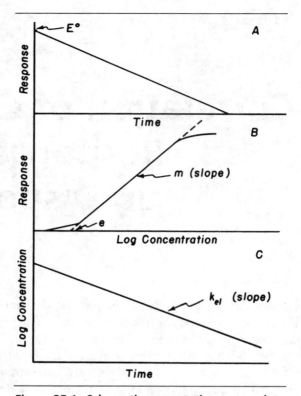

Figure 35-1. Schematic presentation to correlate the pharmacological or clinical effect with the drug's disposition. A = response-time curve; B = log concentration-response curve; C = log concentration-time curve. (For explanation see text.)

This equation is derived from the following:

$$E = m \cdot \log C + c \qquad (2)$$

C = drug concentration in plasma
e = intercept of the straight line segment of the log concentration-response plot with the abscissa [conc.]

Rearrangement of Equation 35.2 results in Equation 35.3:

$$\log C = \frac{E - e}{m} \qquad (3)$$

Since:

$$\log C(t) = \log C(0) - \frac{k_{el} \cdot t}{2.303} \qquad (4)$$

one can substitute the intensity of response for the concentration:

$$\frac{E-e}{m} = \frac{E°-e}{m} - \frac{k_{el} \cdot t}{2.303}$$ (5)

which can be simplified to Equation 35.1.

Combining $\frac{k_{el} \cdot m}{2.303}$ to R, and since $k_{el} = \frac{0.693}{t_{1/2}}$ Equation 35.1 can be rewritten:

$$E = E° - 0.3\frac{m}{t_{1/2}} \cdot t$$ (6)

The time required to decline from the maximum to the minimum effect MEC is the duration of effect t_d:

$$t_d = 3.32 \cdot t_{1/2} \cdot \log\left(\frac{D/V_d}{MEC}\right)$$ (7)

where $D/V_d = C(0)$.

Equation 35.7 clearly indicates that doubling of the dose size does not double the duration of effect, but doubling the half-life will double the duration of effect.

The correlation of clinical response with drug disposition discussed above applies, strictly speaking, only for IV administration, the one-compartment model, with the maximum effect occurring instantly after administration, and first-order kinetics. For other conditions different models have to be used.

Pharmacokinetic-Pharmacodynamic Correlation

One of the major roles of pharmacokinetics in clinical practice is to design dosage regimens which produce the desired pharmacological response while keeping the undesirable effects to a minimum. Unfortunately, it is not usually possible to determine the drug concentration at the site of action (i.e., the receptor). Therefore, attention has been directed to the measurement of drug concentration in plasma or serum. In recent years, an enormous amount of pharmacokinetic data has been generated for many drugs, often at the expense of characterizing the time- and concentration-dependent effect (i.e., pharmacodynamics). To define the relationship of pharmacologic response (i.e., pharmacodynamics) to plasma drug concentration (i.e., pharmacokinetics), three different types of models are generally used. These are: (a) Pharmacodynamic-Pharmacokinetic Models at Steady State; (b) Pharmacodynamic-Pharmacokinetic Models; and (c) Physiologic-Pharmacokinetic Models; all of which are summarized below. For more detailed information, the reader is referred to an excellent handbook on pharmacokinetic-pharmacodynamic correlation by Derendorf and Hochhaus (see Selected References).

Pharmacodynamic-Pharmacokinetic Models at Steady State

These models are based on the assumption that, at steady state, the drug concentration in plasma or serum is a reflection of the drug concentration in the biophase. The following four models can be used.

The **Fixed-Effect Model** relates the drug concentration in plasma or serum to a fixed effect which may be either present or absent, but it may also refer to some degree of effect. The fixed-effect model has only one parameter, i.e., the concentration at which the effect appears (or an undesirable effect disappears). This model has been used to predict the response of digoxin and phenytoin at certain steady state concentrations.

The **Linear Model** assumes a direct proportionality (i.e., a linear relationship) between the plasma or serum concentration of a drug and the intensity of pharmacologic response. An equation of the type $Y = m(X) + C$ represents the model where Y is the intensity of response, X is the serum (or plasma) concentration, and m and C are the slope and intercept, respectively. This model has been used to examine the relationship between quinidine serum concentration and its effect on the heart.

The **Log-Linear Model** is a very common approach and is based upon the empirical plot of response vs. logarithm of dose, plasma concentration, or amount of drug in the body which yields the typical sigmoid dose-response curve. Frequently, the curve is linear between 20 and 80% of the maximum attainable intensity of response and thus cannot be used when the response is <20% or >80%.

The **Nonlinear Model** can enable characterization of drug response through an entire range of plasma drug concentrations. This technique utilizes the Hill equation to relate the intensity of pharmacologic response (R) to the concentration (C) of drug in the body fluids according to the following equation:

$$R = (R_m \cdot Cs)/[(1/Q) + Cs] \qquad (8)$$

where R_m is the maximum intensity of response, Q is a constant related to the affinity of the drug for the receptor, and s is a constant that relates the changes in response to the change in concentration.

Pharmacodynamic-Pharmacokinetic Models

Such models correlate the observed response with the concentration (or amount) of drug in one or more pharmacokinetic compartments. For these models, no assumption of steady state is made. The following five models are used.

The **Central Compartment Response Model** links the drug concentration in the central compartment to the observed pharmacologic effect by substitution of the concentration term with the function describing the change of drug concentration. This approach can be used when a linear relationship (Equation 35.1) or a nonlinear relationship (Equations 35.2 through 35.6) exists between drug concentration and effect (response).

The **Tissue Compartment-Response Model** correlates the concentration of drug in the peripheral compartment (i.e., tissue) with the pharmacologic response. As this concentration is often predicted from plasma pharmacokinetic data, only an approximation of the (tissue) concentration versus effect profile can be achieved. Furthermore, this approach cannot account for equilibration with the biophase when the latter is either faster or slower than equilibration with one of the identifiable pharmacokinetic compartments.

The **Multicompartment Response Model** expresses response as a simple function of the amount of drug in one or more compartments of an appropriate pharmacokinetic model using data from individual subjects rather than mean data from a group of subjects. If the response is allowed to depend upon the drug levels in some or all of the appropriate pharmacokinetic compartments, then the response (R_i) due to the drug amount (X_i) in the ith compartment can be expressed as:

$$R_i = f_i(X_i) \qquad (9)$$

where $f(X_i)$ is some function of the amount of drug in the ith compartment and could be linear, log-linear, or described by the Hill equation.

The **Effect Compartment Model** enables the modeling of response as a function of the drug concentration in an "effect compartment" whose kinetics are related to the central compartment by a first-order process. The hypothetical amount of drug in the effect compartment is then related to the observed effect by a function such as the Hill equation or, alternatively, by a linear or log-linear function. This approach is also referred to as the Sigmoid Emax Model which enables the determination of several clinically useful pharmacodynamic parameter estimates (e.g., EC50 or the concentration which corresponds to a 50% response; Emax or the concentration associated with the maximum effect). This technique has been used to describe the pharmacokinetic-pharmacodynamic relationship for famotidine, methamphetamine, acetaminophen, ibuprofen, and the anticonvulsant effect of the benzodiazepines.

The **Pharmacokinetic Model-Independent Model** assumes a direct relationship between response and the drug concentration in plasma or serum. If the response is measured at the same time as the drug concentration, then no formal pharmacokinetic model is required.

Physiologic-Pharmacokinetic Models

These models are used to describe the effects that are attributed to a drug but are mediated by some indirect mechanism which is located separately from the true site of drug action. In this case, the process that is influenced by the drug must be identified and an attempt made to relate plasma drug concentration to changes in this process. The use of this model has been exemplified by the application of the prothrombin time to predict the anticoagulant effect of warfarin.

In an attempt to simplify approaches to pharmacokinetic-pharmacodynamic correlation, several **In Vitro Response Models** have been proposed. In contrast to the aforementioned approaches, which are prospective in their application, these models utilize a combination of in vitro and in vivo data which is frequently available during the drug development process to predict the concentration versus effect relationship. While these models are of interest to individuals involved in drug development and/or regulatory science, they have not, as yet, been validated. These approaches involve methods of correlation and some examples are provided.

Example 1: Produce a Wagner-Nelson plot to estimate the % of drug absorbed from the amount of drug ultimately available for absorption. Plot the % of drug absorbed vs. the % of drug released *in vitro*. If the fit is nearly perfect, drug release is the absorption limiting step.

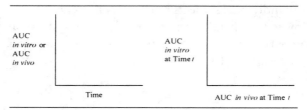

Figure 35-2. In vitro response models: use of AUC in vitro and AUC in vivo. The AUC in vitro and AUC in vivo may be expressed in percent, or a scaling factor may be used.

Example 2: Use intravenous data (same dose as extravascular study or normalize for dose) and by deconvolution of the extravascular data, obtain the % released in vivo. Correlate this with the % released in vitro.

Example 3: As illustrated in Figure 35-2, correlate the AUC of cumulative in vitro release with the AUC determined from blood level data. The AUC data are plotted either versus cumulative time or at time t. This method may be used for slow-release drug products.

Example 4: Convert amount released into a concentration (use the apparent volume of distribution, fraction of drug absorbed, and apparent terminal elimination rate constant from in vivo studies), using, for the absorption rate constant (K_a), the release rate constant either from a sigma minus plot or dA/dt versus midpoint from in vitro release (if the rate of absorption differs at times). Correlate the simulated plasma concentration data with the actual plasma concentration data (see Figure 35-3), performing statistical evaluations for each of the individual points. Alternatively, as illustrated in Figure 35-3, the simulated or actual AUC can be correlated, as can the simulated plasma concentration at time t versus the actual plasma concentration at time t. In this latter case, the smaller the area occupied by the hysteresis loop the better the correlation and hence the greatest predictability from the model.

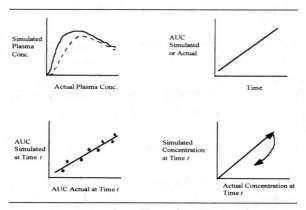

Figure 35-3. In vitro response models: use of simulated and actual concentration data.

Selected References

1. Civiale, C., Ritschel, W. A., Shiu, G. K., Aiache, J. M. and Beyssac, E.: In Vivo-In Vitro Correlation of Salbutamol Release from a Controlled Release Osmotic Pump Delivery System, *Methods Find. Exp. Clin. Pharmacol. 13*:491–498 (1991).

2. Derendorf, H. and Hochhaus, G. (eds.): *Handbook of Pharmacokinetic/Pharmacodynamic Correlation,* CRC Press, Boca Raton, FL (1995).

3. Holford, N. H. G. and Sheiner, L. B.: Understanding the Dose-Effect Relationship: Clinical Application of Pharmacokinetic-Pharmacodynamic Models, *Clin. Pharmacokinet. 6*:429–453 (1981).

4. James, L. P., Marshall, J. D., Heulitt, M. J., Wells, T. G., Letzig, L. and Kearns, G. L.: Pharmacokinetics and Pharmacodynamics of Famotidine in Children, *J. Clin. Pharmacol. 36*:48–54 (1996).

5. Levy, G.: Relationship Between Elimination Rate of Drugs and Rate of Decline of their Pharmacologic Effects, *J. Pharm. Sci. 53*:342 (1964).

6. Levy, G.: Kinetics of Pharmacologic Effects, *Clin. Pharmacol. Ther. 7*:362 (1966).

7. Ritschel, W. A., Koch, H. P. and Alcorn, G. J.: In Vivo-In Vitro Correlations with Sustained-Release Theophylline Preparations, *Methods Find. Exp. Clin. Pharmacol. 6*:609–618 (1984).

8. Ritschel, W. A. and Hussain, A.: Review on Correlation Between Pharmacologic Response and Drug Disposition, *Methods Find. Exp. Clin. Pharmacol. 6*:627 (1984).

36

Bioavailability and Bioequivalence

Bioavailability is defined by the United States Food and Drug Administration (FDA) as the rate and extent to which the active drug ingredient or therapeutic moiety is absorbed from a drug product and becomes available at the site of drug action. It is unfortunate that this official definition is not precise enough.

First, consider the statement with respect to the site of drug action. Although, in general, we assume that the drug concentration in blood, plasma, or serum correlates with the pharmacologic response, it is not applicable to all drugs. Furthermore, the actual bioavailability testing as outlined in the regulation does not attempt to determine the drug concentration at the site of drug action but in systemic circulation. Exception to it is given when it is not possible to measure blood levels; then the bioavailability test is substituted by a pharmacologic or clinical test.

Secondly, this definition does not explicitly include the steadily growing group of prodrugs. As a working hypothesis, we will therefore define bioavailability as follows: bioavailability is both the relative amount of therapeutic moiety in the form of a parent drug, active metabolite, or active moiety of a prodrug from an administered dosage form which enters systemic circulation and the rate the drug appears in it.

Contrary to the belief of many, bioavailability is *not* a criterion of clinical effectiveness *per se.* Clinical effectiveness is so complex (disease states, nutritional status) and the factors influencing absorption so numerous (food intake/fasting, type and amount of food, circadian rhythm, age, etc.) that a test in a small sample size of the population can only be regarded as a *biologic quality control test* under specified conditions.

A **drug product** is defined as a finished dosage form; this means a tablet, capsule, solution, suppository, etc., that contains the active drug ingredient generally, but not necessarily in association with inactive ingredients. One has to assume that prodrugs are included under active drug ingredient, although that is not explicitly stated.

Pharmaceutical equivalents are defined as drug products that contain identical amounts of the identical active drug ingredient, i.e., the same salt or ester of the same therapeutic moiety in identical dosage forms, but not necessarily containing the same inactive ingredients, and that meet the identical compendial or other applicable standard of identity, strength, quality, and purity, including potency and, where applicable, content uniformity, disintegration times, and/or dissolution rates.

Pharmaceutical alternatives are drug products that contain the identical therapeutic moiety or its precursor, but not necessarily in the same amount or dosage form or as the same salt or ester. Each drug product individually meets either the identical or its own respective compendial or other applicable standards of identity, strength, quality, and purity, including potency and, where applicable, content uniformity, disintegration times, and/or dissolution rates.

Whereas **bioavailability** is to demonstrate the amount and rate of drug or active moiety appearing in systemic circulation, and has to be determined for any new drug or new drug product, **bioequivalence** is to demonstrate that other drug products are comparable with respect to biologic performance to an already approved drug product.

A bioequivalence problem may arise when two or more pharmaceutical equivalents or pharmaceutical alternatives, which meet all applicable in vitro standards when administered at the same molar dose of the active therapeutic moiety to the same individuals with the same dosage regimen, result in inequivalent bioavailability. In this case, it could either be that the current in vitro standards for the drug products are not adequate to test and assure bioequivalence or that the products are not appropriately labelled according to their different pharmacokinetic behavior of the dosage form.

It is in the public interest that all products containing the same active ingredient be interchangeable which would require that they are bioequivalent or that for special and desired purposes a different labelling, easily recognizable, is required to immediately indicate a different pharmacokinetic profile.

Bioequivalent drug products are defined as pharmaceutical equivalents or pharmaceutical alternatives whose rate and extent of absorption do not show a significant difference when administered at the same molar dose of the therapeutic moiety, under similar experimental conditions, either single dose or multiple dose.

Some pharmaceutical equivalents or pharmaceutical alternatives may be equivalent in the extent of their absorption but not in their rates and, yet, may be considered bioequivalent because such differences in the rate of absorption are intentional and are reflected in the labelling, are not essential to the attainment of effective body drug concentrations on chronic use, or are considered medically insignificant for the particular drug product.

In order to demonstrate bioequivalence, the Food and Drug Administration has imposed *bioequivalence requirements* for in vitro and/or in vivo testing of specified drug products which must be satisfied as a condition of marketing.

Factors Modifying Bioavailability

In all cases, except when a drug is administered intravenously in the form of a true solution, the drug has to be released from the dosage form and then be absorbed into the systemic circulation by passing through various membranes.

A drug given in different dosage forms or by different routes of administration will yield varying amounts of drug absorbed and, hence, differences in onset, intensity, and duration of the pharmacologic or clinical effect.

These variations are primarily due to differences in the efficiency and rate of absorption which may originate either with the patient or the dosage form. In the first case, we call it a **physiologically modified bioavailability** and in the second case, a **dosage form modified bioavailability.**

In testing of bioavailability and bioequivalence one has to carefully design the study protocol in order to exclude physiologically based modifications of bioavailability. These include age, sex, physical state of the patient, time of administration, stomach emptying rate, type and amount of food, pH and enzyme variations in the gastrointestinal tract, motility of the gastrointestinal tract, blood flow, liver function, kidney function, body weight, and psychological factors such as stress. It is imperative that any design must be able to either exclude such factors or to allow their proper evaluation. The logical consequence is a true cross-over design.

The bioavailability or bioequivalence problems as specified in the new regulation are, therefore, those which depend on the physicochemical characteristics of the drug or the dosage form. These factors are particle size, polymorphic form, presence of a solvate or a hydrate, chemical presentation (salt, ester, ether, complex), pH of dosage forms, environment, solubility characteristics, type and amount of vehicle substances present, the manufacturing method employed for preparing the dosage forms such as type of granulation, change in manufacturing practices, change in blending and mixing practices, improper drying conditions, high-speed tableting, variation in compression force, and instability.

Bioavailability of New Drugs

In the past, clinical pharmacologists and toxicologists have paid too little attention to biopharmaceutical evaluation of new drug products to be tested in man during Phase I studies.

It is well known that the LADMER system (liberation, absorption, distribution, metabolism, elimination, response) applies also to the first administration of a new drug to man with all its implications of physicochemical parameters of the drug and the product. It is very likely that, if one would reanalyze under our present understanding of biopharmaceutics and pharmacokinetics all those drugs which have been abandoned during the past decades as being ineffective in the first clinical trial, one would find quite a number of useful drugs.

The regulation on bioavailability requires that any new drug application submitted in the United States to the FDA must have a complete biopharmaceutical and pharmacokinetic evaluation, including the determination of bioavailability. In the approval process, the generic drug must be a racemate or single enantiomer if the corresponding innovator drug is a racemate or single enantiomer, respectively. This is important given that many important drugs are chiral and that the enantiomers of racemic drugs often differ from one another in their pharmacodynamic and pharmacokinetic properties. If bioequivalence assessments are made using nonstereospecific assays, poor assessments of therapeutic equality may result. This can be particularly true for drugs with complex pharmacokinetics and, most importantly, those that exhibit extensive stereoselectivity in their renal elimination and/or metabolism (e.g., warfarin, albuterol, ibuprofen, ketorolac, verapamil, phenytoin, atenolol, disopyramide). Accordingly, the use of chiral assays and the determination of enantiomer-specific pharmacokinetics provides the most complete and, in many instances, the preferred method of assessing the bioequivalence of racemates.

Bioequivalence Requirements

According to the regulation, the FDA on its own or in the response to a petition by an interested person may identify specific pharmaceutical equivalents or pharmaceutical alternatives that are not or may not be bioequivalent drug products and determine whether to propose or promulgate regulation to establish a bioequivalent requirement for these products.

The criteria and the evidence when bioequivalence requirements have to be established are listed in Table 36-1.

Inspecting Table 36-1, it is quite obvious that for many drugs such a bioequivalent requirement exists *a priori* due to low solubility of the active ingredient or the fact that they appear in the form of polymorphs, in hydrous and anhydrous form, as complexes, solvates, etc.

A bioequivalent requirement may be one or more of the following as specified by the FDA: namely, an in vivo test in humans, an in vivo test in animals other than humans that has been correlated with human in vivo data or in an animal model without correlation with human in vivo data, or an in vitro test which either has been correlated with human in vivo bioavailability or for which no correlation has been established. In vivo bioequivalence requirement in man is mandatory if there is documented evidence that pharmaceutical equivalents or pharmaceutical alternatives do not give comparable therapeutic effects or are not bioequivalent, if the ratio of LD_{50}/ED_{50} is less than 2, or if the ratio of the minimal toxic concentration to the minimal effective concentration is less than 2.

The new regulation also specifies criteria for waiver of evidence of in vivo bioavailability under certain conditions which are listed in Table 36-2.

General Guidelines for the Determination of In Vivo Bioavailability

The in vivo bioavailability of a drug product is demonstrated by both the rate and extent of absorption of the active ingredient or therapeutic moiety. In principle there are four possible approaches to measure the bioavailability:

- Blood level data,
- Urinary excretion data,

Table 36-1. Criteria and Evidence to Establish a Bioequivalent Requirement

1. Difference in therapeutic effects.

2. Bioinequivalence demonstrated.

3. $LD_{50}/ED_{50} < 2$ or $C_{min\ tox}/MEC < 2$.

4. If bioinequivalence would be of serious consequence.

5. If solubility <0.5%, or if <50% dissolved in 30 min, or if particle size is critical, or if drug forms polymorphs, solvates, hydrates, complexes of decreased dissolution, or if drug/excipients <1/5, or if ingredients might interfere with absorption.

6. If absorption from localized site, or f^1 <0.5, or FPE^2, or β^3 or k_m^4 is extremely fast, or if buffers, enteric- or film-coatings are required, or if dose dependent kinetics are in or near therapeutic range.

---

[1] fraction of drug absorbed
[2] first-pass effect
[3] terminal elimination rate constant
[4] rate constant of metabolism

Table 36-2. Criteria for Waiver of In Vivo Bioavailability

1. I.V. solution, solution, topical product for local effect, drugs not intended for P.O. absorption, inhalation product similar to approved one.

2. P.O. (except enteric coated or controlled release) dosage form similar to approved one except for **some** drugs of the following groups:

    antiarrhythmics, anticoagulants, anticonvulsants, antihypertensives, antimalarials, antineoplastics, antithyroids, antituberculars, bronchial dilators, carbonic acid inhibitors, cardiac glycosides, corticoids, estrogens, hypoglycemics, thyroid supplements, tranquilizers, vitamin K.

3. Or otherwise waiver is granted.

- Pharmacologic data, and
- Clinical data.

Whenever possible blood level studies should be carried out and are preferable to all other studies. If such studies are not feasible, they can be substituted by urinary excretion studies. Only if neither one can be done, particularly if the drug cannot be assayed accurately in biological fluid but the pharmacologic response can be measured, a pharmacologic method can be used to substitute for blood level or urinary excretion studies. In the case where it is difficult or impossible to quantify a given pharmacologic response, clinical studies in patients are permissible to substitute for a blood level or urinary excretion study.

The latter approach can also be used for dosage forms intended to deliver the therapeutic moiety locally such as for topical preparations for the skin, ear, eye, mucous membrane, oral dosage forms not intended to be absorbed, and also for bronchodilators administered by inhalation. Although clearly specified in the law, this specific reference seems to be in contradiction to the definition of bioavailability. However, it means that controlled clinical studies may be submitted if low systemic absorption is expected and the bioavailability is substituted by a local availability test where the drug apparently does not enter the systemic circulation.

Selection of a Standard for Bioavailability Testing

The previous practice that the inventor's product is considered as the standard has been abandoned. The change is legitimate because otherwise it might hinder progress. In general, an aqueous true solution of the drug, an aqueous solubilized system of the drug, or an aqueous suspension of the micronized drug will, for most instances, be considered as the standard. However, no strict regulation can be applied since there are drugs which are absorbed solely from the duodenum. In that case, the transition time through the duodenum might be too short for the drug to be quantitatively absorbed.

The selection of the standard for the various categories of bioavailability testing depends on the type of drug product and the questions to be answered. It can be broken down into the following categories: bioavailability testing for a new drug in any new drug product, for any new formulation of a known and marketed product, for a controlled release formulation, for a combination drug product containing two or more drugs, and for any drug product when the drug concentration cannot be determined in biological fluid. The parameters to be determined in each of these categories and the standards and route of administration to be used are listed in Table 36-3. FDA should be consulted prior to applying the standard to any study.

In Vitro–In Vivo Methods for Bioavailability Testing

Possible methods to assess bioavailability include determination of the drug liberation and dissolution at the administration or absorption site, determination of the free drug in systemic circulation, measuring the pharmacologic effect or clinical response, or determination of the urinary excretion of the drug.

The methods of evaluation and examples are listed in Table 36-4.

Table 36-3. Selection of Standard

CATEGORY	PARAMETERS TO BE DETERMINED	STANDARD	ROUTE OF ADMINISTRATION FOR STANDARD
New drug in any drug product	Extent and rate of absorption: elimination half-life, rate of metabolism and/or excretion; dose proportionality after single and multiple dosing	Solution or suspension of drug in single dose study	Same as drug product unless drug is poorly absorbed. In the latter case additional I.V. route
New formulation of marketed product	Extent and rate of absorption; pharmacokinetic parameters of new formulation	Current batch of approved drug product on the market in single dose study	Same as drug product
Controlled release formulation	Extent and rate of bioavailability: pharmacokinetic performance of dosage form	Solution or suspension of drug and/or currently marketed non-controlled release and/or controlled release product in single and multiple dosing study	Same as drug product
Combination drug product	Rate and extent of absorption of one, more or all active drugs	Two or more single-ingredient drug products in single dose study	Same as drug product
Any drug product when drug concentration is not determined in biological fluid	Pharmacologic effect or clinical response	Placebo in single or multiple dose study	Same as drug product

Table 36-4. Possible Methods to Assess Bioavailability

SEQUENCE OF EVENTS UPON ADMINISTRATION OF A DRUG PRODUCT	METHOD OF EVALUATION	EXAMPLE
Drug liberation and dissolution at administration or absorption site	Dissolution rate	In vitro: water, buffer, artificial gastric fluid, artificial intestinal fluid, artificial saliva, artificial rectal fluid
Free drug in systemic circulation	(1) Blood level-time profile (2) Peak blood level (3) Time to reach peak (4) Area under blood level-time curve	In vivo: whole blood, plasma, serum
Pharmacologic effect	(1) Onset of effect (2) Duration of effect (3) Intensity of effect	In vivo: discriminate measurement of pharmacologic effect (blood pressure, blood sugar, blood coagulation time)
Clinical response	(1) Controlled clinical blind or double blind study (2) Observed clinical success or failure	In vivo: evaluation of clinical responses
Elimination	(1) Cumulative amount of drug excreted (2) Maximum excretion rate (3) Peak time of excretion	In vivo: urine

Regarding the question whether or not bioavailability may be measured by some in vitro methods, a personal remark should be voiced. In a true meaning and sense of *bio*availability, no in vitro method can be substituted for a biologic test. An in vitro bioavailability is a contradiction *per se*. However, in vitro methods are necessary to simulate and understand physicochemical processes of absorption, in dosage form development, and as in vitro quality control tests to guarantee batch-to-batch consistency.

Since bioavailability is most precisely determined from either blood level or urinary excretion data, we will discuss the scientific aspects of bioavailability testing based on blood sampling or urine sampling studies only.

Biopharmaceutical Classification System

In recent years, the biological classification system (BCS) suggested by Amidon and coworkers in 1995 has found wide recognition for prognostic evaluation of possible bioavailability problems upon peroral administration of immediate-release (IR) dosage forms, and the system was later modified for extended-release (ER) drug delivery systems. The BCS is based on dissolution, solubility, and gastrointestinal permeability and refers to the likelihood of expected in vitro–in vivo correlation. The BCS is summarized in Table 36-5.

Table 36-5. Biopharmaceutical Classification System for Immediate-Release Drug Products

CLASS	SOLUBILITY	PERMEABILITY	ABSORPTION	EXPECTED IN VITRO- IN VIVO CORRELATION
I	High	High	Very good	Likely
II	Low	High	Dissolution rate limited	Likely
III	High	Low	Permeability rate limited	Less likely
IV	Low	Low	Very poor	Less likely

The relationships between administered dose, dissolution characteristics, drug solubility, and drug absorption can be described by the following three parameters: absorption number (An), dissolution number (Dn), and ratio of dose to dissolved drug (D$_o$):

$$An = (P_{eff}/R) \cdot < Tsi > \tag{1}$$

$$Dn = (3\,D/r^2) \cdot (C_s/\rho) \cdot < Tsi > \tag{2}$$

$$D_o = (M/V_o)/C_s \tag{3}$$

where:

P$_{eff}$ = permeability in units of 10^4 cm/sec
R = gut radius in cm
<Tsi> = the residence time of drug within the intestine
D = the diffusivity
r = the initial radius of drug particle
ρ = the density of dissolved drug
C$_s$ = drug solubility
M = dose of drug
V$_o$ = volume consumed with dose

If P$_{eff} \geq 2.10^{-4}$ cm/sec, drug absorption is complete. For Class I drugs, Dn >1. In this case, the bioavailability, f, can be estimated by:

$$f = 1 - exp\,(-2An) \tag{4}$$

When An > 1.115, the bioavailability is 90% or f = 0.9.

Table 36-6 gives the BCS for extended-release formulations.

Types of Bioavailability

From a scientific point of view, we distinguish between four different types of bioavailability, depending on the purpose of the study and the scientific question to be solved. If new drugs are to be studied probably all four types should be applied, whereas for existing approved drugs only the third or fourth type will be necessary, if a test for bioequivalence is required.

Table 36-6. Biopharmaceutical Classification System for Extended-Release Drug Products

CLASS	SOLUBILITY	PERMEABILITY	SITE DEPENDENCY	EXPECTED IN VITRO-IN VIVO CORRELATION
Ia	High	High	No	Likely
Ib	High	Narrow absorption window	Yes	Less likely
IIa	Low	High	No	Likely
IIb	Low	Narrow absorption window	Yes	Less likely
Va (Bases)	Variable[a]	Variable[b]	Yes	Likely
Vb (Acids)	Variable[b]	Variable[a]	Yes	Less likely

[a] High in upper gastrointestinal tract, low in lower part.
[b] Low in upper gastrointestinal tract, high in lower part.

Absolute Bioavailability or Fraction of Drug Absorbed f

The principle of determining the absolute bioavailability is shown in Figure 36-1. The fraction of drug absorbed f allows determination of the absolute amount of drug absorbed from an extravascularly administered drug product. It is, therefore, essential that the drug be also administered intravenously. However, it is not required to give the same dose IV as is administered extravascularly. For a valid study, both the intravenously and extravascularly administered drug must be given to the same subjects in a cross-over design. The fraction of drug absorbed f is the ratio of the total area under the blood level-time curve upon extravascular route of administration to the total area under the blood level-time curve

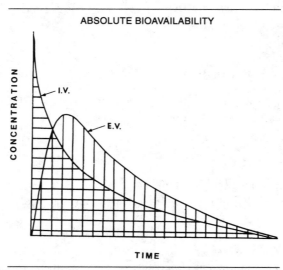

Figure 36-1. Schematic diagram to determine absolute bioavailability from the areas under the curve upon IV and EV administration of identical dose sizes.

upon intravenous administration, corrected for the difference in the dose size as given in Equation 36.5:

$$f = \frac{AUC_{extravascular}^{0\to\infty}[(mg/ml)\cdot h]\cdot D_{I.V.}[mg]}{AUC_{I.V.}^{0\to\infty}[(mg/ml)\cdot h]\cdot D_{extravascular}[mg]} \tag{5}$$

Since the elimination rate constants may vary inter- and intraindividually for the same drug and upon different routes of administration, correction for the observed terminal elimination rate constant data and also for the individual body weight should be made as shown in Equation 36.6:

$$f = \frac{AUC_{extravascular}^{0\to\infty}[(mg/ml)\cdot h]\cdot \dfrac{D_{I.V.}[mg]}{BW_{I.V.}[kg]\cdot \beta_{I.V.}[h^{-1}]}}{AUC_{I.V.}^{0\to\infty}[(mg/ml)\cdot h]\cdot \dfrac{D_{extravasc.}[mg]}{BW_{extravasc.}[kg]\cdot \beta_{extravasc.}[h^{-1}]}} \tag{6}$$

If urinary excretion data are used instead of blood level data, the fraction of drug absorbed f is determined from the ratio of the total amount of unchanged drug excreted into urine upon extravascular administration to that upon intravenous administration, corrected for the dose size as shown in Equation 36.7:

$$f = \frac{Ae_{extravascular}^{\infty}[mg]\cdot D_{I.V.}[mg]}{Ae_{I.V.}^{\infty}[mg]\cdot D_{extravascular}[mg]} \tag{7}$$

Bioavailability in Presence of First-Pass Effect

Drugs showing a first-pass effect may result in considerably lower blood level versus time curves; even though all of the parent drug was absorbed from the site of administration, it did not reach systemic circulation in unchanged form. A drug given IV, IM, SC, or orally will eventually pass through the liver, too. However, it is first distributed in systemic circulation and probably, at least in part, throughout the volume of distribution before being exposed to the liver. At any given time about 80 percent of the blood volume is metabolically inactive.

The fraction of a peroral (PO) or, in part, rectal dose reaching systemic circulation f, under the assumption of otherwise linear kinetics, can be described by Equation 36.8:

$$f = \frac{D_{I.V.}[mg]\cdot AUC_{P.O.}^{0\to\infty}[(mg/ml)\cdot h]}{D_{P.O.}[mg]\cdot AUC_{I.V.}^{0\to\infty}[(mg/ml)\cdot h]} \tag{8}$$

Assuming that only first-pass effect is involved and that the drug is completely absorbed, the fraction of a peroral or rectal dose reaching systemic circulation f is:

$$f = 1 - \frac{D_{I.V.}\cdot f_{m}}{LBF\cdot AUC_{I.V.}^{0\to\infty}\cdot 60\cdot \lambda} \tag{9}$$

f_m = fraction of drug metabolized in the liver
LBF = liver blood flow rate
λ = ratio of the concentration of the drug in whole blood to that in plasma

If the numeric value of f according to Equation 36.8 is less than that obtained with Equation 36.9 then either absorption is incomplete or FPE can be assumed. If the numeric value of f obtained with Equation 36.8 is greater than that obtained with Equation 36.9 it can be assumed that the drug concentration in the portal vein upon PO dosing is high enough to saturate the drug metabolizing enzyme systems.

It is possible to predict the fraction of drug reaching systemic circulation upon PO dosing from IV data. In this case one determines the total area under the curve upon the IV administration and calculates the f according to Equation 36.10, knowing the dose administered IV and assuming a liver blood flow of 1.53 ($1 \cdot min^{-1}$):

$$f = 1 - \frac{D_{I.V.}}{LBF \cdot AUC_{I.V.}^{o \rightarrow \infty} \cdot 60} \tag{10}$$

For differentiation between incomplete absorption and first-pass effect see Chapter 13.

If a drug is administered intrathecally (I.T.) by push or infusion, the CSF (cerebrospinal fluid) bioavailability is 100%. However, if the drug enters the systemic circulation, then the bioavailability in plasma (% f_{plasma}) is:

$$\% \, f_{plasma} = \frac{100 \cdot AUC_{I.T.}/Dose_{I.V.}}{AUC_{I.V.}/Dose_{I.T.}} \tag{11}$$

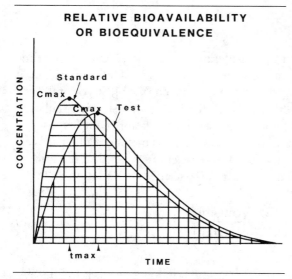

RELATIVE BIOAVAILABILITY OR BIOEQUIVALENCE

Figure 36-2. Schematic diagram to determine relative bioavailability from the areas under the curve from two different drug products given EV by the same route of administration in identical dose sizes.

Relative Bioavailability and Bioequivalence

The principle for determination of relative bioavailability is shown in Figure 36-2.

The relative bioavailability is the *extent* (EBA) and *rate* (RBA) of the bioavailability of a drug from two or more different dosage forms given by the *same* route of administration. According to the FDA regulation the standard used in this procedure is an approved marketed drug product, a solution of the drug, or suspension of the micronized drug.

For determination of EBA and RBA either blood level or urinary excretion data upon single or multiple dosing can be used. For valid studies a crossover design has to be used, whereby differences in clearance and/or terminal disposition rate constants should cancel out. For a single dose blood level study

EBA is calculated according to Equation 36.12 where the indices t.d.p. and s.d.p. mean "test drug product" and "standard drug product," respectively:

$$EBA = \frac{AUC_{t.d.p.}^{0 \to \infty}[(mg/ml) \cdot h] \cdot D_{s.d.p.}[mg]}{AUC_{s.d.p.}^{0 \to \infty}[(mg/ml) \cdot h] \cdot D_{t.d.p.}[mg]} \cdot 100 \qquad (12)$$

In case of multiple dosing EBA can be determined from the blood level-time curve within a complete dosing interval τ at steady state using Equation 36.13:

$$EBA = \frac{AUC_{t.d.p.}^{\tau_n \to \tau_{n+1}}[(mg/ml) \cdot h] \cdot D_{s.d.p.}[mg]}{AUC_{s.d.p.}^{\tau_n \to \tau_{n+1}}[(mg/ml) \cdot h] \cdot D_{t.d.p.}[mg]} \cdot 100 \qquad (13)$$

In the case of urinary excretion data, the total amount of unchanged drug excreted into urine upon single dose administration is used applying Equation 36.14 to determine EBA:

$$EBA = \frac{Ae_{t.d.p.}^{\infty}[mg] \cdot D_{s.d.p.}[mg]}{Ae_{s.d.p.}^{\infty}[mg] \cdot D_{t.d.p.}[mg]} \cdot 100 \qquad (14)$$

In the case of urinary excretion data from multiple dosing Equation 36.15 is applicable:

$$EBA = \frac{Ae_{t.d.p.}^{\tau_n \to \tau_{n+1}}[mg] \cdot D_{s.d.p.}[mg]}{Ae_{s.d.p.}^{\tau_n \to \tau_{n+1}}[mg] \cdot D_{t.d.p.}[mg]} \cdot 100 \qquad (15)$$

Bioequivalence is given if there is no significant difference in extent and rate of relative bioavailability of a test product when compared to the approved standard.

Relative Optimal Bioavailability

The term *relative optimal bioavailability* was suggested in 1970 for optimizing extent and rate of bioavailability for a drug product during the development phase. For determination of $EBA_{rel.\ opt.}$ the active drug is administered in aqueous solution without addition of any further excipient by the same route which is intended for the drug product under development. In case the drug is not water soluble, an aqueous-organic solvent, such as glycerol, propylene glycol, alcohol, or polyethylene glycol-water mixture, is used. The total AUC and the absorption rate constant k_a are determined from blood level-time data.

The $EBA_{opt.\ rel.}$ is termed optimal because the first step in the sequence of events responsible for bioavailability, the drug liberation, is omitted since the drug is already in aqueous solution, hence, in absorbable optimal form. However, it is relative because the bioavailability might be further increased by the addition of buffers to either prevent decomposition or inactivation or to increase the nonionized moiety or by addition of sorption promoting agents. It is further relatively optimal because the assumption that a drug in aqueous solution is always "better" absorbed may not be valid in all cases. It is well known that if a drug is absorbed exclusively from the duodenum the transit time of the drug in solution might be too short to permit complete absorption.

The absorption rate constant obtained with the solution is termed "true" rate constant for this particular route of administration, whereas the rate constant for absorption obtained with the drug product will only be an *apparent* one which is overlapped by the process of drug liberation and dissolution. If one determines the blood level-time profiles and absorption rate constants upon administration of the drug in solution, then the drug in powder form filled into gelatin capsules, then the drug in powder form with the addition of the anticipated excipients filled into gelatin capsules, followed by administration of the granules filled into gelatin capsules, and finally of the tablet, or any other dosage form, it is possible to pinpoint whether a bioavailability problem may be associated with the drug, the excipients, or the manufacturing method.

The $EBA_{rel.\ opt.}$ is determined according to Equation 36.16:

$$EBA_{rel.opt.} = \frac{AUC^{o \to \infty}_{(drugs;\ +vehicle;\ granules;\ tablet)}}{AUC^{o \to \infty}_{(solution)}} \cdot 100 \qquad (16)$$

The method of optimal relative bioavailability will definitely be determined in animal models and not in man. It constitutes a useful tool in drug product development.

For determination of area under the concentration-time curve see Chapter 20.

Determination of Rate of Bioavailability

The rate of bioavailability (RBA) is actually the apparent absorption rate constant of the drug from the drug product. Even if the extent of bioavailability is identical for two or more products it does not necessarily mean that they result in comparable blood level curves, because it is the rate which determines the time and height of the peak in case of complete absorption and constant elimination rate as shown in Figure 36-3.

All three curves in Figure 36-3 have the same area under the curve. However, only curves I and II will be clinically effective, since at least a portion of the blood level curve is above the minimum effective MEC or minimum inhibitory concentration MIC, whereas curve No. III does not even reach this minimum therapeutic concentration. Also onset and duration may depend on the rate of bioavailability. The determination of RBA is model dependent, since the blood level-time curve upon extravascular administration is a composite of at least a biexponential or higher exponential process. A number of methods have been described for determination of the RBA. The residual method only will be discussed as a typical example and the most widely used method.

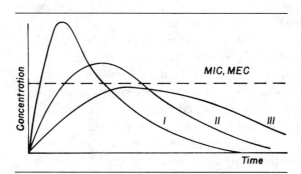

Figure 36-3. Extent of bioavailability and clinical effectiveness. All three curves have identical AUCs, yet one curve does not reach the required minimum effective concentration.

The drug concentration data are plotted on a log scale versus time. In the case of a one-compartment open model (see Figure 36-4, top) the mono-

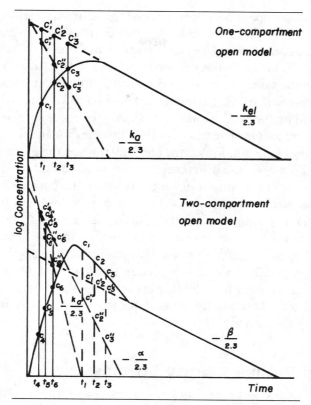

Figure 36-4. Determination of rate of bioavailability by the residual method.

Top:

C_{index} = actual blood concentrations during absorptive phase at corresponding sampling times t_{index}

C'_{index} = concentrations on back-extrapolated k_{el} slope at times t_{index}

C''_{index} = differences between C'_{index} and C_{index}

k_{el} = elimination rate constant

k_a = absorption rate constant

Bottom:

$C_{1,2,3}$ = actual blood concentrations during distributive phase at corresponding sampling times $t_{1,2,3}$

$C'_{1,2,3}$ = corresponding concentration values on back-extrapolated terminal disposition slope β

C''_{index} = difference between C'_{index} and $C_{1,2,3}$

$C_{4,5,6}$ = actual blood concentrations during absorptive phase at corresponding sampling times $t_{4,5,6}$

$C'_{4,5,6}$ = corresponding concentrations on fast disposition slope α

$C''_{4,5,6}$ = difference between $C'_{4,5,6}$ and $C_{4,5,6}$

β = terminal disposition rate constant

α = hybrid distribution rate constant

k_a = absorption rate constant

exponential elimination slope is back-extrapolated to the ordinate. Using the intercept B the differences between the actual blood level points during the absorptive phase and the concentrations on the back-extrapolated monoexponential line at the same time are plotted on the same graph. Combining these different points a straight line is obtained by using a least square fit, and the slope of this line is the absorption rate constant k_a.

In case the two-compartment open model is applicable, first the fast disposition slope α is determined by the residual method as the differences between the descending curved part of the curve and the back-extrapolated monoexponential terminal slope data and the corresponding concentrations at the identical time on the β slope. Then the residuals are determined between the differences of the actual blood level data during the absorptive phase and the concentrations on the α-slope, the corresponding concentrations on the α-slope at the same times, as shown in Figure 36-4, bottom graph. A least square fit of the difference points will yield the absorption rate constant k_a.

The same procedure for determination of absorption rate constant can also be applied to a plot of log mean excretion rate versus midpoint time obtained from a cumulative urinary excretion study. The mean excretion rate versus midpoint time plot is the identical image to the corresponding blood level curve and is suitable for determination of terminal disposition rate constant, time of peak for the drug concentration in the blood, and determination of absorption rate constant.

Evaluation of Bioavailability Studies

The most precise evaluation of extent and rate of bioavailability is obtained from single dose or multiple dose blood level studies followed by single dose or multiple dose urinary excretion studies.

Single Dose Studies

In case of blood level studies the following three parameters characterize rate and extent of bioavailability:

- Area under curve ($AUC^{o \to \infty}$);
- Actual peak height (C_{max}); and
- Time to reach the peak (t_{max}).

In case of urinary excretion studies the three parameters characterizing the rate and extent of bioavailability are the following:

- Total amount of drug excreted in infinite time in unchanged form (Ae^{∞});
- Actual peak height (C_{max}) determined from the log excretion rate *versus* midpoint time curve; and
- Time to reach the peak (t_{max}) determined from a log excretion rate *versus* midpoint time plot.

Considering only the AUCs from blood level studies or only Ae^{∞} from urinary excretion studies is not appropriate since two different drug products may result in the same

AUC or Ae$^\infty$ and yet may not be therapeutically equivalent. A hypothetical example is given in Figure 36-5.

As seen in Figure 36-5, all drugs give the same areas under the curve. Yet drug product I is clearly superior since the peak is above the MEC, whereas drug product III does not even reach the minimum effective concentration. The two drug products differ in C_{max} and t_{max}. Drug product II may even be superior to product I although $C_{max\,II}$ is less than $C_{max\,I}$ but still above the MEC. However, the duration is longer than with product I, as seen at top of Figure 36-5. The corresponding amount of drug Ae$^\infty$ totally excreted at time T$^\infty$ is the same for all three drug products as seen on bottom of Figure 36-5. However, the course of the different curves has to be used for determination of the rate of bioavailability.

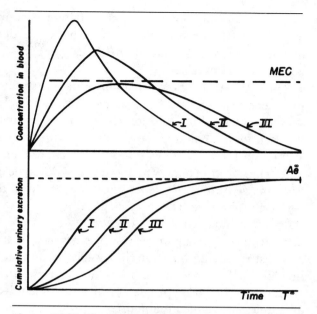

Figure 36-5. Blood level versus time curve for three drug products with identical extent of bioavailability but different rates of bioavailability (top), and the corresponding cumulative urinary excretion curves (bottom): Ae$^\infty$ = total amount of unchanged drug eliminated in urine at infinite time T$^\infty$.

Multiple Dose Studies

Multiple dose studies are carried out for one dosing interval at steady state. Two parameters characterize rate and extent of bioavailability:

- Area under curve during dosing interval AUC$^{\tau_n \rightarrow \tau_{n+1}}$; and
- Percent fluctuation.

The fluctuation is given by:

$$\% \text{ Fluctuation} = 100 \cdot \left(\frac{C_{max}^{ss} - C_{min}^{ss}}{C_{min}^{ss}} \right) \qquad (17)$$

Steady state should be verified by taking trough levels on two consecutive days at the same time. It is not advisable to take trough levels of two consecutive dosing intervals (if <24 h) because a difference may occur due to circadian rhythm even when steady state is reached. Switching from one product to another, the new steady state should be verified.

In case of urinary excretion studies the urine is collected for one entire dosing interval at steady state.

The AUCs can be determined either from the blood level equation after curve-fitting or by the trapezoidal rule (see Chapter 20).

Bioavailability should be evaluated by 90 percent confidence interval based on the two one-sided t-test approach. This approach involves determination of confidence interval for the ratio of means using a modified t-test method. The previously used 75/75 decision rule is no longer acceptable.

In evaluation of bioavailability data one should not plot all data from all volunteers together and determine the parameters as an average from all cumulative data. Instead, one should evaluate either the blood level data or cumulative urinary excretion data separately for each individual and compare these with those of the standard, then determine the average and standard deviation for each parameter.

The question of how many subjects should be used is a difficult one to answer. There is no magic number. It depends on the statistical design of the study and the degree of variations obtained. However, in general, 12 to 18 volunteers will be sufficient to make a statistical evaluation.

From a clinical point of view we may ask: what is the clinical significance of bioavailability studies? This question clearly goes beyond the scope of bioavailability testing as outlined in the FDA regulation but is, nevertheless, a very valid question. Without doubt we should strive for drug products which are bioequivalent and are, therefore, interchangeable unless it is stated that a drug product might not be indicated for a desired purpose. Bioavailability should not be considered as a test which generates an imaginary number for a given drug in a given dosage form for a given route of administration, but it should be a guarantee for in vivo quality.

For most of the drugs we assume that the drug concentration in blood, plasma, or serum is directly related to the therapeutic response. Even if the biophase, the locus of interaction between the drug and the cell or cell component, is not in the systemic circulation but somewhere in the tissue, the drug concentration in systemic circulation may correlate with the therapeutic response since the transfer of free, nonprotein bound drug from the circulation to the tissue depends on the concentration gradient and can be described mathematically. Exceptions are cases where active transport is involved.

The question of bioavailability should also be considered from a point of view of drug-receptor interaction. (For receptor theories see Chapter 5.)

In relation to bioavailability we may therefore conclude that if a drug exerts its pharmacologic effect according to the occupation theory, then one could assume that the amount of drug available systemically would be the most important parameter. If a drug exerts its pharmacological effect according to the rate theory, then one could assume the rate and extent of bioavailability would be the most decisive parameters. However, the rate of bioavailability is also important when the drug follows the occupation theory. This is true because the extent of bioavailability may be the same for different products and yet one may be ineffective due to a low rate of bioavailability which may not permit the drug to reach a concentration in blood above threshold or minimum effective level.

From a point of view of bioavailability, drugs can be classified according to two basic response patterns:

- The response is based on the log dose-response curve; or
- The response is based on the minimum effective or minimum inhibitory concentration.

The two patterns are shown in Figure 36-6.

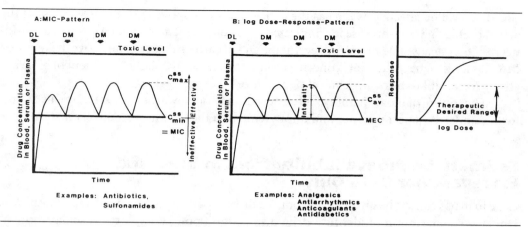

Figure 36-6. Schematic diagram for pharmacokinetic classification with respect to dosage regimen calculation and bioavailability evaluation for drugs following the MIC pattern (A) or the log dose-response pattern (B).

DL = loading dose
DM = maintenance dose
MIC = minimum inhibitory concentration
MEC = minimum effective concentration
C_{max}^{ss} = maximum blood level at steady state
C_{min}^{ss} = minimum blood level at steady state
C_{av}^{ss} = average steady state blood level (18)

For the log dose-response pattern it is desirable to maintain the drug concentration within the therapeutic range. The higher the EBA is within this range the greater will be the intensity of the pharmacologic effect.

Levy demonstrated that a given degree of change of extent of drug absorption will not necessarily be directly proportional to the change in pharmacologic effect due to the approximately log-linear character of most dose-response relationships as seen from Figure 36-7.

The loss of pharmacologic effectiveness increases disproportionally the steeper the log dose-response curve is and the deeper the therapeutic dose is located on that curve.

For the MIC pattern it is desired to maintain the drug concentration during the entire course of therapy above the minimum inhibitory or minimum effective concentration which will differ with each type of microorganism and its sensitivity.

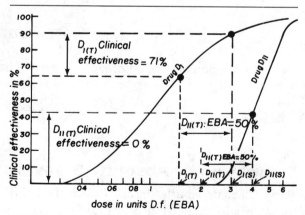

Figure 36-7. Schematic diagram demonstrating disproportional decrease in clinical effectiveness with decrease in extent of bioavailability for drugs following the log dose-response pattern. D_I, D_{II} log dose-response curves for drugs I and II; $D_{I(S)}$, $D_{II(S)}$ = doses of standard for drugs I and II; $D_{I(T)}$, $D_{II(T)}$ = doses of test product showing only 50% extent of bioavailability; EBA = extent of bioavailability = D·f.

The drug will be effective as long as the concentration is above the MIC, regardless of the actual peak height. In this case it is indicated to estimate whether or not a given drug product results at steady state in a blood level at the end of each dosing interval above the required MIC. As long as the steady state concentration is above the MIC the actual extent of bioavailability seems not to be of any clinical significance.

The testing of bioavailability adds a new dimension towards the development of uniform standards of performance and improvement of the health care delivery system.

Estimate on Bioavailability from In Vitro and Extravascular Data Only

Certain drugs cannot be given intravenously, or IV blood level-time data are not available. Under the assumption of identical drug disposition upon IV and extravascular route of administration and absence of dose dependency, it should be possible to predict the fraction of drug absorbed, f, by comparing the $AUC^{0\to\infty}$ from the EV administration with the generated $AUC^{0\to\infty}$ for IV administration based on the relationship between volume of distribution, apparent partition coefficient, and extent of protein binding (Ritschel-Hammer method). For more on this relationship see Chapter 16.

The $AUC^{0\to\infty}$ for the hypothetical IV administration can be estimated for the one- and two-compartment model according to Equations 36.18 and 36.19 using k_{el} and k_{13}, respectively, from the extravascular concentration-time profile:

$$AUC_{I.V.}^{0\to\infty} = \frac{D}{(0.0955 \cdot APC + 1.2232) \cdot (1-p) \cdot BW \cdot k_{el}} \tag{18}$$

$$AUC_{I.V.}^{0\to\infty} = \frac{D}{(0.0397 \cdot APC + 0.0273) \cdot (1-p) \cdot BW \cdot k_{13}} \tag{19}$$

The fraction of drug absorbed is calculated by Equation 36.20:

$$f = \frac{AUC_{extravasc.}^{0\to\infty}}{AUC_{I.V.}^{0\to\infty}} \tag{20}$$

Estimation of Absolute Bioavailability from Peroral Data

As described previously, the calculation of absolute bioavailability for a given drug requires that it be administered directly into the vascular space (e.g., intravenously). An alternate approach has been proposed whereby only peroral data are used to estimate absolute bioavailability. In contrast to approaches to determine the true absolute bioavailability of a drug, this alternate method requires that information on postdose drug concentrations in both plasma and urine be available. The basis of this alternative method is simple. Assuming first-order kinetics, the constancy of f, and independence of a possibly existing nonrenal clearance (CL_{NR}) from renal function, plots of the oral total clearance against renal clearance are constructed. In subjects with varying renal function, these plots can be fitted to linear function in accord with:

$$(D/AUC)_{P.O.} = CL_{NR}/f + (1/f)CL_R, \text{ or} \tag{21}$$

$$(D/AUC)_{P.O.} = (1/f)CL_R \tag{22}$$

dependent upon whether the drug in question is cleared nonrenally and renally or only by renal mechanisms. Estimates of mean absolute bioavailability and nonrenal clearance after peroral administration can be obtained from the reciprocal of the slope and y-axis intercept of this plot, respectively.

Selected References

1. Amidon, G. L., Lennernas, H., Shah, V. P. and Crison, J. R.: A Theoretical Basis for a Biopharmaceutic Drug Classification: The Correlation of in vitro Drug Product Dissolution and in vivo Bioavailability. *Pharm. Res. 12*:413–420 (1995).

2. *APhA Guidelines for Biopharmaceutical Studies in Man,* American Pharmaceutical Association Academy of Pharmaceutical Sciences. Washington, D.C., 1972.

3. APhA: *The Bioavailability of Drug Products,* American Pharmaceutical Association, Washington, D.C., 1975.

4. Brest, A. N.: *The Scientific Evaluation of Drug Equivalency,* Proceedings of a Colloquium, Excerpta Medica, Amsterdam-Geneva-London-Princeton, 1974.

5. Brodie, B. B. and Heller, W. M.: *Bioavailability of Drugs,* Proceedings of the Conference on Bioavailability of Drugs, S. Karger, Basel-Munich-Paris-London-New York-Sydney, 1972.

6. Cabana, B. E.: Importance of Biopharmaceutics and Pharmacokinetics in Clinical Medicine, *Arzneim. Forsch. 26*:151 (1976).

7. Chodes, D. J. and DiSanto, A. R.: *Basics of Bioavailability,* The Upjohn Company, Kalamazoo, 1973.

8. Daddario, E. Q. and Desimone, D.: *Drug Bioequivalence,* A Report of the Technology Assessment Drug Bioequivalence Study Panel, U.S. Government Printing Office, Washington, D.C., 1974.

9. Department of Health, Education, and Welfare, Public Health Service, Food and Drug Administration, HEW Publication No. (FDA) 76-3009, 1976.

10. Dittert, L. W. and DiSanto, A. R.: The Bioavailability of Drug Products, *J APhA NS 13*:421 (1973).

11. *Federal Register. 42* F.R. 1624–1653 (Jan. 7) 1977.

12. Grahnén, A.: Design of Bioavailability Studies, *Pharm. Int. 5*:100 (1984).

13. Hinderling, P. H. and Shi, J.: Absolute Bioavailability Estimated from Oral Data. *J. Pharm. Sci. 84*:385–386 (1995).

14. Hirtz, J.: La Disponibilité Biologique des Médicaments, *Labo. Pharma. Probl. Techn. 20*:63 (1972).

15. Jamali, F.: Stereochemistry and Bioequivalence, *J. Clin. Pharmacol. 32*:930–934 (1992).

16. Kaplan, S. A. and Jack, M. L.: Utility of Bioavailability Studies in Drug Development, *Drug Develop. Ind. Pharm. 3*:39 (1977).

17. Levy, G.: *Bioavailability; Clinical Effectiveness and the Public Interest,* Conference on Bioavailability of Drugs, Washington, D.C.: (Nov. 22) 1971.

18. Levy, G.: Bioavailability *versus* Pharmacologic Availability, *Rev. Can. Biol. 32*:124 (1973).

19. Lobenberg, R. and Amidon, G. L.: Modern Bioavailability, Bioequivalence and Biopharmaceutical Classification System: New Scientific Approaches to International Regulatory Standards. *Eur. J. Pharm. Biopharm. 50*:3–12 (2000).

20. Nerukar, S. G., Dighe, S. V. and Williams, R. L.: Bioequivalence of Racemic Drugs. *J. Clin. Pharmacol. 32*:935–943 (1992).

21. Orzechowski, G.: Biologische Verfügbarkeit (Bioavailability), *Dtsch. Apoth. Ztg. 25*:659 (1973).

22. Oser, B. L., Melnick, D. and Hochberg, M.: Physiological Availability of the Vitamins. Study of Methods for Determining Availability in Pharmaceutical Products, *Ind. Eng. Chem. Anal. Educ. 17*:401 (1945).

23. Proceedings, Food and Drug Administration Bioequivalence Hearing, Department of Health and Human Services, Maple Glen, PA, 1987.

24. Report by the Bioequivalence Task Force on Recommendations from the Bioequivalence Hearing Conducted by the Food and Drug Administration, FDA, Rockville, MD, Jan. 1988.

25. Rietbrock, N.: Therapeutische Gleichwertigkeit und Ungleichwertigkeit chemisch identischer Stoffe, *Arzneim. Forsch. 26*:135 (1976).

26. Ritschel, W. A.: Bioavailability in the Clinical Evaluation of Drugs, *Drug Intell. Clin. Pharm. 6*:246 (1972).

27. Ritschel, W. A.: Bioavailability of Peroral Dosage Forms, *Boll. Chim. Farm. 112*:137 (1973).

28. Ritschel, W. A.: Bioavailability Testing and Clinical Significance, *Pharm. Acta Helv. 49*:77 (1974).

29. Ritschel, W. A.: Physicochemical and Pharmaceutical Properties of Drugs and Dosage Forms Influencing the Results of Phase I Studies. In: *Advances in Clinical Pharmacology*, Edited by Kuemmerle, H. P., Shibuya, T. and Kimura, E., Urban and Schwarzenberg, Munich-Baltimore, 1977, Vol. 13.

30. Ritschel, W. A.: Pharmacists and Bioavailability: The American Perspective, *Labo. Pharma. Probl. Tech. 272*:40 (1978).

31. Ritschel, W. A.: The Scientific Basis of Bioavailability, *Labo. Pharma. Probl. Tech. 276*:395 (1978).

32. Ritschel, W. A. and Hammer, G. V.: Prediction of the Volume of Distribution From in vitro Data and Use for Estimating the Absolute Extent of Absorption. *Int. J. Clin. Ther. Tox. 18*:298 (1980).

33. Ritschel, W. A.: What Is Bioavailability? Philosophy of Bioavailability Testing, *Methods Find. Exp. Clin. Pharmacol. 6*:777 (1984).

34. Ritschel, W. A.: Bioavailability: A Critical Evaluation. In: *Biotechnology in Health Care, Proceedings of the 37th Indian Pharmaceutical Congress,* New Delhi, Printorium Press, Ahmedabad, India, 1987, pp. 111–142.

35. Ritschel, W. A.: Aspects for Bioavailability and Bioequivalence Revision: Possible Implications on Clinical Pharmacology, *Methods Find. Exp. Clin. Pharmacol. 9*:453–459 (1987).

36. Schneller, G. H.: Status Report on Drug Bioavailability, *Am. J. Hosp. Pharm. 27*:485 (1970).

37. Schnieders, B.: Bioverfügbarkeit, Wirksamkeitsnachweis und Folgerungen für die Arzneimittelgasetzgebung. *Arzneim. Forsch. 26*:158 (1976).

38. Smolen, V. F.: *Pharmacokinetic Engineering Approach to Drug Delivery System Design and the Optimization of Drug Effects,* Proceedings of the International Conference on Cybernetics, Washington, D.C.: 340 (1976).

39. Wagner, J. G.: Pharmacokinetics and Bioavailability, *Triangle 14*:101 (1975).

40. Wagner, J. G.: An Overview of the Analysis and Interpretation of Bioavailability Studies in Man, *Arzneim. Forsch. 26*:105 (1976).

41. Wagner, J. G.: *Biopharmaceutics and Relevant Pharmacokinetics,* Drug Intelligence Publications, Hamilton, Illinois: 297 (1971).

42. Wermeling, D., Drass, M., Ellis, D., Mayo, M., McGuire, D., O'Connell, D., Hale, V. and Chao, S.: Pharmacokinetics and Pharmacodynamics of Intrathecal Ziconotide in Chronic Pain Patients. *J. Clin. Pharmacol. 43*:624–636 (2003).

43. Westlake, W. J.: Use of Statistical Methods in Evaluation of In Vivo Performance of Dosage Forms, *J. Pharm. Sci. 62*:1579 (1973).

44. Young, D. B., Devane J. G. and Butler, J.: In vitro-in vivo correlation. Plenum Press, New York, NY 1997.

37

Body Surface Areas

For most drugs, dosing is based on mg drug per kg body weight. However, there are some toxic drugs, such as aminoglycosides and cancer chemotherapeutic agents, which preferentially are based on mg per body surface area, SA, using either the total surface area in m², or normalized in mg/m². In pediatrics, SA is also used to calculate dose size if the drug's apparent volume of distribution is less than 0.3 (see Table 24-2).

The "normal" adult SA is generally accepted to be 1.73 m² as the reference value for the average patient. For instance, in case of renal failure a correction for altered glomerular filtration rate or creatinine clearance is made. The GFR or creatinine clearance is based on 1.73 m²; hence, for dosing of drugs in renal failure (see Chapter 17, section on Factors Influencing Renal Clearance, and Equations 28.30 and 28.31) one needs to estimate the patient's individual SA.

The most widely used method to estimate the total body surface area is that by DuBois and DuBois:

$$SA = \frac{BW\,[kg]^{0.425} \cdot H\,[cm]^{0.725} \cdot 71.84}{10,000}[m^2] \tag{1}$$

or:

$$SA = \frac{167.2 \cdot \sqrt{BW}\,[kg] \cdot \sqrt{H}\,[cm]}{10,000}[m^2] \tag{2}$$

where BW is body weight and H is body height.

In case of amputation or loss of body parts, an estimate of the modified surface area in the amputee needs to be made, SA_{Amp}. Table 37-1 lists body parts along with the mean percentage of total body surface area.

Other Surface Areas

Often it is instructive to explain processes by considering the physiologic and/or anatomic aspects involved. For instance, the fast absorption of compounds from the GI tract becomes

Table 37-1. Surface Area of Body Parts Expressed as Percentage of Total Body Surface Area

BODY PARTS	MEAN PERCENT OF SA$_{PART}$	RANGE
Index Finger	0.34	0.28–0.40
Hand + 5 Fingers	2.80	2.36–3.35
Lower Arm (includes hand but not fingers)	4.00	3.55–4.44
Upper Arm	5.90	4.73–6.88
Thigh	11.89	9.77–15.50
Lower Leg	6.04	5.11–7.15
Foot	3.11	2.54–3.93

very plausible in that the tube system of 9 m length and 2.5–7 cm in diameter does not result in a surface area of about 4 m^2, rather having a surface area of about 120–200 m^2 due to the folds, macrovilli, and particularly microvilli present in the lumenal site. Table 37-2 lists surface areas of some anatomic sites.

In order to estimate the SA in an amputee, first the "normal" SA is calculated by Equation 37.1. In case of both legs being amputated, the H prior to amputation is used. Then the mean percent of SA$_{Part}$ is taken from Table 37-1, and, if necessary, multiplied by num-

Table 37-2. Surface Areas in m^2 of Anatomic Sites

ANATOMIC SITE	SURFACE AREA IN m^2
Skin	1.73
Head	0.097
Trunk	0.6
Lung	70
GI Tract	120–200
Mouth Cavity	0.02
Stomach	0.1–0.2
Small Intestine	120–200
Large Intestine	0.5–1
Rectum	0.05
Glomeruli (both kidneys)	1.16
Capillaries in Placenta	
Day 100	1.2
Birth	14.0

ber of parts (i.e., $0.34 \cdot 3$ for 3 fingers). The surface area in the amputee, SA_{Amp} is estimated by Equation 37.3:

$$SA_{Amp} = SA - \left(SA \cdot \frac{\% \, SA_{Part}}{100} \right) [m^2] \tag{3}$$

It seems that the weight-height formula by DuBois and DuBois underestimates the surface area in newborns. Hence, for newborns the following equation is suggested:

$$SA_{newborns} = 0.0224265 \cdot BW^{0.5378} \cdot H^{0.3964} \, [m^2] \tag{4}$$

Selected References

1. DuBois, D. and DuBois, E. F.: A Formula to Estimate the Approximate Surface Area if Height and Weight be Known, *Arch. Intern. Med. 17*:863–871 (1916).

2. Haycock, G. B., Schwartz, G. J. and Wisotsky, D. H.: Geometric Method for Measuring Body Surface Area: A Height-Weight Formula Validated in Infants, Children, and Adults, *J. Pediatr. 93*:62–66 (1978).

3. Colangelo, P. M., Welch, D. W., Rich, D. S. and Jeffrey, L. P.: Two Methods for Estimating Body Surface Area in Adult Amputees, *Am. J. Hosp. Pharm. 41*:2614–2655 (1984).

38

Extracorporeal Methods of Drug Removal

Across the United States more than 200,000 adults and children receive long-term dialysis as treatment for end-stage renal disease. The majority of such individuals maintained on dialysis receive three times a week hemodialysis or daily peritoneal dialysis. Hemodialysis can also be used in the acute care setting to remove selected drugs/chemicals from the body in case of poisoning. As well, the various forms of hemofiltration and hemoperfusion are ordinarily reserved for acute care settings, the former (hemofiltration) to restore fluid and electrolyte balance and the latter (hemoperfusion) to remove toxicants.

Principles of Dialysis

In essence, dialysis is the exchange of solute and water across a semipermeable membrane. All dialysis systems operate on the principles of diffusion, osmosis, hydrostatic pressure, and convection. Diffusion is the movement of a solute from a region of high to low solute concentration. Osmosis is the process by which fluid moves from a solution of lower to a solution of higher osmolality. Hydrostatic pressure relates to the pressure of fluids within a compartment (e.g., blood vessel). When hydrostatic pressure across a membrane is unequal, fluid tends to move from an area of higher to lower pressure. Finally, solute movement across a membrane that occurs simply because it is trapped in the flow of water is coined convection.

During dialysis, the patient's blood and dialysis fluid are partitioned on opposing sides of a semipermeable membrane usually flowing in opposite directions. This is illustrated by Figure 38-1 which schematically depicts hemodialysis and the countercurrent flow which results from blood and dialysate moving in opposite directions. As blood and dialysis fluid interface across the semipermeable membrane, fluid tends to flow from the blood compartment to the dialysis fluid as a result of increased pressure in the blood compartment (i.e., hydrostatic pressure) or increased osmotic pressure in the dialysis fluid compartment (i.e., osmosis). In a similar manner, solutes move across the semipermeable membrane in response to concentration differences (i.e., diffusion) or as a result of being trapped in the fluid that moves across the membrane (i.e., convection).

Due to their large molecular weight and size, circulating plasma proteins and blood cells do not pass through the semipermeable membrane and therefore remain in the blood. The rate of diffusion (i.e., clearance) for a particular solute, such as "uremic toxins" or drugs, varies with the size (i.e., molecular weight) of the solute, the extent of plasma protein

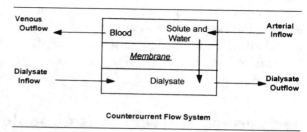

Figure 38-1. Schematic representation of hemodialysis.

binding, membrane permeability (e.g., composition of the membrane and pore structure/size, all of which are the determinants of the sieving coefficient), and the extent of the concentration gradient across the membrane. Of these factors, the degree of protein binding and the extent of the concentration gradient across the semipermeable membrane are the most important, the latter being governed by the rate of dialysis fluid and blood flow as well as the solute composition of the dialysis fluid. A relevant example is seen with urea, an end product of nitrogen metabolism that accumulates in the blood of patients with renal failure and is not present in dialysis fluid. When blood and dialysis fluid pass on opposite sides of the semipermeable membrane, urea diffuses from the blood to the dialysis fluid because the concentration on the blood side is greater than the dialysis fluid concentration. Moreover, the extent of the concentration gradient and, hence, dialysis efficiency are also determined by the velocity of dialysis fluid and blood flow. At rapid blood and dialysis fluid flow rates, the solute gradient across the semipermeable membrane is continually regenerated and there is insufficient time for the solute to equilibrate, a state that decreases solute clearance.

During many extracorporeal procedures (e.g., hemodialysis, CAVHD, CVVHD), blood flows or is pumped from the patient through a dialyzer where fluid and solute exchange takes place before the "cleansed" blood is returned to the patient. The dialyzer is a device encased by a plastic housing that contains thousands of thin capillaries made of semipermeable membrane through which the patient's blood flows. Dialysis fluid is pumped through a separate port into the plastic housing and bathes the outside of the capillary tubes. The dialysis fluid usually flows in a direction opposite the blood flow (i.e., countercurrent flow as depicted in Figure 38-1) in order to maintain the solute concentration gradient. With hemodialysis, significant amounts of fluid and accompanying solutes (e.g., creatinine) can be removed from the patient in a process known as ultrafiltration as depicted in the schematic representation contained in Figure 38-2. Simply, ultrafiltration is governed by the difference in the hydrostatic pressure generated by blood flow (i.e., positive pressure) and dialysate flow (i.e., negative pressure) across the membrane. This pressure difference across the membrane is referred to as transmembrane pressure (TMP). During the process of ultrafiltration, the source of "plasma water" is most commonly

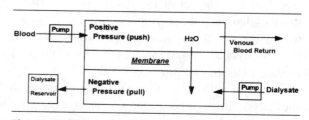

Figure 38-2. Schematic of ultrafiltration during hemodialysis.

the extracellular fluid space which is reduced consequent to rapid reestablishment of an equilibrium between the vascular and extracellular fluid pools. The principles of dialysis are relatively unchanged in peritoneal dialysis with the exception that the dialysis membrane is endogenous as described below and that ultrafiltration results from osmotic as opposed to hydrostatic forces.

Techniques and Methods Capable of Extracorporeal Drug Removal

As the circulating free fraction of a drug or toxin is "dissolved" in plasma water and will attain a distributional equilibrium between the plasma compartment and other body water/tissue compartments, any procedure that produces a removal of plasma water and solutes can theoretically produce an increase in the plasma clearance and hence extracorporeal drug removal. The efficiency of a given extracorporeal procedure to remove a drug or toxin is dependent upon the physicochemical characteristics and concentration of the drug/toxin, the physical characteristics of the dialysis procedure (e.g., the dialyzer, blood and dialysis flow rates), and the duration of time over which the procedure is applied. The different techniques that can result in extracorporeal drug removal are summarized as follows.

Hemodialysis is the process of pumping blood from the patient to a dialyzer where dialysis fluid and blood pass in opposite directions resulting in solute and fluid exchange. The circuit is completed with the return of "cleansed" blood to the patient. In hemodialysis the flow of dialysis fluid is so rapid (i.e., 500 ml/min) that the rate limiting factors in solute clearance are blood flow and membrane characteristics. A typical hemodialysis "session" provides a urea clearance of 3–4 ml/kg/min. However, it should be noted that different types of dialyzers have different physical characteristics (e.g., coil dialyzers, plate dialyzers, hollow fiber dialyzers) and inconsistent efficiencies for the removal of specific substrates. Comparison of the efficiency of different types of dialyzers is usually accomplished by comparing the clearance of a small molecular weight solute (e.g., urea); this information is provided by the manufacturer of a given dialyzer.

Peritoneal dialysis is a form of dialysis which occurs inside the body. In peritoneal dialysis, the blood and dialysis fluid are partitioned across the peritoneal membrane, a highly vascularized semipermeable membrane that lines the abdominal organs and anterior abdominal wall, enclosing a space known as the peritoneal cavity. The "driving forces" for peritoneal dialysis are the rate of blood flow through the circulation of the abdominal cavity (i.e., mesenteric blood flow which approximates 20% of the cardiac output) and the osmolality of the dialysate as determined by its solute composition and concentrations. To initiate the procedure, dialysis fluid is placed into the peritoneal cavity where it remains for a predetermined length of time (i.e., dwell time), ranging anywhere from 30 minutes to six hours. During the dwell of dialysis fluid in the peritoneal cavity, solute and fluid are exchanged across the peritoneal membrane which acts as a naturally occurring dialyzer. At the conclusion of the dwell, the dialysis fluid containing the solutes and fluid removed from the blood is drained and discarded. Once the spent dialysis fluid (i.e., dialysate) is drained, the process is repeated with fresh dialysate. In peritoneal dialysis, fluid moves from the blood to the dialysis fluid because the dialysis fluid contains a large amount of glucose which creates an osmotic gradient across the peritoneal membrane, that is, the osmolality of the peritoneal dialysate fluid is much higher than blood. Solute exchange results from diffusion and convection.

The solute (including drugs and toxins) and fluid removal observed in peritoneal dialysis is much less efficient (e.g., ml/min) than hemodialysis. Because peritoneal dialysis is usually carried out continuously (i.e., daily), as compared to the relatively short, intermittent hemodialysis sessions (i.e., thrice weekly), the net clearance of solutes in peritoneal dialysis achieved over a one week period approximates that observed in hemodialysis. In contrast to hemodialysis, common complications of peritoneal dialysis (e.g., peritonitis caused by infection) can alter the characteristics of the peritoneal membranes and hence the efficiency of this procedure.

Hemofiltration is similar to hemodialysis with the following important exceptions: (1) a countercurrent flow of dialysis fluid is not included in the circuit, (2) the flow rate of blood into the dialyzer is generally less, and (3) the surface area of the dialyzer membrane is smaller. As a result, solute and fluid removal occur consequent to hydrostatic pressure and convection, respectively. Hemofiltration is generally used acutely for fluid removal in the unstable patient with renal compromise. However, if performed optimally, the clearance of low molecular weight solutes (e.g., urea, creatinine) does occur. As solute clearance is dependent upon convection, the process is much less efficient than either hemodialysis or peritoneal dialysis, and it is dependent upon the amount of fluid removed. In order to optimize solute clearance, large volumes of fluid must be removed from the patient. This is accomplished by providing the patient with a large amount of replacement fluid, which offsets the large amount of fluid removed by hemofiltration, resulting in net loss of only a small amount of fluid from the patient but enhanced solute clearance.

Hemodiafiltration constitutes a variation of hemofiltration where dialysis fluid is run across the membrane in a countercurrent direction to blood as is accomplished during hemodialysis (Figure 38-1). The major differences between hemodialysis and hemodiafiltration are that the dialysis fluid and blood flow rates are typically much slower in hemodiafiltration and the membrane surface areas are smaller. As a result, hemodiafiltration is much less efficient at removing both solutes (including drugs and toxins) and fluid because the concentration gradient between the blood and dialysis fluid is not optimally maintained.

Variations of both peritoneal dialysis, hemofiltration, and hemodiafiltration are used clinically to afford enhanced solute clearance, improve patient compliance, and/or because of the relative ease by which they can be initiated. These are summarized in Table 38-1.

Hemoperfusion describes a process of passing blood through columns of adsorptive material (e.g., activated charcoal, Amberlight XAD-4 resin) maintained as a matrix in a stationary phase. A hemoperfusion circuit is schematically depicted in Figure 38-3. This procedure is used exclusively in emergency toxicology applications as it is intended to acutely remove organic substances from the intravascular space. Compared to hemodialysis, peritoneal dialysis, or hemoperfusion, hemoperfusion is the most efficient extracorporeal technique for this application in that it can remove drugs/toxins which are both free and bound to either red blood cells or circulating plasma proteins consequent to higher binding affinity (for the drug) to the stationary matrix in the hemoperfusion canister.

Hemoperfusion is most efficient for removing those drugs/toxins which are distributed to the body water spaces consequent to the high efficiency of removal from blood which produces rapid reequilibration of the free drug from the extravascular to the intravascular "compartment." In these instances, the clearance of selected drugs (i.e., those with a $V_d <$ 0.7 L/kg) resulting from hemoperfusion is generally 1.2- to 5-fold higher than intrinsic

Table 38-1. Specific Methods for Peritoneal Dialysis, Hemofiltration, and Hemodiafiltration

METHOD	CHARACTERISTICS
Peritoneal Dialysis	
CAPD	Involves 4 to 5 exchanges of dialysate per day, each lasting 4 to 6 hours with a prolonged nocturnal dwell.
IPD	Intermittent sessions of dialysis typically done in four, 10-hour sessions with rapid exchanges (i.e., one per hour). Rarely used at present.
APD	Refers to peritoneal dialysis performed with the aid of an automated machine to facilitate exchanges. Includes applications of Continuous Cycling Peritoneal Dialysis (CCPD), Nocturnal Intermittent Peritoneal Dialysis (NIPD), and Tidal Peritoneal Dialysis (TPD).
Hemofiltration	
CAVH	Arterial blood pressure used as driving force for blood across membrane with blood return to venous circulation.
CVVH	Identical to CAVH with exception that blood obtained from venous circulation, driven across membrane using a pump and returned to the venous circulation.
Hemodiafiltration	
CAVHD	CAVH with countercurrent circulation of dialysate across membrane.
CVVHD	Identical to CAVHD with exception that venous blood is utilized as described for CVVH.

Abbreviations include: CAPD, continuous ambulatory peritoneal dialysis; IPD, intermittent peritoneal dialysis; APD, automated peritoneal dialysis; CAVH, continuous arterio-venous hemofiltration; CAVHD, continuous arterio-venous hemodiafiltration; CVVH, continuous veno-venous hemofiltration; and CVVHD, continuous veno-venous hemodiafiltration

clearance and 2- to 5-fold higher than observed with hemodialysis. For drugs with large apparent volumes of distribution (e.g., >2–3 L/kg) consequent to extensive tissue binding (e.g., digoxin, phenothiazines, tricyclic antidepressants, methaqualone), hemoperfusion may not result in a significant net reduction in the amount of drug removed from the body. In these instances, the expected benefits from applying this procedure often do not exceed the risks associated with it (e.g., thrombocytopenia, hemorrhage consequent to heparinization, leukopenia, air embolism, hypocalcemia, hypoglycemia, hypotension, and hypothermia). In all instances, the application of either hemoperfusion or hemodialysis in emergency toxicology should only be used when intrinsic clearance mecha-

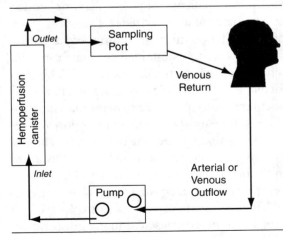

Figure 38-3. Schematic of a hemoperfusion circuit.

nisms (e.g., renal and hepatic) are limited/insufficient for timely removal of the toxicant and when the relative risk for serious adverse events (e.g., seizures, acidosis, organ dysfunction) associated with persistent elevations of a given toxicant in the blood (or tissues) is high. The use of these techniques in emergency toxicology is optimized by prudent evaluation of plasma drug concentrations.

Plasmapheresis describes a procedure whereby blood is removed in a manner analogous to hemodialysis but is not passed through a membrane. Rather, a centrifugation procedure separates blood into its constituent parts, the serum and its proteins (e.g., albumin, alpha-1-acid glycoprotein, globulins, steroid binding proteins, etc.) are removed, and the cellular components/fractions are returned to the patient. While plasmapheresis is capable of acutely reducing the plasma concentration of extensively bound drugs, it is quantitatively not an efficient method to remove drugs from the body with the possible exception of those substances which are extensively bound to albumin (or other circulating plasma proteins) and whose apparent volume of distribution is largely confined to the intravascular volume (e.g., warfarin, heparin).

Cardiopulmonary Bypass is an extracorporeal technique which is used to substitute for cardiac and pulmonary function during cardiac surgery. Blood is cooled (to approximately 27°C), anticoagulated with heparin, diluted with saline to a hematocrit in the mid-20s, and circulated through the bypass circuit where it is oxygenated and returned to patient via a series of roller pumps in a relatively nonpulsatile pattern of flow. Drug distribution can be altered by changes in blood flow and by hemodilution, with a decrease in plasma protein binding. During the procedure, a reduction in the elimination of some drugs may occur consequent to impairment of renal or hepatic clearance due, to a great degree, to lowered perfusion and hypothermia. The procedure, *per se,* can remove selected drugs (e.g., fentanyl, thiopental) consequent to binding to the cardiopulmonary bypass circuit.

Extracorporeal Membrane Oxygenation (ECMO) is a technique which enables oxygenation of the blood pumped across a membrane oxygenator via nonpulsatile flow. ECMO is generally reserved for use in infants and small children with acute, potentially reversible pulmonary failure. While ECMO frequently produces physiological changes that can alter drug pharmacokinetics (e.g., reduced renal clearance of filtered drugs secondary to reduced glomerular filtration rate from nonpulsatile blood flow, expanded extracellular fluid space with a potential for an increased V_d of selected drugs), the procedure itself can reduce plasma drug levels via extracorporeal drug loss. This occurs consequent to adhesion of the drug to the circuit components and/or loss of drug in the circulating blood volume during changes in the equipment. Specific drugs (e.g., benzodiazepines, propofol) are largely sequestered within the ECMO circuit. Serum concentrations of heparin, morphine, fentanyl, furosemide, phenytoin, and phenobarbital are also reduced by these mechanisms. The pharmacokinetics of drugs can be further influenced by ECMO when other extracorporeal methods (e.g., hemodialysis, hemofiltration) intended to remove endogenous toxins are connected into the circuit.

Exchange Transfusion is a technique generally reserved for small infants whereby venous blood containing a potentially harmful solute (e.g., bilirubin) is removed and replaced by donor blood which contains either less or normal amounts of the solute. The efficiency of exchange transfusion in removing drugs is limited by the volume of blood which can be safely removed and the fact that a relatively low amount of the total body burden of a given drug resides within the intravascular space.

Efficiency of Extracorporeal Drug Removal by Dialysis

For those extracorporeal techniques which utilize a dialyzer or membrane (e.g., hemodialysis, CAVHD, CVVHD, peritoneal dialysis), performance (i.e., efficiency) is dependent upon: (1) solute removal or mass transfer, (2) fluid removal, (3) flow resistance, and (4) compliance of the blood compartment. Performance can be conceptualized by considering the schematic hemodialysis circuit depicted in Figure 38-4 and the following determinants.

A. Mass Transfer: As depicted in Figure 38-4, the rate of solute flux across the membrane is determined by the physical properties of the membrane and by the concentration gradient across the membrane. Thus, the flux (denoted by "R" in Figure 38-4) has two components, that due to diffusion and that due to ultrafiltration (i.e., convection). Diffusion depends upon the properties of the membrane, the molecular size of the solvent, and the concentration gradient. Solutes of small molecular size are removed primarily by diffusion but, as molecular size increases, so does the importance of ultrafiltration. Also, the capacity of a dialyzer will rise as available dialysis surface area increases and as the blood-dialysate concentration gradient increases. Major factors which limit mass transfer are: (1) membrane resistance produced by the thickness of the dialysate fluid film bounding the dialysis membrane (which can be decreased by increasing the velocity of the dialysate flow), (2) the ability of the blood to deliver solute to the membrane, (3) the ability of the dialysate to remove solute away from the membrane, and (4) the intrinsic ability of the membrane to transfer solute (e.g., porosity, molecular weight cut-off).

B. Fluid Removal: This results from ultrafiltration of blood with net removal of water to the dialysate. Ultrafiltration is the product of the fluid filtration rate, the blood solute concentration, and the sieving coefficient.

C. Flow Resistance: This determines the operating pressure required to achieve a given blood flow rate. Flow resistance can be altered by physical constraints of the dialyzer or dialysis circuit and/or intrinsic "factors" (e.g., blood pressure, size/volume of arterial/venous circulation at point of vascular access).

D. Compliance: The compliance of the system can be defined as the degree of change in internal (i.e., blood compartment) volume per unit time in transmembrane pressure which is the pressure difference across the membrane, measured by the difference between the average pressures in the blood and dialysate compartments.

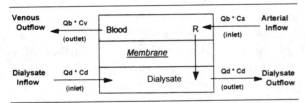

Figure 38-4. Dynamic schematic of a hemodialysis circuit. Abbreviations include: Qb, blood flow rate; Qd, dialysate flow rate; Cv, venous solute concentration; Ca, arterial solute concentration; Cd, dialysate solute concentration. "R" denotes mass transfer of solute and/or fluid (i.e., ultrafiltration).

As stated previously, the efficiency of any extracorporeal technique in removing solutes from the blood is dependent upon the characteristics of the solute, the characteristics (i.e., both physical and patient-related) of the technique/procedure, and the duration of its application (i.e., acute vs. chronic, time of a given procedure). With the exception of charcoal/resin hemoperfusion, the relative efficiency of the commonly used extracorporeal techniques in removing drugs or other xenobiotics from the blood is as follows: hemo-dialysis > continuous peritoneal dialysis > intermittent peritoneal dialysis > hemodiafiltra-tion (e.g., CAVHD and CVVHD) > hemofiltration (CAVH, CVVH) > plasmapheresis > exchange transfusion. Data concerning the efficiency of hemodialysis and hemoperfusion for removing specific drugs and toxins can be found in specific references (see Pond, 1991; Winchester JF, et al., 1977 and specific product information) which should be consulted when these techniques are applied clinically.

Evaluation of Pharmacokinetics during Extracorporeal Therapy

As denoted previously, the provision of extracorporeal therapy has the potential to enhance the removal of not only toxicants but also therapeutic drugs from the body. In this latter instance, failure to recognize the extent of drug removal and, in many cases, to effectively replace the amount of drug (i.e., the fraction of the dose) lost can potentially result in under-dosing and subsequent compromise of therapeutic efficacy. In those instances where the concentration of a drug can be accurately and readily measured in blood (plasma) and dialysate, it is possible to determine the pharmacokinetics of a given drug as altered by the extracorporeal procedure and hence approximate the efficiency of the procedure's ability to remove drug. The resultant data then enable the determination of a replacement dose in those instances when drug removal is deemed to be clinically significant (i.e., generally >20% of a dose). Given the additivity of clearance terms, it must be recognized that intrin-sic clearance (e.g., Cl_{renal} and $Cl_{hepatic}$) of a drug or toxin continues during an extracorporeal procedure and between application of a given procedure at rates which, generally speaking, are considered to be independent of the procedure *per se*.

Several different approaches for examining the pharmacokinetics of dialysis have been reported. Potentially useful equations which have been applied during the therapeutic use of **hemodialysis** are denoted as follows.

Dialysis clearance (Cl_d) can be *determined* with knowledge of the arterial solute con-centration (Ca), the venous solute concentration (Cv), and the blood flow rate (Qb) according to Equation 38.1:

$$Cl_d = [(Ca - Cv)/Ca] \cdot Qb \qquad (1)$$

Alternatively, Cl_d can be *estimated* using Equation 38.2 where t is the length of the dialysis period in hours:

$$Cl_d = \frac{\text{Total Amount of Solute in Dialysate}}{(\text{Mid-dialysis Ca}) \cdot (t)} \qquad (2)$$

When a difference is expected between the partitioning of a drug between the plasma and plasma water (i.e., as with ultrafiltration), Cv can be corrected using Equation 38.3 when the venous and arterial concentrations of relevant drug binding proteins (i.e., V_{prot} and A_{prot}, respectively) are known:

$$Cv_{actual} = Cv_{observed}[1 - (V_{prot} - A_{prot})/V_{prot}] \qquad (3)$$

As well, Cl_d can be corrected using Equation 38.4 for alterations in plasma protein binding (% Free) and hematocrit (H), both of which can occur in patients with uremia:

$$Cl_{d\,corrected} = Cl_{d\,uncorrected} \cdot (\%\,Free) \cdot (1-H) \tag{4}$$

When ultrafiltration is measurable, Cl_d can be determined according to Equation 38.5:

$$Cl_d = [(Ca - Cv)/Ca] \cdot Qb + (Cv/Ca) \cdot QF \tag{5}$$

where the ultrafiltration rate $(QF) = KuF \cdot (Pm - Posm)$ where KuF is the ultrafiltration coefficient or capacity and $(Pm - Posm)$ is the effective transmembrane pressure.

In those instances where the removed substance(s) accumulate in the dialysate bath (Figure 38-2) over time so that the concentration gradient is constantly decreasing, removal of a solute (drug) is expressed as dialysance (D) which can be calculated according to Equation 38.6:

$$D = [Qb\,(Ca - Cv)]/(Ca - B) \tag{6}$$

where B is the concentration of the solute in the dialysate bath. It should be noted that both D and Cl_d reflect the efficiency of a given dialyzer or hemodialysis procedure to remove drug at a given time during the procedure. Given the fact that B changes during dialysis, D may change as well (i.e., efficiency can change during dialysis).

During dialysis, the total plasma clearance (Cl) of a drug is equal to the sum of the renal drug clearance (Cl_{renal}), the nonrenal (e.g., hepatic) drug clearance (Cl_{nr}), and the dialysis clearance (Cl_d). Likewise, the overall elimination rate constant during dialysis (k_{el}) can be expressed according to Equation 38.7:

$$k_{el} = k_r + k_{nr} + k_d \tag{7}$$

where k_r is the renal elimination rate constant, k_{nr} is the nonrenal (metabolic) elimination rate constant, and k_d is the dialysis elimination rate constant. k_{nr} (Equation 38.8) and k_d (Equation 38.9) can be estimated as follows if the apparent volume of distribution (V_d) of the drug is known or can be calculated:

$$k_{nr} = Cl_{nr}/V_d \tag{8}$$

$$k_d = Cl_d/V_d \tag{9}$$

k_{el} can also be estimated during a dialysis period (i.e., intradialysis) according to Equation 38.10:

$$k_{el} = (\ln Cd_1 - \ln Cd_2)/(td_2 - td_1) \tag{10}$$

where Cd_1 and Cd_2 represent declining plasma drug concentrations obtained at two discrete time periods (i.e., td_1 and td_2) during the dialysis procedure. As well, the intradialysis elimination half-life ($t_{1/2d}$) can be estimated according to Equation 38.11:

$$t_{1/2d} = 0.693/k_d \tag{11}$$

To estimate k_d, the interdialysis elimination rate constant ($k_{el\,interdialysis}$) can be first estimated using Equation 38.12 as follows:

$$k_{el\,interdialysis} = (\ln C_1 - \ln C_2)/(t_2 - t_1) \tag{12}$$

where C_1 and C_2 represent declining plasma drug concentrations obtained following reequilibration of body water spaces and plasma drug concentrations following the completion of hemodialysis (i.e., generally >2 hours postdialysis) obtained at two discrete time points (t_1 and t_2) during a time period when the patient is not receiving hemodialysis. In this instance, $k_{el\,interdialysis}$ represents the sum of k_{nr} and k_r and reflects drug elimination in the absence of dialysis. k_d is then simply calculated from the difference of k_{el} and $k_{el\,interdialysis}$ as illustrated by Equation 38.13:

$$k_d = k_{el} - k_{el\,interdialysis} \tag{13}$$

As well, the apparent elimination half-life of the drug between dialysis periods ($t_{1/2\,interdialysis}$) can be estimated according to Equation 38.14:

$$t_{1/2\,interdialysis} = 0.693/k_{el\,interdialysis} \tag{14}$$

To further estimate the efficiency of the hemodialysis procedure as an extracorporeal route for drug clearance, the fraction of drug lost during dialysis (Fd) can be approximated using Equation 38.15 as follows:

$$Fd = 1 - e^{-(k_{el} \cdot t)} \tag{15}$$

where t represents the time (usually in hours) of the hemodialysis period. Alternatively, the fraction of the drug in the body at the onset of hemodialysis that is removed by the dialysis machine alone (F'd) can be estimated using Equation 38.16:

$$F'd = [k_d/k_{el}] \cdot [1 - e^{-(k_{el} \cdot t)}] \tag{16}$$

In contrast to the pharmacokinetics of hemodialysis which can be described as denoted above, **peritoneal dialysis** represents a unique challenge. The inability to accurately estimate blood flow rate(s) makes the calculation of Cl_d or D virtually impossible. In patients receiving intermittent forms of peritoneal dialysis, repeated assessment of plasma drug concentrations during dialysis and between dialysis periods enables the estimation of both $k_{el\,interdialysis}$ and k_d as described above (Equations 38.10, 38.12, and 38.13) and their corresponding values of $t_{1/2}$. Equation 38.15 can then be used to approximate the fraction of drug lost during a discrete peritoneal dialysis procedure/interval. The respective elimination rate constants can also be used in a monoexponential expression to predict the plasma drug concentration either between (i.e., interdialysis) or within (i.e., intradialysis) dialysis periods according to Equation 38.17 as follows:

$$Cp_{tx} = Cp \cdot e^{-(K' \cdot tx)} \tag{17}$$

where Cp_{tx} is the plasma concentration at a specific time point (i.e., tx), Cp is the initial plasma drug concentration either between dialysis periods or during a dialysis period and

K′ represents either the apparent elimination rate constant during dialysis (i.e., k_{el}) or between dialysis periods (i.e., $k_{el\,interdialysis}$).

Alternatively, the fraction of drug dose removed by peritoneal dialysis (F_{pd}) can be approximated by direct measurement of the amount of drug in the dialysate ($A_{dialysate}$) according to Equations 38.18 and 38.19:

$$A_{dialysate} = C_{dialysate} \cdot V_{dialysate} \qquad (18)$$

$$F_{pd} = (A_{dialysate}/Dose) \cdot 100 \qquad (19)$$

where $C_{dialysate}$ is the concentration of drug in the dialysate, $V_{dialysate}$ is the volume of the dialysate during a discrete period of peritoneal dialysis, and Dose represents the amount of drug administered during a given period of peritoneal dialysis (i.e., that corresponding to $A_{dialysate}$).

Several calculations involving **hemofiltration** (i.e., CAVH or CVVH) or **hemodiafiltration** (i.e., CAVHD, CVVHD) are potentially useful in examining extracorporeal drug removal by these procedures. The sieving coefficient (Si) of a substance is the relationship between drug concentration in the ultrafiltrate (C_{uf}) and the average drug concentration in the plasma calculated from the arterial (Ca) and venous (Cv) concentrations as reflected by Equation 38.20:

$$Si = C_{uf}[(Ca + Cv)/2] \qquad (20)$$

During hemofiltration, the Si corresponds well with the free fraction of the drug. However, if dialysate is circulated across the membrane in a countercurrent fashion to increase efficiency (i.e., the use of hemodiafiltration), the saturation (Sa) of the combined dialysate and ultrafiltrate with a particular drug is no longer identical after sieving. Nonetheless, Sa can also be calculated by Equation 38.20 if Si is substituted by Sa.

Extracorporeal clearance of a solute during hemodiafiltration (Cl_{hf}) can be calculated using Equation 38.21 as follows:

$$Cl_{hf} = Sa \cdot (Qd + Quf) \qquad (21)$$

where Qd and Quf are the flow rates of dialysate and ultrafiltration, respectively. As well, the fraction (i.e., %) of a drug dose eliminated by hemodiafiltration (F_{hf}) can be estimated from the relationship of Cl_{hf} to the total body clearance (Cl) as denoted in Equation 38.22:

$$F_{hf} = (Cl_{hf}/Cl) \cdot 100 \qquad (22)$$

Generally speaking, extracorporeal elimination by hemofiltration or hemodiafiltration is not considered to be clinically significant unless F_{hf} is >25%.

Percent of drug in the body eliminated by dialysis, F_{dial}, can be calculated by:

$$F_{dial}[\%] = 100\% \cdot [(t_{1/2} - t_{1/2\,HD})/t_{1/2}] \times [1 - e^{(-0.693 \cdot t/t_{1/2\,HD})}] \qquad (23)$$

where:

$t_{1/2}$ = elimination half-life

$t_{1/2\ HD}$ = elimination half-life during hemodialysis based on concentrations in samples collected entering dialyses

t   = time on dialysis

Reloading after dialysis is done by a reloading dose, D_{RELOAD}:

$$D_{RELOAD} = F_{dial} \cdot V_d \cdot C_{ss\ av} \tag{24}$$

Clinical Applications

As with hemodialysis and peritoneal dialysis, the aforementioned equations can be applied only if the drug of interest can be routinely (and quickly) measured with accuracy in the relevant biological fluids. In the absence of this ability, selected references (Bressolle, F., et al., 1994; Reetze-Bonorden, P., et al., 1993) can be consulted to determine if hemofiltration or hemodiafiltration would be expected to produce significant drug removal and also how drug therapy might be altered (e.g., replacement dosing) to "compensate" for extracorporeal drug loss. General information regarding the potential impact of both hemodialysis and peritoneal dialysis on extracorporeal drug removal and its therapeutic implications can be obtained by examination of the primary medical literature, selected references (see Winchester et al., 1977; Bekersky 1987; Bennett, W. M., et al., 1983; Lee and Marbury, 1984; Taketomo, C. K. et al., 1997) and specific product information supplied by the drug manufacturer.

Selected References

1. Bekersky, I.: Renal Excretion, *J. Clin. Pharmacol. 27*:447–449 (1987).

2. Bennett, W. M., Aronoff, G. R., Morrison, G., Golper, T. A., Pulliam, J., Wolfson, M. and Singer, I.: Drug Prescribing in Renal Failure: Dosing Guidelines for Adults, *Am. J. Kidney Dis. 3*:15–193 (1983).

3. Bressolle, F., Kinowski, J-M., de la Coussaye, J. E., Wynn, N., Eledjam, J-J. and Galtier, M.: Clinical Pharmacokinetics During Continuous Haemofiltration, *Clin. Pharmacokinet. 26*:457–471 (1994).

4. Buck, M. L.: Pharmacokinetic Changes During Extracorporeal Membrane Oxygenation: Implications for Drug Therapy of Neonates. *Clin. Pharmacokinet. 42*:403–417 (2003).

5. Buylaert, W. A., Herregods, L. L., Mortier, E. P. and Bogaert, M. G.: Cardiopulmonary Bypass and the Pharmacokinetics of Drugs: An Update, *Clin. Pharmacokinet. 17*:10–26 (1989).

6. Dagan, O., Klein, J., Gruenwald, C., Bohn, D., Barker, G. and Koren, G.: Preliminary Studies of the Effects of Extracorporeal Membrane Oxygenator on the Disposition of Common Pediatric Drugs, *Ther. Drug Monitor.* 15:263–266 (1993).

7. Gibson, T. P., Matusik, E., Nelson, L. D. and Biggs, W. A.: Artificial Kidneys and Clearance Calculations, *Clin. Pharmacol. Ther. 20*:720–726 (1976).

8. Lazarus, J. M. and Hakin, R. M.: Medical Aspects of Hemodialysis, In *The Kidney,* 4th Edition, B. M. Brenner and F. C. Rector (editors.), W. B. Saunders, Philadelphia, PA, pp. 2223–2298 (1991).

9. Lee, C-s. C. and Marbury, T. C.: Drug Therapy in Patients Undergoing Haemodialysis: Clinical Pharmacokinetic Considerations, *Clin. Pharmacokinet. 9*:42–66 (1984).

10. Parker, P. R. and Parker, W. A.: Pharmacokinetic Considerations in the Haemodialysis of Drugs, *J. Clin. Hosp. Pharm. 7*:87–99 (1982).

11. Pond, S. M.: Extracorporeal Techniques in the Management of Poisoned Patients, *Med. J. Aust. 154*:617–622 (1991).

12. Randinitis, E. J. et al.: Pharmacokinetics of Pregabalin in Subjects with Various Degrees of Renal Function. *J. Clin. Pharmacol. 43*:277–283 (2003).

13. Reetze-Bonorden, P., Bohler, J. and Keller, E.: Drug Dosage in Patients During Continuous Renal Replacement Therapy: Pharmacokinetic and Therapeutic Considerations, *Clin. Pharmacokinet.* *24*:362–379 (1993).

14. Rippe, B. and Krediet, R. T.: Peritoneal Physiology—Transport of Solutes, In *The Textbook of Peritoneal Dialysis,* R. Gokal and K. D. Nolph (editors), Kluwer Academic Publishers, Norwell, MA, pp. 69–113 (1994).

15. Taketomo, C. K., Hodding, J. H. and Kraus, D. M. *Pediatric Dosage Handbook,* 4th Edition, Lexi-Comp, Hudson, OH, 1997.

16. Winchester, J. F., Gelfand, M. C., Knepshield, J. H. and Schreiner, G. E.: Dialysis and Hemoperfusion of Poisons and Drugs—Update, *Trans. Am. Soc. Artif. Intern. Organs 23*:762–842 (1977).

39

Pharmacogenetics and Pharmacogenomics

Pharmacotherapy has benefited from knowledge of pharmacogenetic principles acquired over the past 40–50 years. Completion of the Human Genome Project brings the considerable hope that morbidity and mortality will be decreased through the development of more effective strategies to diagnose, treat, and prevent human disease, including the promise of truly individualized and targeted drug therapy. The purpose of this chapter is to introduce the concepts of pharmacogenetics, pharmacogenomics, pharmacoproteomics (and other "-omic" fields of endeavor spawned in the genome era) as they relate to pharmacokinetics and pharmacodynamics.

Historical Considerations

In 1959, Friedrich Vogel coined the term *pharmacogenetics* to describe the study of genetically determined variations in drug response. Through a series of twin studies conducted during the late 1960s and early 1970s, Elliott Vesell illustrated the importance of genetic variation in drug disposition by observing that the half-lives of several drugs were more similar in monozygotic twins than in dizygotic twins. With the discovery of the debrisoquin/sparteine hydroxylase polymorphism due to inherited defects in the cytochrome P450 2D6 gene (CYP2D6) and mephenytoin hydroxylase deficiency (CYP2C19), the importance of genetic polymorphisms in drug-metabolizing enzymes has become increasingly apparent. This is particularly true in recent years due to an enhanced awareness of the number of clinically useful drugs that are metabolized by polymorphically expressed enzymes and the recognition that pharmacogenetic differences between patients can produce marked differences in drug disposition and response ranging from ineffective treatment to toxicity with administration of "usual" recommended drug doses.

The introduction of therapeutic drug monitoring programs is considered by many to represent the first application of personalized medicine. It provided recognition that all patients were unique and that serum drug concentration data for an individual patient theoretically could be used to optimize pharmacotherapy: this recognition is a significant advance over the concept of "one dose fits all." At a molecular level, the pharmacokinetic properties of a drug are determined by the genes that control its disposition (e.g., absorption, distribution, metabolism, excretion) with drug-metabolizing enzymes and transporters assuming particularly important roles. Over the past 25 years, the functional consequences of genetic variation in several drug-metabolizing enzymes have been described in subjects representative of different ethnic groups. It has also become more apparent in recent years that the concentration-effect relationship (*pharmacodynamics*) can be determined as a consequence of genetic control of drug receptors and other target proteins (e.g., membrane transporters, receptors involved in signal transduction) which may not only be affected by a given drug but also may be a function of disease pathogenesis. However, the most important concept is that the drug response, encompassing both facets of drug disposition and action, is in many instances a polygenic event involving multiple genes. Therefore, for a particular individual, polymorphisms in a single gene are unlikely to be solely predictive of response.

In 1987, the term *genomics* was introduced to describe the study of the structure and function of the entire complement of genetic material–the genome–including chromosomes, genes, and DNA. Information from the Human Genome Project revealed that the genome consists of 3 gigabases (3 billion bases) of DNA sequence that code for approximately 30,000 genes, far fewer than was originally expected. However, it appears that this number of genes encodes 100,000 proteins through the process of alternative splicing whereby a gene's exons or coding regions are spliced together in different ways to produce variant mRNA molecules that are translated into different proteins or isoforms of the same protein. Thus, the vast amounts of genomic data generated by the Human Genome Project have laid the foundation for an "-omic" revolution that includes but is not limited to *pharmacogenomics* and, most recently, the hybrid field of *metabonomics* which is the study of the changes in the global pool of intermediary metabolites present in target tissues or biofluids following pathophysiologic stimuli.

Basic Concepts and Definitions

Genetic variability results from gene mutation and the exchange of genetic information between chromosomes that occurs during meiosis. With the exception of sex-linked genes (genes occurring on the X or Y chromosome), every individual carries two copies of each gene they possess. All copies of a specific gene present within a population may not have identical nucleotide sequences and these genetic *polymorphisms* contribute to the variability observed in that population. The presence of different nucleotides at a given position within a gene is called a *single nucleotide polymorphism* (SNP) and SNPs are rapidly becoming an important component of the genomics lexicon. More recently, focus has shifted to characterizing *haplotypes,* collections of SNPs and other allelic variations that are located close to each other and inherited together. In genes where polymorphisms have been detected, alternative forms of the gene are called *alleles.* When the alleles at a particular gene locus are identical, a *homozygous* state exists whereas the term *heterozygous* refers to the situation where different alleles are present at the same gene locus. The term *genotype* refers to an individual's genetic constitution while the observable characteristics or physical manifestations constitute the *phenotype,* which is the net consequence of genetic and environmental effects.

Pharmacogenetics, the study of the role of genetic factors in drug disposition, response, and toxicity, essentially relates allelic variation in human genes to variability in drug responses at the level of the individual patient. The field of pharmacogenetics classically has focused on the phenotypic consequences of allelic variation in single genes but often in the past there was confusion between genotypic and phenotypic definitions of "polymorphism." Thus, there was a need to clarify the relationship between genetic concepts and the clinical relevance of a given phenotype. A *pharmacogenetic polymorphism* can be defined as a monogenic trait caused by the presence in the same population of more than one allele at the same locus and more than one phenotype in regard to drug interaction with the organism. The frequency of the least common allele should be at least 1 percent. According to this definition, the key elements of pharmacogenetic polymorphisms are heritability, the involvement of a single gene locus, and the fact that distinct phenotypes are observed within the population only after drug challenge.

The vast majority of current understanding of pharmacogenetic polymorphisms involves enzymes responsible for drug biotransformation. Clinically, individuals are classified as being "fast," "rapid," or "extensive" metabolizers at one end of the spectrum, and "slow" or "poor" metabolizers at the other end of a continuum that may, depending on the particular enzyme, also include an intermediate and/or ultrarapid metabolizer group. *Pediatric pharmacogenetics* involves an added measure of complexity since fetuses and newborns may be phenotypically slow or poor metabolizers for certain drug-metabolizing enzymes (or transporters) that as a consequence of normal developmental immaturity, are functionally deficient when their activity is compared to that in normal, healthy adults.

Although some authors use the terms pharmacogenetics and pharmacogenomics interchangeably, the latter term represents the marriage of pharmacology with genomics and is therefore considerably broader in scope. *Pharmacogenomics* can be defined as the study of the genome-wide response to small molecular weight compounds administered with therapeutic intent. In contrast to the focus of pharmacogenetics on single gene events, pharmacogenomics involves understanding how interacting systems or networks of genes influence drug responses. This definition is particularly appealing to the development of an integrated concept of disease and drug response since the concept of many genes acting in concert captures the essence of the multifactorial processes (e.g., development, diet, environment, concomitant therapy/xenobiotic exposure, sex, race, concomitant disease processes) that not only produce intersubject variability in drug response but also serve as the basis for individualization of drug treatment as a therapeutic goal. Representative examples of genetic polymorphisms in disease- or treatment-modifying genes that can influence drug response are provided in Table 39-1.

Pharmacogenetic and Pharmacogenomic Tools

Completion of the Human Genome Project was facilitated by several technological advances including the development of cloning systems to accommodate large DNA inserts, dideoxy nucleotide sequencing and its automation, and the polymerase chain reaction (PCR). Progress was further accelerated with the development of automated, capillary-based DNA sequencers with fluorescence detection and software to analyze and compile DNA sequence data. Indeed, the demands of pharmacogenetic and pharmacogenomic analyses have driven the development of an industry dedicated to the discovery and refinement of technologies to conduct high-throughput measurement of gene and protein expression and genotyping of SNPs. These technologies are not limited to

Table 39-1. Representative Examples of Polymorphisms in Disease- or Treatment-Modifying Genes Capable of Influencing Drug Response (adapted from Evans and McLeod 2003)

GENE OR GENE PRODUCT	DISEASE OR RESPONSE ASSOCIATION	MEDICATION	INFLUENCE OF POLYMORPHISM ON DRUG EFFECT OR TOXICITY
Adducin	Hypertension	Diuretics	Myocardial infarction or strokes
Apolipoprotein E	Atherosclerosis	Statins	Enhanced survival
HLA	Toxicity	Abacavir	Hypersensitivity reactions
Ion channels (HERG)	Long QT syndrome	Erythromycin, quinidine, terfenadine	Increased risk of drug-induced torsade de pointes
LTC_4 synthase, ALOX5	Asthma	Montelukast	Anti-inflammatory effect
β_2-Adrenoreceptor	Asthma, hypertension	Albuterol, metoprolol	Reduced drug activity
D_2 receptor, 5-HT2A serotonergic receptor	Depression	Clozapine, SSRIs	Possible reduced drug activity
CYP3A5	Hypertension	Calcium channel blockers	Possible reduced activity

use in research laboratories but at present have been adapted to facilitate their clinical use in hospitals and other health-care institutions.

Historically, pharmacogenetic analyses were dependent upon phenotyping studies to estimate enzyme activity in vivo at a specific time point as well as genotyping strategies to identify and characterize SNPs and other forms of allelic variation. Phenotyping studies are best conducted with a probe compound (usually a drug that can be used therapeutically) carefully selected to ensure that its biotransformation is primarily dependent upon a single target enzyme and varies quantitatively with the level of protein expression (i.e., phenotyping data correlate with the level of enzyme activity in vitro, the fractional clearance of the probe and other substrates of the target enzyme in vivo, and biotransformation of the probe is increased or decreased in the presence of inducers or inhibitors, respectively). An ideal phenotyping probe should involve noninvasive sampling strategies, such as collection of urine or expired air rather than blood samples, especially when phenotyping studies are to be conducted in infants and children. Finally, candidate phenotyping probes should be widely available (nonprescription status, preferably), have a wide margin of safety, not produce undesirable adverse effects at the dose used for phenotype assessment, and be free from interaction with other drugs and/or conditions. For pediatric studies, the phenotyping probe should be selected from compounds that are likely to be administered to children and perceived as safe by parents, caregivers, and ethical committees (e.g., dextromethorphan as opposed to debrisoquin or sparteine for CYP2D6). Representative pharmacologic compounds that have been used to assess the activity of specific polymorphically expressed enzymes are given in Table 39-2.

Table 39-2. Representative Pharmacologic Agents Used for Phenotyping

ENZYME	PROBE COMPOUNDS
CYP2A6	Coumarin
CYP2D6	Debrisoquin, dextromethorphan, sparteine
CYP2C9	Diclofenac, phenytoin, tolbutamide, S-warfarin
CYP2C19	S-Mephenytoin, omeprazole
CYP3A4/5	Alfentanil, cisapride*, dapsone, erythromycin, lidocaine, midazolam, nifedipine
CYP2E1	Chlorzoxazone
CYP1A2	Caffeine
NAT2 (N-acetyltransferase)	Caffeine
TPMT (thiopurine methyltransferase)	(determined from red blood cell lysates)
XO (xanthine oxidase)	Caffeine
UGT2B7 (glucuronosyltransferase)	Morphine
UGT1A6	Acetaminophen
SULT1A1 (sulfotransferase)	Acetaminophen

* Denotes CYP3A5 specific substrate.

In most instances, pharmacologic phenotyping involves either the determination of the plasma clearance of the model substrate and its primary metabolite (i.e., the one where formation is catalyzed by the enzyme under study) or alternatively, the amount (expressed as fractional recovery) of these substances excreted into urine over a suitable time following administration of the phenotyping probe. The assessment of phenotype is then made based upon examining the data from a given subject in comparison to population frequency distributions where an antimode has been previously determined to separate the population into respective phenotypes (e.g., ultrarapid, extensive, intermediate, and poor metabolizers). This approach is illustrated by examination of the urinary ratios of dextromethorphan (DM) and its primary metabolite, dextrorphan (DX) to assess CYP2D6 phenotype (Figure 39-1).

In contrast to pharmacogenetic studies that typically target single

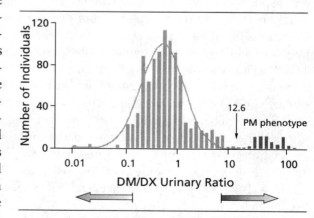

Figure 39-1. Evaluation of CYP2D6 phenotype using dextromethorphan (DM) and dextrorphan (DX) urinary ratios.

genes, pharmacogenomic analyses are considerably broader in scope since they focus on complex and highly variable drug-related phenotypes (e.g., valproic acid hepatotoxicity or weight gain; tumor response to cancer chemotherapy; drug response in asthma, epilepsy, attention deficit, and hyperactivity disorders). As an example, systematic surveys of gene expression in different cell types (tumor cells versus "normal" cells; cells obtained from patients with the disease of interest, such as epilepsy) are often conducted with the hope of identifying new targets for pharmacotherapeutic intervention. Similarly, cataloging differential gene expression before and after drug exposure has the potential to correlate gene expression with variable drug responses and possibly uncover the mechanisms of tissue-specific drug toxicities. These types of studies utilize *microarray* or "*gene-chip*" *technology* to monitor global changes in expression of thousands of genes simultaneously, thereby enabling "global gene profiling." In essence, a microarray consists of a matrix of DNA fragments (probes) precisely positioned (i.e., coordinates are known) at high density on a solid support, such as a glass slide or a filter. The probes serve as molecular detectors for mRNA in the sample. Common experimental designs involve labeling mRNA (or cDNA) from a control sample with one fluorescent dye and mRNA or cDNA from the disease/treatment sample with a second fluorescent dye, using an experimental strategy that allows expression to be compared between the sample pair. In this manner, the expression pattern of thousands of genes can be analyzed in a single sample with the underlying hypothesis that the measured intensity for each arrayed gene represents its relative expression level. Because of the massive amounts of data generated in these experiments, sophisticated computational methods and data-mining tools are necessary to reveal patterns of expression.

Influence of Polymorphisms in Drug-Metabolizing Enzymes on Pharmacokinetics

Clinical observation of patients with high drug concentrations/excessive or prolonged drug responses together with the realization that the biochemical traits (subsequently identified as proteins involved in drug biotransformation) were inherited provided the origins of the concept of pharmacogenetics. Indeed, with few exceptions, the major consequence of pharmacogenetic polymorphisms in drug-metabolizing enzymes is concentration-dependent toxicity due to impaired drug clearance (e.g., excessive anticoagulant response to warfarin in a CYP2C9 poor metabolizer, life-threatening neutropenia with 6-mercaptopurine in a patient with TPMT deficiency) and, to a lesser extent, reduced conversion of prodrugs to therapeutically active compounds (e.g., conversion of codeine to morphine by CYP2D6). Alternatively, extensive activity of a drug-metabolizing enzyme conveyed by a pharmacogenetic polymorphism (e.g., multiple copies of the CYP2D6 gene) can markedly diminish systemic exposure to a normal "therapeutic dose" of a drug and as a consequence lead to therapeutic failure. The association between a pharmacogenetic polymorphism in a drug-metabolizing enzyme and the dose-exposure profile for a drug is illustrated by the pharmacokinetics of nortriptyline (a CYP2D6 substrate) when examined as a function of the CYP2D6 genotype (Figure 39-2).

Chapter 13 (Drug Biotransformation) summarizes the important considerations regarding pharmacogenetic determinants of drug-metabolizing enzyme activity and provides specific examples of some pharmacokinetic implications of polymorphically expressed enzymes. Also, continuously updated, internet-based information regarding pharmacogenetics, enzyme-substrate interactions, and potential clinical consequences of genetic polymorphisms are available (see *http://medicine.iupui.edu/ flockhart/*). Salient features of the more common polymorphisms of clinically relevant drug-metabolizing enzymes and transporters are summarized in Table 39-3.

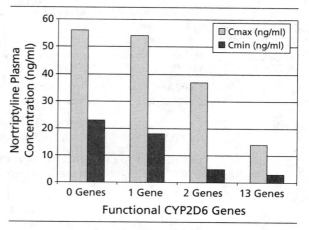

Figure 39-2. Relationship of CYP2D6 polymorphism to nortriptyline pharmacokinetics following a single 25-mg oral dose (adapted from Dalen et al. 1998).

Pharmacogenomic Association between Disease and Drug Therapy

As denoted previously, pharmacogenetic polymorphisms have been described for a host of drug receptors (Table 39-1) and drug-metabolizing enzymes and transporters (Table 39-2). Interpreted in isolation, these biological "facts" as they pertain to a given person could appear to be without therapeutic meaning or potential. However, through the application of pharmacogenetic and pharmacogenomic strategies, the potential of "personalized medicine" can begin to be realized. These strategies are now being employed to investigate specific disease processes with respect to their origin and/or possible response to treatment. The latter is exemplified by the examination of cells from cancer tissue (e.g., carcinoma of breast, large intestine) to detect the presence of specific characteristics (allelic variants) that can either influence prognosis (via determination of malignant potential) and/or treatment (e.g., drug selection in breast cancer treatment based upon genotype of the estrogen receptor).

Another example is seen with the treatment of acute lymphoblastic leukemia (ALL). Patients with ALL who have one wild-type allele for TPMT and thus intermediate activity of this enzyme tend to have a better response to 6-mercaptopurine therapy than patients with two wild-type alleles which convey full activity. However, reduced TPMT activity also places patients at risk of developing irradiation-induced secondary brain tumors and etoposide-induced acute myeloid leukemias. In the approximately 20 percent of patients with ALL that do not respond to conventional chemotherapy, gene expression (microarray) studies in ALL blasts are able to discriminate among phenotypic subtypes and identify some individuals at risk for further treatment failure. Finally, recent studies examining the impact of pharmacokinetics and pharmacogenomics on treatment with the antirejection drug tacrolimus have demonstrated that polymorphisms in CYP3A4, CYP3A5, the CYP3AP1 pseudogene, and MDR1 work in a coordinated fashion and serve as determinants of the critical drug dose necessary to ensure efficacy.

The application of pharmacoproteomic strategies may also help to understand the impact of ontogeny on the incidence of specific adverse drug reactions (e.g., Reye's

Table 39-3. Consequences and Frequencies of Polymorphisms in Selected Drug-Metabolizing Enzymes

ENZYME OR TRANSPORTER	PREDOMINANT ALLELIC VARIANT	FUNCTIONAL CONSEQUENCES	ALLELIC FREQUENCY (%)		
			CAUCASIAN	ASIAN	AFRICAN
CYP2A6	CYP2A6*2	Inactive enzyme	1–3	0	
	CYP2A6del	No enzyme	1	15	
CYP2C9	CYP2C9*2	Reduced affinity	8–13	0	
	CYP2C9*3	Reduced activity	6–9	2–3	
CYP2C19	CYP2C19*2	Inactive enzyme	13	23–32	13
	CYP2C19*3	Inactive enzyme	0	6–10	
CYP2D6	CYP2D6*2×N	Increased activity	1–5	0–2	2
	CYP2D6*4	Inactive enzyme	12–21		
	CYP2D6*5	No enzyme	2–7	1	2
	CYP2D6*10	Unstable enzyme	1–2	51	4
	CYP2D6*17	Reduced affinity	0		21
	CYP2D6*29	Reduced activity	0		7
CYP3A5	CYP3A5*3A	Reduced activity	70	65–80	27–50
	CYP3A5*3B	Reduced activity	95	27	
	CYP3A5*3C	Reduced activity			70
UGT2B7	UGT2B7*1	Reduced activity	51	73	
	UGT2B7*2	Reduced activity	49	27	
	UGT2B15*1	Reduced activity	48		
	UGT2B15*2	Reduced activity	52		
UGT1A6	UGT1A6*2	Reduced activity	34		
TPMT	TPMT*3A	Reduced activity	4		3–4
	TPMT*3C	Reduced activity	5		52
OATP	OATPC*15	Reduced activity	16–60	14–30	
MDR	MDR1 (C3435T)	Reduced activity			

Frequency data represent approximate values from the literature. Designation of relative activity for allelic variants reflects comparison to homozygous, wild-type genotype (adapted from Tribut et al. 2002).

syndrome associated with aspirin use, valproate hepatotoxicity, and lamotrigine-induced cutaneous events) that occur predominantly or at a considerably higher frequency in children. Since patterns of gene expression and the nature of the gene interactions contribute to the pathogenesis of many diseases, they thereby serve as potential targets for pharmacologic intervention that, in some instances, may only be discernible at specific critical points in the entire spectrum of development (i.e., pediatric through geriatric).

The aforementioned example of ALL demonstrates how both a disease and its response to treatment may be polygenically determined. While gene expression profiling and proteomic studies represent strategies for identifying genes that may influence drug response, the pharmacogenomic association between disease, drug effect, and therapeutic outcome can only be discerned through a process that integrates knowledge in the domains of clinical pharmacology (including mechanism of action, pharmacokinetics, pharmacodynamics) and clinical medicine (pathophysiology and expression of disease). A potential model for exploring pharmacogenomic associations is illustrated by Figure 39-3.

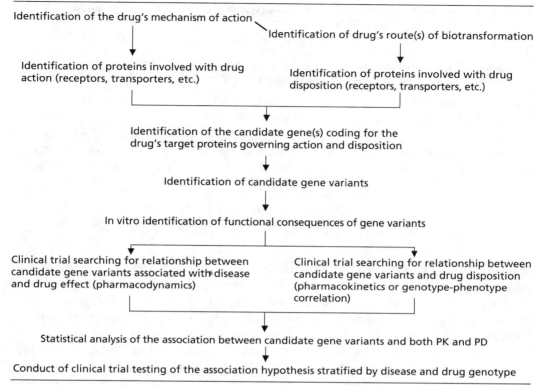

Figure 39-3. Model for exploring pharmacogenetic associations and their potential clinical relevance (adapted from Tribut et al. 2002).

Practical Clinical Interpretation of Pharmacogenetic Information

As denoted in Table 39-2, many of the model substrates are drugs that are commonly used in the treatment of children and adults. In some instances, therapeutic drug monitoring and the application of clinical pharmacokinetic principles are used to guide and individualize therapy (e.g., phenytoin, caffeine). In other instances, the observed clinical effect of the drug (i.e., its pharmacodynamics) is used as an indirect measure of the exposure-response relationship which in turn is used to guide therapeutic dose selection [e.g., use of international normalized ratio (INR) for adjustment of warfarin therapy, use of intragastric pH or histologic evidence of healing for determination of omeprazole dose regimens, use of degree of sedation for midazolam therapy]. In those instances, the application of clinical pharmacokinetic principles provides an estimate of drug clearance for a compound that is predominantly metabolized by a single enzyme; a direct assessment of phenotype is apparent as is an indirect assessment of genotype. Conversely, the concordance observed between genotype and phenotype for a given enzyme enables prediction of phenotype (and thus, relative clearance of drug substrates for the enzyme) in most instances from a single genotype determination. The exception is when genotype-phenotype discordance is present which can occur when the activity of a given drug-metabolizing enzyme is altered consequent to development (e.g., as in neonates and young infants) or drug-drug/drug-enzyme interactions

Table 39-4. Examples of Clinical Utility Associated with Genotyping for Drug-Metabolizing Enzymes (DMEs)

APPLICATION	EXAMPLE DMEs AND THERAPEUTIC DRUGS
Evaluation of adverse drug reactions	CYP2C9 (warfarin, phenytoin), CYP2D6 (SSRIs), CYP2C19 (omeprazole), TPMT (6-mercaptopurine, azathioprine)
A priori selection of therapeutic dose range	CYP2C9 (warfarin), CYP2D6 (SSRIs, atomoxetine), TPMT (6-mercaptopurine, azathioprine)
Interpretation of variability in pharmacokinetic and/or pharmacodynamic data	CYP2C19 (proton pump inhibitors), CYP2D6 (tricyclic antidepressants, SSRIs, codeine), CYP3A4/5 (midazolam, alfentanil, nifedipine, cisapride), UGT2B7 (morphine), UGT1A6 (salicylates, β-blockers, methyldopa, acetaminophen), UGT2B15 (oxazepam), TPMT (6-mercaptopurine, azathioprine), NAT2 (isoniazid, procainamide, hydralazine), COMT (levodopa)

(e.g., inhibition of CYP2D6 activity by terbinafine, converting extensive metabolizers to poor metabolizers). When performed properly, genotype assessment for a given drug-metabolizing enzyme may be of value in the interpretation of pharmacokinetic and/or pharmacodynamic data, either prospectively or retrospectively. As reflected by the examples contained in Table 39-4, the greatest clinical utility of genotyping for drug-metabolizing enzymes (or transporters in the case of MDR1) at the current time resides with the interpretation of pharmacokinetic data (e.g., examination of AUC, clearance, and/or elimination half-life relative to genotype) as a means to critically evaluate the reasons for intersubject variability in drug disposition.

Clinical Applications

The postgenomic era represents an unprecedented opportunity to translate the increasing volume of untapped genomic, proteomic, and metabonomic data into discoveries that favorably impact the treatment of patients. Currently, pharmacogenetic and pharmacogenomic information is being used in the drug development process and, as a consequence, for regulatory decision making; such actions enhance the understanding of pharmacokinetics and the exposure-response relationship for many drugs. However, it must be recognized that focus on the influence of a single gene or gene product is likely to be of limited value in terms of understanding the consequences of genetic potential/variability on the pharmacokinetics or pharmacodynamics of a given drug. Rather, practitioners must be able to utilize pharmacogenetic and pharmacogenomic information to augment their understanding of drug disposition and action and thereby enable greater individualization (i.e., personalization) of drug therapy in a given patient than might be possible by using only response and/or serum concentration data. There is reason to be optimistic that new strategies and technologies will help to further unravel the apparent complexities of pharmacogenomics and to transform this "new biology" into a therapeutic tool for routine clinical use.

Selected References

1. Burchell, B.: Genetic Variation of Human UDP-glucuronosyltransferase. Implications in Disease and Drug Glucuronidation. *Am. J. Pharmacogenomics.* 3:37–52 (2003).

2. Dalen, P., Dahl, M. L., Ruiz, M. L. B., Nordin, J., and Bertilsson, L.: 10-Hydroxylation of Nortriptyline in White Persons with 0, 1, 2, 3 and 13 Functional CYP2D6 Genes. *Clin. Pharmacol. Ther.* *63*:444–452 (1998).

3. Donato, M. T. and Castell, J. V.: Strategies and Molecular Probes to Investigate the Role of Cytochrome P450 in Drug Metabolism. Focus on In Vitro Studies. *Clin. Pharmacokinet.* *42*:153–178 (2003).

4. Eichelbaum, M., Spannbrucker, N., Steincke, B., and Dengler, H. J.: Defective N-Oxidation of Sparteine in Man: A New Pharmacogenetic Defect. *Eur. J. Clin. Pharmacol.* *6*:183–187 (1979).

5. Evans, W. E. and McLeod, H. L.: Pharmacogenomics—Drug Disposition, Drug Targets and Side Effects. *N. Engl. J. Med.* *348*:538–549 (2003).

6. Givens, R. C., Lin, Y. S., Dowling, A. L., Thummel, K. E., Lamba, J. K., Schuetz, E. G., Stewart, P. W., and Watkins, P. B.: CYP3A5 Genotype Predicts Renal CYP3A Activity and Blood Pressure in Healthy Adults. *J. Appl. Physiol.* *95*:1297–1300 (2003).

7. Johnson, J. A.: Drug Target Pharmacogenomics: An Overview. *Am. J. Pharmacogenomics.* *1*:271–281 (2001).

8. Kahn, P.: From Genome to Proteome: Looking at a Cell's Proteins. *Science.* *270*:369–370 (1995).

9. Kim, R. B.: MDR1 Single Nucleotide Polymorphisms: Multiplicity of Haplotypes and Functional Consequences. *Pharmacogenetics.* *12*:425–427 (2002).

10. Lamba, J. K., Lin, Y. S., Schuetz, E. G., and Thummel, K. E.: Genetic Contribution to Variable Human CYP3A-Mediated Metabolism. *Adv. Drug. Deliv. Rev.* *54*:1271–1294 (2002).

11. Lee, C. R., Goldstein, J. A., and Pieper, J. A.: Cytochrome P450 2C9 Polymorphisms: A Comprehensive Review of the in-vitro and Human Data. *Pharmacogenetics.* *12*:251–263 (2002).

12. Leeder, J. S.: Pharmacogenetics and Pharmacogenomics. *Pediatr. Clin. North Am.* *48*:756–781 (2001).

13. Leeder, J. S.: Developmental and Pediatric Pharmacogenomics. *Pharmacogenomics.* *4*:331–341 (2003).

14. Lesko, L. J., Salerno, R. A., Spear, B. B., Anderson, D. C., Anderson, T., Brazell, C., et al.: Pharmacogenetics and Pharmacogenomics in Drug Development and Regulatory Decision Making: Report of the First FDA-PWG-PhRMA-DruSafe Workshop. *J. Clin. Pharmacol.* *43*:342–358 (2003).

15. Lin, J. H. and Yamazaki, M.: Role of P-Glycoprotein in Pharmacokinetics: Clinical Implications. *Clin. Pharmacokinet.* *42*:59–98 (2003).

16. Mancinelli, L., Cronin, M., and Sadee, W.: Pharmacogenomics: The Promise of Personalized Medicine. *AAPS Pharm.* Sci. *2*:1–12 (2002).

17. Nishizato, Y., Ieiri, I., Suzuki, H., Kimura, M., Kawabata, K., Hirota, T., Takane, H., et al.: Polymorphisms of OATP-C (SLC21A6) and OAT3 (SLC22A8) Genes: Consequences for Pravastatin Pharmacokinetics. *Clin. Pharmacol. Ther.* *73*:554–565 (2003).

18. Pauli-Magnus, C. and Meier, P. J.: Pharmacogenetics of Hepatocellular Transporters. *Pharmacogenetics.* *13*:189–198 (2003).

19. Streetman, D. S., Bertino, J. S., and Nafziger, A. N.: Phenotyping of Drug-Metabolizing Enzymes in Adults: A Review of in vivo Cytochrome P450 Phenotyping Probes. *Pharmacogenetics.* *10*:187–216 (2000).

20. Thummel, K. E., O'Shea, D., Paine, M. F., et al.: Oral First-Pass Elimination of Midazolam Involves Both Gastrointestinal and Hepatic CYP3A-Mediated Metabolism. *Clin. Pharmacol.* Ther. *59*:491–502 (1996).

21. Tribut, O., Lessard, Y., Reymann, J-M., Allain, H., and Bentue-Ferrer, D. Pharmacogenomics. *Med. Sci. Monitor.* *8*:152–163 (2002).

22. Venter, J. C., Adams, M. D., Myers, E. W., et al.: The Sequence of the Human Genome. *Science.* *291*:1304–1351 (2001).

23. Vesell, E. S.: Twin Studies in Pharmacogenetics. *Hum. Genet.* *1*:19–30 (1978).

24. Vogel, F., Moderne Problem der Humangenetik. *Ergib Inn Kinderheild.* *12*:52–125 (1959).

25. Wall, A. M. and Rubnitz, J. E.: Pharmacogenomic Effects on Therapy for Acute Lymphoblastic Leukemia in Children. *Pharmacogenomics J.* *3*:128–135 (2003).

26. Watkins, P. B.: Role of Cytochromes P450 in Drug Metabolism and Hepatotoxicity. *Semin. Liver Dis.* *10*:235–250 (1990).

27. Weinshilboum, R.: Inheritance and Drug Response. *N. Engl. J. Med.* *348*:529–537 (2003).

28. Witzman, F. A. and Grant, R. A.: Pharmacoproteomics in Drug Development. *Pharmacogenomics J.* *3*:69–76 (2003).

Appendix
Pharmacokinetic Parameters of Important Drugs

Pharmacokinetic data have become an integral part of the pharmacologic characterization of a drug. Regulatory agencies require determination of pharmacokinetic data in Phase I studies and submission of pharmacokinetic drug data as part of a New Drug Application.

For research and development, pharmacokinetic drug data are used in design of new chemical entities based on structure-activity relationships, and for design of proper dosage forms to result in the desired therapeutic concentrations.

Clinically, pharmacokinetic data are used for the design of dosage regimens in drug-naive patients, for drug monitoring, and for dosage regimen adjustment. Furthermore, pharmacokinetic data give information or indications whether a drug may be excreted in milk (pK_a), whether the half-life may change in renal impairment or advanced age (F_{el}), and whether protein binding may be of clinical importance regarding displacement, hypo- and hyper-albuminemia (if EPB > 80 percent), etc.

Data listed in the appendix have been compiled and extracted from more than a thousand publications. Hence, it is not possible for reasons of space to give a listing of references. The data have been listed as *mean* data. Reports are often conflicting, contradictory, or at least show wide variations among investigators. This, in part, is due to different analytical methods employed for drug assay, different population groups, and different experimental conditions.

Only the elimination half-life ranges are listed for many drugs. This should be indicative that a calculated dosage regimen based on literature mean data may not result in a desired therapeutic concentration and hence, drug monitoring becomes more important. Also, most of the pharmacokinetic data refer to healthy, young adults. However, many physiologic and pathologic conditions may greatly influence the pharmacokinetics of a drug. Again, drug monitoring in such situations may become important.

The following symbols are used:

$t_{1/2}$	= elimination (terminal) half-life
k_{el} or β	= terminal disposition rate constant
V_d	= apparent volume of distribution ($V_{d\beta}$ or $V_{d\,area}$)

367

F_{el}	= fraction of unchanged drug excreted in urine
f	= fraction of drug absorbed = absolute bioavailability. Unless otherwise indicated, f refers to *peroral* administration.
EPB	= extent of protein binding in plasma
Ther. Range or MEC	= therapeutic range or minimum effective concentration
	Note: For antimicrobial agents the MEC or MIC (minimum inhibitory concentration) depends on the sensitivity of the microorganism. Hence, a sensitivity test may be more appropriate than a listed mean value.
URA	= usual route of administration. This listing is not exhaustive. Even if not listed, the drug may be used by other routes.
D	= dose size *usually* employed as maintenance dose. Loading doses are not listed.
τ	= dosing interval for multiple dosing
t_{max}	= time to reach the peak upon extravascular administration
NA	= Not applicable
—	= Data not available
a	= V_d/f
b	= C_{max} or C_{max}^{ss}
c	= C_{min} or C_{min}^{ss}
d	= if required, repeat dose after 2 h
e	= $\mu mol/L$
f	= poor metabolizer
g	= effective concentration 50% = EC_{50}

Pharmacokinetic Parameters of Important Drugs

DRUG	$t_{1/2}$ [h]	k_{el} or β [h⁻¹]	V_d [l/kg]	F_{el}	f	EPB [%]	pk_a	Ther. Range or MEC [µg/ml]	URA	D [mg]	τ [h]	t_{max} [h]
Acarbose	2	0.347	—	0.89	0.02	—	—	—	PO	25–100	8	1
Acebutolol	2.9 (2.4–3.5)	0.239	2.9	0.4	0.4	84	B: 9.4	0.5–2.0	PO	300	8	2
Acetaminophen	2.5 (2–4)	0.277	1.1	0.05	0.85	<5	A: 9.51	10–20	PO	325–650	4	1
Acetazolamide	3.5	0.198	0.2	0.9	1.0	93	A: 7.2	5–20	IV,PO,IM	125–500	6–24	2
Acetohexamide	5.3 (1.3–7)	0.13	—	—	—	88	B: 6.8	20–60	PO	250–500	12–24	2
Acetyldigoxin	53.0	0.013	4.2	0.2	0.8	12	—	0.001–0.0015	PO,IV	0.25–1	24	1
Acetylprocainamide	9.5 (6–12)	0.0729	1.4	0.85	0.85	11	—	2–22	PO	—	—	1
Acetylsalicylic Acid	0.25	2.77	0.21	0.01	1.0	72	A: 3.5	20–300	PO	325–650	4	0.75
Acyclovir	2.5 (2.1–3.5)	0.28	0.6	0.15	0.2 (0.15–0.3)	25	A: 2.27	0.2–5	PO	200–400	4–12	2
Adefovir Dipivoxil (active: Adefovir)	7.5	0.092	0.37	0.45	0.59	4	—	0.18b	PO	10	24	1.75 (0.5–4)
Alendronate	>10 years	NA	0.4	0.5	0.7	78	—	<0.005	PO	5–40	24	—
Alfentanil	22 (0.8–3.6)	0.53	1.03	0.01	NA	88.5	B: 6.5	0.2–0.5	IV	1,2,5,8	—	—
Alfuzosin	10 (5–20)	0.069	7.7a	0.11	—	—	—	0.05–0.2	PO	2.5	8	1
Allopurinol	1.3	0.5	0.2	0.1	0.9	2	B: 10.2	0.006–2.5	PO,IV	100–200	8–12	2
Almotriptan	3.5	0.2	2.7	0.65	0.7	25	—	0.05–0.7	IV,PO	6.25–12.5	—d	1.5–3
Alosetron HCl	93	0.0074	1.1 (0.9–1.4)	—	0.6	82	—	0.05b	PO	1	24	1
Alprazolam	11.0 (6.3–15.8)	0.063	1.16	0.11	0.8	71	B: 2.4	0.005–0.02	PO	0.25–4.5	8	—
Alprenolol	2.7 (2–3)	0.257	3.4	0.01	0.01	11	B: 9.6	0.025–0.1	PO	100–200	8–12	2
Amantadine	11.8 (9.7–14.5)	0.0587	3.5	0.9	0.95	67	B: 9	0.2–0.9	PO	200–400	12–24	6
Amifostine	0.256	2.7	0.46	—	NA	—	—	105e	IV	200 mg/m²	NA	NA

(Continued)

Pharmacokinetic Parameters of Important Drugs (*Continued*)

DRUG	$t_{1/2}$ [h]	k_{el} or β [h^{-1}]	V_d [l/kg]	F_{el}	f	EPB [%]	pk$_a$	Ther. Range or MEC [µg/ml]	URA	D [mg]	τ [h]	t_{max} [h]
Amikacin	2.5	0.277	0.21	0.94	0	5	—	5–30	IV,IM	5–7.5 mg/kg	6–8	0.75–2
Aminopyrine	2.3	0.301	0.67	0.007	1	17	B: 5	1–25	PO	130–300	4	1
p-Aminosalicylic Acid	0.85	0.815	0.23	0.25	0.9	65	A: 3.25	0.6–4	PO	2000–3000	6	3
Amiodarone	4.3 h to 14 days	2.06 · 10^{-3} –0.16	1.3–12.9	0.05	0.2–0.58	93–97	B: 7.4	0.7–3.4	IV PO	IV 5–25/day PO 100–600/day	24 —	— 2–12
Amitriptyline	17 (15–30)	0.0407	8.8	0.05	0.65	96	B: 9.4	0.05–0.2	PO	30–300	24	3
Amobarbital	21	0.033	1.1	0	1	34	A: 7.7	1–8	PO,IV,R	15–100	8	1–5
Amodiaquine	50	0.0138	36	—	1	90	—	0.015	PO	400	168	—
Amoxapine	8	0.0866	—	0.05	0.95	91	B: 7.6	0.2–0.4	PO	200–300	24	1.5
Amoxicillin	1.2	0.578	0.47	0.7	0.92	17	A: 2.4, 7.4,9.6	2–8	PO	500	6	1.5
Amphetamine	12.2	0.078	4.0	0.65	1	—	B: 9.77	0.01–0.03	PO	5–30	12	1.5
Amphotericin B	360	0.00193	4.0	0.003	0.05	90	B: 5.7, 10.0	0.2–2.0	IV	1 mg/kg or 5–20	24 48	NA
Ampicillin	0.9	0.77	0.52	0.9	0.5	20	A: 2.54, 7.2	2–8	PO,IV,IM	250–500	6	2
Amprenavir	8.8 (7–10.6)	0.079	6.1	0.01	—	90	—	0.3–7.6	PO	1200	12	1.5
Anakinra	5 (4–6)	0.138	—	—	0.95	—	—	—	SC	100	24	3–7
Antipyrine	11.5 (5–35)	0.06	0.62	0.1	1	10	B: 2.2	—	PO	500–1000	Test	1.5
Aprindine	21 (15–30)	0.033	3.7	0.01	0.9	90	—	1–3	PO	10–150	12	—
Aripiprazole	75	0.009	5.7	0.2	0.87	>99	—	—	PO	10–30	24	4
Atenolol	6.1 (4.5–8)	0.113	1.23	0.4	0.6	<5	B: 9.6	0.2–1.3	PO	100–200	8–12	2

Drug												
Atomoxetine	5.2	0.133	0.85	0.03	0.63 0.94f	98	—	0.17b	PO	0.5–1.2 mg/kg	24	1.5
Atorvastatin	14	0.05	3.8	0.02	0.14	98	—	—	PO	10–80	24	2–4
Atrasentan	22.5	0.031	5–10.8a	0.05	—	—	—	0.130b 3.4b	PO	23.25 139.5	—	1 1.7
Atropine	2.5	0.277	3	0.4	0.75	50	B: 9.8	—	PO,SC	0.3–1.2	4–6	1
Auranofin	1920 (1000–3000)	0.00036	3.6	0.15	0.25	90	—	0.2–1.1	PO	3	12	6
Avitriptan	8	0.087	1.12	—	—	—	—	0.4–1.2	IV Inf	12–38	—	NA
Azathioprine	0.2 (0.16–0.47)	3.465	0.8	0	0.4	30	—	0.05–2	IV,PO	1–3 mg/kg (IV) 50–100 (PO)	24	NA
Azidocillin	0.8	0.866	0.28	0.6	0.3	85	A: 2.8	0.01–0.8	PO,IV,IM	500–1500	6	0.75
Azidothymidine	1	0.7	1.6	0.14	0.65	34	A: 9.68	0.12–1	PO,IV	PO 100 IV 1–2/kg	4	1
Azimilide	85 (72–120)	0.0081	13	0.1	—	94	—	0.5g	INF	4.5–9 mg/kg	NA	NA
Azithromycin	53	0.013	125a	—	—	—	—	—	IV Inf PO	500 500	24 24	NA 3
Azlocillin	1.0	0.693	0.2	0.65	0	30	A: 2.82	50–500	IV	2000	6	NA
Aztreonam	1.75	0.4	0.2	0.7	1 (IM)	60	A: 0.7, 2.75, 3.91	0.4–130	IM,IV	1000–2000	8–12	1
Bacitracin	1.5	0.462	—	0.3	0.01	—	—	—	Topical	—	—	—
Baclofen	3.5 (3–4)	0.198	0.85	0.8	0.95	30	A: 3.87, 9.62	0.08–0.4	PO	10–20	4–6	2–3
Beclomethasone	0.5	1.38	—	0.15	0.2	87	—	—	Nasal Inhal	0.042 in each nostril	6–12	—
Benazepril (Benazeprilat)	10	0.07	0.12	0.2	0.37	—	—	—	PO	20–40	12–24	0.5

(Continued)

Pharmacokinetic Parameters of Important Drugs (*Continued*)

DRUG	$t_{1/2}$ [h]	k_{el} or β [h⁻¹]	V_d [l/kg]	F_{el}	f	EPB [%]	pk_a	Ther. Range or MEC [µg/ml]	URA	D [mg]	τ [h]	t_{max} [h]
Betaxolol	15–17	0.043	4.76	0.20	0.85	45–60	B: 9.38	0.005–0.1	Ophthalmic	10–40	24	2.4–3
Bosentan	5.4	0.128	0.26	0.03	0.6	98	—	0.7–1.4	PO	62.5–125	12	4
Bretylium	15 (5–17)	0.045	—	0.75	0.2	3	—	0.5–2.4	IV,IM,PO	100–400	8	1–9
Bromazepam	35	0.02	1.7ª	—	—	—	—	0.034[b] 0.055[b]	PO R	3 —	24 —	1 2.7
Brompheniramine	24.9 (11–35)	0.0278	11.7	0.05	0.8	—	B: 3.59, 9.12	0.005–0.015	PO,IV,IM	5–20	4–12	2–5
Budesonide	2.1	0.33	2.85	0.67	0.1 PO	88	—	0.5[b] ng/ml	Inhal PO	0.4 9	24 24	10 2
Bumetanide	1.2	0.6	0.2	0.5	0.7	95	A: 0–3, 4,10	0.0002–40	PO,IV,IM	0.5–2	24	1.5
Buprenorphine	3.0	0.23	2.7	0.15	0.55	96	B: 8.42	0.001–0.125	IV, Buccal, IM	4–20 µg/kg	6–8	2.5
Bupropion	20	0.035	59ª	0.005	—	84	—	0.115[b]	PO	100–150	8–12	2
Buspirone	2.5	0.28	5.3	0.4	0.9	—	B: 1.2, 7.3	0.001–0.003	PO	20–30	12	0.75
Butabarbital	37.5	0.0185	0.8	0.08	1	26	A: 8.16	1–5	PO	15–50	8	7
Butorphanol	4.7	0.15	7.9	0.75	0.72	80	B: 8.6	0.04–0.08	IM,IV,PO, Nasal	1–4	3–4	0.5–1
Candesartan	9	0.77	0.13	0.33	0.15	99	—	—	PO	16	24	3–4
Captopril	3 (2–4)	0.23	2.0	0.5	0.65	25	A: 3.7	0.05–0.5	PO	25–50	8–12	1
Carbamazepine	37 (24–48)	0.018	1.2	0.01	0.9	72	—	4–12	PO	200–400	8	4
Carbenicillin	0.8	0.866	0.15	0.8	0.5	50	A: 2.6	10–125	IM,IV	4000–5000	4	1
Carbenoxolone	16.3 (13–18)	0.0425	0.1	0.01	1	99.9	A: 6.7, 7.1	5–20	PO	50	8	2–8

Drug												
Carboplatin	4 (2.6–5.9)	0.17	0.23	1	NA	0	—	—	IV Inf	300–500 mg/m²	4 weeks	—
(Platinum in ultrafiltered plasma)	35	0.02	4.9	—	—	—	—	—	—	—	—	—
Carisoprodol	8.0	0.0866	0.6	0.01	1	55	B: 4.2	10–30	PO	350–700	6	4
Carvedilol	8 (7–10)	0.086	1.9	<0.02	0.3	98	—	40–100	PO,IV	6.25–50	12	1.5
Caspofungin Acetate	45	0.015	—	0.014	NA	97	—	—	IV Inf	35	24	NA
Cefaclor	0.8 (0.6–1)	0.866	0.24	0.6	0.9	40	—	0.5–10	PO	250	8	1
Cefadroxil	1.3	0.533	0.15	0.95	1.0	10	—	0.5–10	PO	500–1000	12	1
Cefamandole	0.8	0.866	0.16	0.7	0.95	74	A: 2.3	0.5–5	IV,IM	1000–2000	6	—
Cefazolin	1.6	0.433	0.17	0.85	0	86	—	0.1–6.3	IM	250–500	8	—
Cefdinir	1.7	0.416	—	0.18	0.2	65	—	1.6[b]	PO	300	12	3
Cefditoren Pivoxil	1.6	0.433	0.13	—	—	88	—	1800[b]	PO	200–400	12	1.5–3
Cefepime	2.1	0.32	0.3	0.84	1 (IM)	20	—	0.015–32	IM,IV	1000–2000	8–12	1.25 (IM)
Cefixime	3 (2–4)	0.23	0.29	0.3–0.35	0.45	—	A: 1.9, 2.7, 4.1	—	PO	500–1000	8.2	4
Cefmenoxime	1	0.7	0.25	0.7	1 (IM)	77	—	0.8–45	IV,IM	1000–2000	4–6	0.75 (IM)
Cefmetazole	1.25	0.6	0.14	0.75	NA	85	—	6–140	IM,IV	2000	6–12	1.5 (IM)
Cefonicid	4.5	0.154	0.11	0.99	NA	90	—	220[b]	IV,IM	1000	24	1 (IM)
Cefoperazone	2	0.346	0.16	0.3	NA	80	A: 2.55	4–60	IV,IM	1000–2000	12	1.5 (IM)
Ceforanide	2.8	0.248	0.19	0.9	—	80	—	—	—	—	—	—
Cefotaxime	1.2 (0.9–1.5)	0.578	0.38	0.65	0	40	A: 3.4	0.2–8	IV,IM	1000–2000	8–12	—
Cefotetan	3.5	0.2	0.17	0.75	0.9 (IM)	90	—	0.6–65	IM,IV	1000–2000	12	1.5 (IM)
Cefoxitin	0.7	0.99	0.15	0.85	0	60	—	1–10	IV,IM	1000	6	—

(Continued)

Pharmacokinetic Parameters of Important Drugs (Continued)

DRUG	$t_{1/2}$ [h]	k_{el} or β [h⁻¹]	V_d [l/kg]	F_{el}	f	EPB [%]	pk_a	Ther. Range or MEC [µg/ml]	URA	D [mg]	τ [h]	t_{max} [h]
Cefpodoxime (Proxetil)	2.4	0.3	0.5	0.3	0.5	30	—	0.1–3	PO	100–400	12	2.5
Cefprozil	1.3	0.53	0.2	0.6	0.95	36	—	—	PO	250–500	12	—
Cefsulodin	1.5	0.46	0.25	0.6	NA	30	—	0.2–100	IM,IV	1000	6	0.3 (IM)
Ceftazidime	1.8	0.385	0.25	0.88	0.05	17	—	—	—	—	—	—
Ceftibuten	2.4	0.29	0.21	0.95	—	65	—	—	PO	400	24	—
Ceftizoxime	1.2 (0.9–1.4)	0.578	0.25	0.7	0	48	—	2–64	IV,IM	1000	8	—
Ceftriaxone	6.5	0.1	0.2	0.5	NA	90	—	0.03–8	IM,IV	1000–2000	12–24	2.5 (IM)
Cefuroxime	1.4	0.495	0.28	0.95	0	35	A: 2.5	1–50	IV,IM	750–1500	8	—
Celecoxib	11	0.063	5.7	0.27	0.2–0.4	97	—	0.7 (100 mg)	PO	100–200	12	3
Cephacetrile	1.0 (0.5–1.4)	0.693	0.18	0.85	0	25	A: 1.97	3	IV,IM	500–1000	6–8	—
Cephalexin	0.9	0.77	0.26	0.9	0.9	15	A: 5.25, 7.3	6–50	PO	250	6	1
Cephaloridine	1.2	0.578	0.23	0.85	0.05	20	A: 2.25	0.1–16	IM,IV	500–1000	6–8	—
Cephalothin	0.6	1.155	0.26	0.52	0	65	A: 2.5	0.1–6.3	IM,IV	500–1000	6	—
Cephapirin	0.75	0.924	0.15	0.7	0.05	45	A: 2.15	1–12	IV,IM	500–1000	4–6	—
Cephradine	0.76	0.912	0.32	0.9	1	15	A: 2.63, 7.27	0.5–12	PO,IV,IM	250–500	6	1
Cerivastatin	2.5	0.28	—	0.24	0.6	>99	—	—	PO	0.1–0.8	24	2.5–3
Cetrorelix	45 (13–68)	0.015	2.4–3.7[a]	—	—	—	—	0.0014[9]	SC	0.25–1	24	—
Cevimeline HCl	5	0.138	6	0.16	—	20	—	—	PO	30	8	1.5
Chloral Hydrate (active: Trichloroethanol)	8 (6–10)	0.0866	0.6	0	0	40	—	5–20	PO	500–1500	24	0.5

Drug											
Chloramphenicol	2.7 (2–3)	0.257	0.57	0.05	0.85	60	B: 5.5	5–40	PO	250	4	2
Chlordiazepoxide	15.0 (5–30)	0.046	0.3	0	1	94	B: 4.66	1–3	PO,IV,IM	5–10	6–8	3
Chloroguanide	15	0.0462	19.2	0.4	1	70	—	0.035	PO	100	24	3
Chloroquine	127 (43–312)	0.00545	93.6	0.6	1	55	B: 8.1	0.01–0.28	PO	300	168	6
Chlorothiazide	1.5 (0.75–2)	0.462	0.2	0.95	0.14	65	B: 6.8, 9.4	—	IV,PO	500–2000	12–24	—
Chlorphenesin Carbamate	3.1	0.223	1.3	0	1	—	—	—	PO	400	6	1–3
Chlorpheniramine	20 (2–43)	0.0346	4.3	0.23	0.4	70	B: 9.16	0.005–0.01	PO,IV,IM	4–40	4–24	3
Chlorpromazine	30 (15–59)	0.023	21.0	0.01	0.32	96	B: 9.3	50–300	PO,IM,R	10–1000	24	3.5
Chlorpropamide	32 (30–36)	0.0216	0.15	0.2	1.0	72	A: 4.8	50–150	PO	100–250	12–24	3
Chlortetracycline	5.6	0.124	1.74	0.18	0.7	54	B: 3.3, 9.3	0.5–6	PO,IV	250–500	6	3
Chlorthalidone	49 (40–60)	0.014	11.0	0.8	0.64	75	A: 9.4	2–10	PO	25–400	12–48	12
Cicletanine	10	0.07	0.5	0.004	0.6	—	—	0.4–2	PO	50	24	0.8
Cidofovir (with co-administration of Probenecid)	4.6	0.152	0.54	0.72	NA	6	—	19[b]	IV Inf	5 mg/kg	NA	NA
Cilostazol	12	0.058	—	0	—	98	—	—	PO	100	12	2–4
Cimetidine	2.0	0.346	1.8	0.7	0.8	19	B: 7.11	0.25–1	PO,IV,IM	300	4	1
Ciprofloxacin	4.0 (3–6.5)	0.25	2.25	0.3–0.5	0.65–0.8	20–40	A: 6	0.03–8.0	PO,IV	100–500	12	0.7–1.8
Cisapride	5.8	0.12	5.65[a]	—	—	98	—	0.05[b]	PO	20	24	1–2
Cisplatinum	89 (58–120)	0.0077	0.5	0.8	NA	90	A: —	1–5	IV	50–120 mg/m^2	3–4 weeks	NA
Citalopram	33	0.021	0.2	0	0.80	80	—	—	PO	20–40	24	4
Citrorelix	74	0.0093	13.4	—	—	—	—	0.02–0.45[b]	SC	5–10	168	1–2
Clemastine	21 (10–32)	0.03	11	0.05	0.4	—	—	0.002–0.003	PO	1	12	3.5 (2–5)
Clenbuterol	30	0.0023	4.0	—	1.0	45–68	B: 9.57	50–90 pg/ml	PO	0.01–0.02	6–12	3

(Continued)

Pharmacokinetic Parameters of Important Drugs (Continued)

DRUG	$t_{1/2}$ [h]	k_{el} or β [h⁻¹]	V_d [l/kg]	F_{el}	f	EPB [%]	pk_a	Ther. Range or MEC [µg/ml]	URA	D [mg]	τ [h]	t_{max} [h]
Clinafloxacin	5.6	0.124	1.9	0.7	0.85	—	—	1.2[b]	PO	200–400	12	1.5 (1–3)
Clindamycin	2.8 (2–3)	0.248	1.1	0.1	0.9	90	B: 7.72	0.002–0.5	PO	150–450	6	1
	11	0.062	—	—	0.3	—	—	0.2[b]	VAG ovula	100	24	4.6
	14	0.048	—	—	0.04	—	—	0.02[b]	VAG cream	100	24	8
Clodronate	27	0.026	98.9[a]	<0.03	—	—	—	0.8[b] (2 × 400 mg) 1.0[b] (2 × 800 mg) 4.4[b] (2 × 1600 mg)	PO	400–1600	12	0.5–1
Clofibrate	16.7 (6.4–25)	0.041	0.12	0.15	1	95	A: 2.95	80–150	PO	500	4–6	4
Clonazepam	40 (19–60)	0.017	1.5–4.4	0.02	0.75	47–82	B: 1.5	0.01–0.08	PO	1–2	8–12	2
Clonidine	8 (6–23)	0.086	3.5	0.3	0.8	20	B: 8.3	0.0002–0.002	PO	0.15–0.3	6–8	3
Clopidogrel	8	0.086	—	0	0.5	98	—	—	PO	75	24	1
Clorazepate	47	0.0147	1.1	—	1	—	—	0.6	PO	15–60	24	—
Cloxacillin	0.6	1.155	0.35	0.4	0.5	94	A: 2.9	7–14	PO	500	6	1
Clozapine	55 (11–105)	0.0126	3.5 (2–5)	—	—	90	—	—	PO	12.5–450	24	3–4
Cocaine	0.95 (0.6–1.3)	0.73	2.1	0.7	1	40	B: 8.6	0.03–0.3	PO,IV	5–30	single	1
Codeine	3.3 (3–4)	0.21	3.45	0.1	0.5	10–25	B: 8.1	0.025	PO,IM,SC	30	6–8	1.25
Colchicine	30	0.02	6.7	0.15	0.44	40	B: 1.7, 12.4	0.007–0.02	PO,IV	0.5–1	24	1 (0.5–2)
Colistimethate	3	0.231	0.5	0.75	1 I.M.	20	—	1–5	PO,IV,IM	2.5–5 mg/kg	6,12	2
Colistin Sulfate	3	0.231	0.55	0.8	1 I.M.	20	—	1–5	IM,PO	1.5 mg/kg	12	—
Coumarin	0.8 (0.5–1.5)	0.8662	1.7	0	0.04	35	NA	0.02	PO,IV	IV 10–25 PO 30	8 12	— 0.1

Creatine	2.7	0.257	0.47a	0.8	0.38	0	—	160b	PO	5000	6	2
Cromolyn Sodium	1.35	0.52	—	0.02	0.01	69	A: 2	NA	Inhal	0.08 per spray	NA	NA
Cyclobenzaprine	18.4	0.038	2.1	0.01	0.55	—	—	0.025b	PO	10	8	4
Cyclophosphamide	7.6 (6.4–8.7)	0.0912	0.8	0.15	1	12	NA	10–25	PO,IV	1–5 mg/kg	24	1
Cyclosporine	20	0.035	7.5	0.01	0.3	90	—	0.1–0.5	IV,PO	IV 7 mg/kg PO 12 mg/kg	8,24	— / 4.5
Cytarabine	0.22	3.15	2.2	0.07	1	13	B: 4.5	0.01–0.1	IV	2 mg/kg	24	0.3–1
Dalteparin	2.5	0.28	0.05	0.05	0.9	—	—	0.4–0.6	IV	2500–5000 IU	24	NA
Dapsone	29 (22.5–39.3)	0.0239	1.9	0.23	0.95	77	B: 13	1–7	PO	50–300	24	2–8
Demeclocycline	12 (8–14)	0.057	1.6	0.5	0.6	65	B: 3.3	0.05–10	PO	150–300	6–12	3–4
Demethylchlortetracycline	13.6	0.051	1.8	0.4	0.7	75	B: 3.34, 7.2,9.3	0.5–3	PO	300	12	3
Deramciclane	28	0.025	18.5a	—	—	—	—	0.016c–0.033b (10 mg bid) 0.047c–0.091b (30 mg bid) 0.075c–0.160b (60 mg bid)	PO	10–60	12	2–3
Desipramine	17	0.0401	41.9	0.1	1	8.3	B: 10.2	0.15–0.3	PO	50	8	3
Deslanoside	44	0.0157	4.4	0.6	0.8	97	NA	—	IV,IM	0.2	12	—
Dexamethasone	3.5 (1.8–5.3)	0.198	1.04	0.77	0.81	84	B: 25	0.005–0.01	IV,PO,IM	0.4–16	24	1
Dexloxiglumide	2.7	0.257	1.1a	0.02	—	—	—	2.4b (100 mg) 15.3b (400 mg)	PO	100–400	8	1.5
Dextromethorphan	2.7 (2–4)	0.2566	1.1	0.2	0.75	—	B: 8.3	0.2–0.35	PO	30	6–8	2
Dezocine	2.4	0.3	10.1	0.01	NA	—	—	0.005–0.009	IM,IV	5–20	3–6	0.15–1.5 (IM)
Diazepam	32.9 (27–37)	0.021	2.0	0.4	1	97	B: 3.4	0.1–1	PO,IV,IM	2–10	6–8	1
Diazoxide	30 (20–40)	0.023	0.2	0.4	1.0	91	A: 9.0	15–25	PO,IV	75–500	8–12	4

(Continued)

Pharmacokinetic Parameters of Important Drugs (Continued)

DRUG	$t_{1/2}$ [h]	k_{el} or β [h⁻¹]	V_d [l/kg]	F_{el}	f	EPB [%]	pk_a	Ther. Range or MEC [µg/ml]	URA	D [mg]	τ [h]	t_{max} [h]
Diclofenac Sodium	1.1	0.63	0.17	0.1	0.52	99.7	A: 3.9	0.05–3	PO	100–150	8–12	2.5
Dicloxacillin	0.8	0.866	0.29	0.7	0.8	96	A: 2.67	15–18	PO	500	6	1
Dicumarol	8.2	0.085	0.13	0.01	0.8	99	A: 4.4,8	5–10	PO	25–200	24	—
Dicyclomine	1.8	0.385	3.65	—	0.5	—	B: 9	0.025	PO,IM	10–20	4–8	—
Didanosine	1.5	0.462	1.08	0.18	0.42	—	—	—	PO	200	12	1
Diflunisal	10 (8–12)	0.069	0.1	0.1	1.0	99	A: 3	50–100	PO	500	8–12	2.5
Digitoxin	164 (118–190)	0.0042	0.6	0.08	0.9	93	NA	0.01–0.035	PO,IV	0.1–0.2	24	10
Digoxin	43 (33–51)	0.0161	6.3	0.76	0.62	23	NA	0.0008–0.002	PO,IV,IM	0.25–0.75	24	4
Dihydrocodeine	6.0	0.11	3.5	0.1	0.21	—	B: 8.68	0.05–0.25	PO	0.8–1.7 mg/kg	12	0.7
Diltiazem	4.0	0.173	0.77	0.35	0.5	80	—	0.03–0.2	PO	60	6	1.5
Diphemanil Methylsulfate	8.4	0.08	212	0.5	low	—	—	0.008–0.06	PO	250	24	3
Diphenhydramine	5.2 (4–7)	0.133	3.7	0.03	0.5	98	B: 8.98	0.01–0.1	PO	25–50	6–8	3
Dipyridamole	13 (11.5–15)	0.053	1.75 (1–2.5)	0	NA 0.4–0.7	99	—	4.6	IV Inf PO	0.57 mg/kg 75–100	NA 6	NA 1.25
Dirithromycin	44	0.016	11.5	0.02	0.1	20	—	1–22	PO	500	24	4
Disopyramide	7.8 (6–10)	0.0888	0.8	0.55	0.9	68	B: 9.6	2–8	PO	100–200	6	1.25
Distigmine Bromide	60	0.0116	1	0.06	0.047	—	—	0.0044	PO	5	—	1.5
Disulfiram	4.8	0.144	23	0.5	0.9	50	—	0.6	PO	125–500	24	4
Dobutamine	0.033	20.79	0.2	0.01	0	—	B: 9.4	0.04–0.17	IV	2.5–10 µg/kg/min	Infusion	NA
Docetaxel	11	0.063	2.3	0.08	NA	94	—	—	IV Inf	60–100 mg/m²	3 wks	NA

Drug												
Donepezil	70	0.01	12	0.17	1	96	—	0.05	PO	5–10	24	3.5
Dopamine	0.15 (0.1–0.2)	4.62	0.93	0.03	0	—	B: 8.9	0.01–0.1	IV	1.5–5 µg/kg/min	Infusion	NA
Doxazosin	22	0.0315	2.5a	0.01	0.65	98	—	0.012b (2 mg)	PO	1–8	24	2–3
Doxepin	16.8 (8.2–24.5)	0.0413	20.2	—	0.27	80	B: 8	30–50	PO	25 / 75	8 / 24	2 / 2
Doxorubicin	33 (20–48)	0.021	20–30	<0.05	NA	75	—	—	IV Inf	20 mg/m2	168	NA
Doxycycline	20 (14–22)	0.0347	1.5	0.55	0.8	82	B: 3.4, 7.7	1–2	PO	100	24	3
Dronabinol	3 (2–4)	0.03	10.6	<0.01	0.1–0.2	95	B: 10.6	—	—	5 mg/m2	4	1–3
Droperidol	2.2 (2–2.4)	0.315	1.75	0.01	—	87	B: 7.6	—	IV,IM	2.5–10	—	—
Duloxetine	12.5	0.055	27.7	—	—	95	—	0.005–0.02	PO	20–40	12	6
Eletriptan HBr	4.5	0.15	2.7	—	0.5	85	—	0.06b (20 mg) 0.12b (40 mg)	PO	20–40	d	1
Enalapril (Enalaprilat measured)	35	0.02	1.3	0.54	0.55–0.75	55	B: 5.4	0.07–0.125	PO	10–40	24	3.5
Eniporide	2.17	0.32	1.45	0.4	NA	—	—	—	IV	2–100	—	NA
Enoxacin	4.5 (3–6)	0.15	1–6	0.4	0.9	40	—	0.06–16	PO	400–1000	12–24	2 (1–3)
Entacapone	2.5 (1.5–3.5)	0.277	—	0.1	0.45	—	—	—	PO	200	with each levodopa dose	1–2
Eprosartan	7 (5–9)	0.099	4.4	0.07	0.13	98	—	—	PO	600	24	1–2
Ergonovine (Ergometrine)	1.2 (0.5–2)	0.6 (0.3–1.4)	1	0	0.8	—	—	0.004–3	PO,IV	0.2–0.4	6–12	1.25
Ertapenem	4	0.173	0.12	0.38	1 (IM)	95	—	1–160	IV Inf, IM	1000	24	2.3 (IM)
Erythromycin	1.4 (1.3–3)	0.495	0.6	0.15	0.4	73	B: 8.8	0.5–2.5	PO,IM,IV,R	250	6	2.5
Esomeprazole	1.3	0.533	0.37	—	0.9	97	—	—	PO	20–40	24	1–2

(Continued)

Pharmacokinetic Parameters of Important Drugs (Continued)

DRUG	$t_{1/2}$ [h]	k_{el} or β [h⁻¹]	V_d [l/kg]	F_{el}	f	EPB [%]	pk_a	Ther. Range or MEC [µg/ml]	URA	D [mg]	τ [h]	t_{max} [h]
Estazolam	17 (10–24)	0.04	0.35 (0.15–0.65)	0.05	—	93	—	30–160	PO	0.5–2	24	2
Etanercept	102	0.0068	0.34[a]	—	—	—	—	1.1[b]	SC	25	72	69
Ethacrynic Acid	1.25 (0.5–2)	0.55	0.1	0.22	1.0	95	A: 3.5	0.05–0.1	IV,PO	50–200	12	6–8
Ethambutol	3.5 (2.5–5.5)	0.198	2.3	0.85	0.8	39	B: 6.6,10	1.5	PO	15 mg/kg	24	3
Ethchlorvynol	25	0.0277	3.7	0.001	1	—	—	2–15	PO	500	24	1–2
Ethinamate	2.3	0.301	1.6	0	1	1	—	5–10	PO	500–1000	24	—
Ethinyl Estradiol	16.7	0.044	13.1[a]	—	—	—	—	0.02	PO	0.02	24	1.5
Ethionamide	2	0.347	—	0.01	1	30	—	1–5	PO	15–20 mg/kg	24	—
Ethosuximide	50 (40–60)	0.0139	0.62	0.3	0.9	0	A: 9.3	50–100	PO	250–500	12–24	2
Etodolac	7.5	0.09	0.4	0.01	0.8	99	A: 4.65	20–40	PO	200–400	6–8	1.3
Etoposide	8	0.087	0.35	NA / 0.8		—	—	0.14[b] / 0.08[b] (µg/ml) /(mg/m²)	IV Inf / PO	50 mg/m² / 50 mg/m²	24 / 24	NA / 1.5
Etoricoxib	27	0.0257	1.6	—	1.0	—	—	3.5[b]	PO	120	24	1.5
Everolimus	34	0.02	11.9[a]	—	—	—	—	0.017[b] (2 mg)	PO	1–2	24	0.5
Ezetimibe	22	0.054	—	0.09	0.03	>90	—	0.05	PO	10	24	4–12
Famciclovir	2.3	0.3	1.5	0	0.77	20	—	3.3[b]	PO	500	8	0.9
Famotidine	3 (2–4)	0.23	1.2	0.7	0.45	—	B: 7.1	0.01–0.07	PO	20–40	12–24	3 (1–4)
Fampridine	3.5	0.2	3.34[a]	—	—	—	—	>0.05[b] (10 mg)	IV / PO	0.3 mg/kg / 10–25	— / 12	NA / 1
Felbamate	21	0.033	0.75	0.45	1	25	—	30–50	PO	300–900	6	2
Felodipine	13 (10–16)	0.05	10	0.5	0.2	99	—	1.5–7.5	PO	5–20	24	3

Drug											
Femoxetine	16	0.04	90	0.02	0.7	—	—	0.05–0.1	PO	400–600	24	6 (4–8)
Fenfluramine	19 (18–20)	0.0365	14	0.4	0.65	40	B: 9.1	0.04–0.12	PO	20	8	1–2
Fenofibrate (active: Fenofibric Acid)	18	0.038	0.56[a]	0.5	—	99	—	—	PO	67–201	24	5–8
Fenoprofen	2.5	0.28	—	0.035	0.85	99	A: 4.5	30–110	PO	300–600	6	1.5
Fentanyl	2.4	0.289	1.25	0.06	0.3	70	B: 8.43	0.02–0.025	IV,IM	0.05–0.1	—	—
Fibroblast Growth Factor-2	7.6	0.09	0.24	—	—	—	—	0.1–0.27[b] / 0.0015–0.3[b]	IV Inf Intra-coronary	18–36 µg/kg / 0.33–48 µg/kg	NA / —	NA / —
Fiduxosin	20	0.035	6.4[a]	<0.01	—	—	—	0.03[c]–0.17[b] (30 mg) / 0.08[c]–0.57[b] (60 mg) / 0.14[c]–0.73[b] (90 mg)	PO	30–90	24	4.5
Finasteride	5	0.14	1.1	0.005	0.8	90	—	0.001–0.04	PO	5	24	2
Flecainide Acetate	20 (12–27)	0.04	7	0.3	1	40	B: 93	0.2–1	PO	50–100	12	3
Fleroxacin	10	0.07	1.7	0.5	0.9	26	—	2.5–10	PO	400–1000	12–24	4
Floxuridine	0.2	3.46	0.55	0.6	NA	—	A: 8	—	IV	0.1–0.6/kg	24	NA
Flucloxacillin	0.8	0.866	0.12	0.55	0.5	96	A: 2.7	0.4	PO	500	6	1–2
Fluconazole	22	0.032	0.71	0.46	0.9	11	B: 3.7	0.06–6	PO	1/kg	24	2
Flucytosine	4.8 (3.5–6.2)	0.144	0.6	0.8	0.85	4	A: 2.9, 10.7	35–70	PO	50–150 mg/kg	24	2
Fludarabine Phosphate (active: Fluoro-Ara-A)	19 (15–23)	0.036	2.4	0.23	NA / 0.6 (PO)	—	—	—	IV Inf / PO	25 mg/m² / 40	NA / 24	NA / —
Fludrocortisone	5	0.14	0.79	0.2	1.0	40	—	0.001–0.002	PO	0.1–0.2	24	1.7
Flumazenil	54 (41–79)	0.013	1 (0.8–1.6)	0.01	NA	50	—	0.02–0.1	IV	0.2–1	As needed	NA
Flunisolide	1.5	0.262	1.8	0.5	0.5	—	—	—	Nasal	0.1	12	—
Flunitrazepam	30 (25–35)	0.023	4.5	—	0.8	—	B: 1.84	0.001–0.05	PO	1–2	24	—

(Continued)

Pharmacokinetic Parameters of Important Drugs (Continued)

DRUG	$t_{1/2}$ [h]	k_{el} or β [h⁻¹]	V_d [l/kg]	F_{el}	f	EPB [%]	pk_a	Ther. Range or MEC [μg/ml]	URA	D [mg]	τ [h]	t_{max} [h]
Fluoxetine	50 (24–72)	0.0139	0.57	0	0.94	94.5	—	0.015–0.05	PO	20–80	24	6–8
Flurbiprofen	5.7	0.12	0.15	0.7	—	99	—	—	PO	50–100	8	1.5
Fluticasone	3	0.231	3.68	0.05	0.02	91	—	—	Nasal Inhal	0.2	24	—
Fluticasone Propionate	5.1	0.136	92.4ᵃ	—	—	—	—	0.06ᵇ ng/ml	Inhal	0.2	24	1.5
Fluvastatin	1.2	0.6	0.49	0.02	0.24	>98	—	0.06–0.7	PO	20–40	12–24	1.25
Fluvoxamine	15	0.046	0.36	0.94	0.53	80	—	0.08–0.55	PO	50–300	24	2–8
Foscarnet	5	0.14	0.5	0.85	NA	15	—	35–175	IV	80–120	8–12	NA
Fosinopril (Fosinoprilat measured)	12	0.06	0.16	0	0.36	95	—	0.07–0.27	PO	10	24	3
Frovatriptan	25.7	0.027	3.5	—	0.3	15	—	4.2ᵇ (males) 7.0ᵇ (females)	PO	2.5	—ᵈ	3
Furosemide	1.5 (0.5–2)	0.462	0.2	0.75	0.6	99	A: 4.7	1–6	PO,IV,IM	20–40	6–8	1
Gabapentin	5.5	0.126	0.9	0.8	0.8	3	—	>2	PO	300–1800	8–24	2
Galantamine HBr	7 (4–10)	0.099	0.93	0.32	0.99	18	—	—	PO	16–32	24	1
Gallopamil	4.3	0.16	2	0.02	0.23	93	—	0.02–0.1	PO	50	8	1.75
Ganciclovir	4 (3–5)	0.173	0.74	0.05	0.09	2	—	— / 1ᵇ	IV Inf / PO	5 mg/kg / 1000	12 / 8	NA / 2–3
Gatifloxacin	7.8	0.089	1.8	0.8	0.96	20	—	4ᵇ	PO / IV Inf	400 / 200–400	24 / 24	1.5 / NA
Gemtuzumab Ozogamicin	72.4	0.0096	0.26	—	NA	—	—	—	IV Inf	9 mg/m²	336	—
Gentamicin	2	0.347	0.25	0.9	0	10	B: 5.9	0.5–10	IM	1 mg/kg	8	0.5–1.5
Gliclazide	10.4	0.07	0.2	0.01	—	90	A: 5.98	0.5–15	PO	40–160	12–24	4 (2–8)

Drug										
Glipizide	3.3 (2–4)	0.210	0.1	1	98.5	A: 90.5	0.11–0.33	PO	2.5–20	12–24	1.5
Glutethimide	8.7 (5.3–11.6)	0.079	0.002	1	54	B: 4.52	0.2–0.8	PO	125–250	8	1–6
Glyburide	9 (6–12)	0.077	0.0	1	95	A: 5.3	—	PO	2.5–10	12	2–4
Granisetron	9 (1–31)	0.08	0.12	—	65	—	0.02–0.175 / 0.001–0.04	IV Inf / PO	0.04/kg / 1	24 / 12	NA / 1
Griseofulvin	14 (10–24)	0.095	0.01	0.5	—	NA	0.3–1.3	PO	250	2	4
Guanabenz	8.5 (6–10)	0.0815	0.01	0.7	90	—	>0.01	PO	4–48	12	2–5
Guanethidine	43	0.016	0.5	0.7	—	—	>0.008	PO	10–400	24	—
Haloperidol	20 (10–24)	0.0347	0.01	0.6	92	B: 9,12	0.001–0.015	PO,IM	0.5–5	8–12	5
Hetacillin	1.3	0.533	0.9	—	20	A: 2.5, 7.3	1.6–6.2	PO,IM,IV	200–450	6	1
Hexobarbital	4.1	0.169	0	1	—	A: 8.2	2–4	IV	500–1000	once	1
Histamine Dihydrochloride	0.183	3.78	—	NA	—	—	0.038e	SC	1	—	—
Human Growth Hormone	3.8	0.18	—	0.75	—	—	0.05b	SC	0.1 mg/kg	NA	7.5
Hydralazine fast acetylator	4 (2–6)	0.173	0.02	0.22	87	A: 7.1	0.5–1.5	PO	50	6–12	1
slow acetylator	5 (2–8)	0.139	—	0.38	87	A: 7.1	0.5–1.5	PO	50	6–12	1
Hydrochlorothiazide	10.2 (5.6–14.8)	0.0679	0.95	0.67	50	A: 7.9, 8.6	0.1–0.4	PO	25–76	8–12	3
Hydrocortisone	1.75 (1.5–2)	0.396	0.01	1	95	NA	0.05–0.25	PO	10–200	6–8	1
	—	—	—	0.05	—	—	0.02–0.04b	R	100	8–24	1.5
Hydroflumethiazide	16.6 (11–27)	0.0417	0.47	0.52	75	A: 8.9, 10.7	—	PO	25–100	12–24	—
Hydromorphone	2.6	0.266	0.06	0.6	7.8	B: 8.09, 9.47	0.001–0.03	IV,IM,PO	IV,IM: 1–1.5 / PO: 2–4	4–6 / 4	1 / 0.5
Hydroxychloroquine	72	0.00962	0.67	1	55	—	0.01–0.02	PO	310	168	—
Ibuprofen	2.2	0.315	0.01	1	99	A: 4.8	5–50	PO	200–600	6–8	1.25

(Continued)

Pharmacokinetic Parameters of Important Drugs (*Continued*)

DRUG	$t_{1/2}$ [h]	k_{el} or β [h^{-1}]	V_d [l/kg]	F_{el}	f	EPB [%]	pk$_s$	Ther. Range or MEC [μg/ml]	URA	D [mg]	τ [h]	t_{max} [h]
Imatinib	18	0.038	2.9	0.05	98	95	—	—	PO	400–600	24	2–4
Imipenem	1	0.0693	—	0.5	N/A 0.75	20	—	10–80	IV Inf IM	250–1000 500–750	6–8 12	NA 2
Imipramine	7	0.099	15	0	0.5	96	B: 8	0.15–0.5	PO	25–50	8	1
Indinavir	1.8	0.385	—	0.10	—	60	B: 3.7	—	PO	800	8	0.8
Indomethacin	6.1 (3–11)	0.11	0.9	0.15	1	97	A: 4.5	0.5–3	PO	25–50	8–12	1.5
Insulin	1.75 (1.5–2)	0.396	0.6	0.05	0	5	—	10–20 μU/ml	IV,IM,SC	16–20	12	0.25–1
Interferon Alfa-2a	5.1 (3.7–8.5)	0.136	0.4	—	0.8	—	—	1.5–2.6b ng/ml 1.25–2.3b ng/ml (36 million U)	IM SC	3–36 million U 3–36 million U	48 —	3.8 7.3
Interferon Alfa-n3	4.4 (3.3–6.3)	0.157	0.97	—	—	—	—	700 U/ml 50 U/ml 50 U/ml	IV Inf IM SC	10 million U 10 million U 10 million U	— — —	NA 6 8.5
Interferon Gamma-1b	0.63 5.9 2.9	1.09 0.117 0.239	— —	— — —	NA 0.89 0.89	— — —	— — —	— — —	IV SC IM	50 mcg/m² 50 mcg/m² 50 mcg/m²	48 48 48	NA 7 4
Interleukin-10	2.23	0.31	0.048	—	NA	—	—	0.6b	IV	0.02 mg/kg	—	NA
Irbesartan	13 (11–15)	0.053	1.04 (0.75–1.33)	0.2	0.85	90	—	—	PO	150–300	24	1.5
Irinotecan	6	0.12	0.03	0.15	NA	50	—	0.35–1.2	IV Inf	125/m²	168	NA
Isoniazid fast acetylator	1.1 (0.6–2)	0.63	0.6	0.3	0.9	15	B: 2.0, 3.85	0.5–15	PO,IM	100	8	1.5
slow acetylator	3.6 (2–4)	0.194	0.6	0.5	0.9	15	B: 2.0, 3.85	0.5–15	PO,IM	100	8	1.5
Isosorbide Dinitrate	0.5 (0.4–1)	1.39	5	0	0.2	30–70	NA		Oral PO	5–10 10–40	2–3 6	0.5

Isosorbide-5-mononitrate	5 (4–6)	0.14	0.64	0.02	1.0	3.5	NA	0.2–0.5	PO	20	6–12	1
Isotretinoin	21	0.033	8.3	0	—	—	—	0.86[b]	PO	0.25–0.5 mg/kg	12	5
Isoxicam	29 (24–34)	0.023	0.17	0.02	1.0	96	3.6	5–12	PO	200	12–24	4–10
Itraconazole	21	0.03	12	0.03	0.6	99	A: 3.7	0.2–0.6	PO	200–400	8–12	4.5
Ivermectin	16	0.043	2.18[a]	<0.01	—	—	—	0.05[b]	PO	0.15–0.2 mg/kg	3–12 months	4
Kanamycin	2	0.347	0.25	0.81	0 / 0.7 IM	0	B: 7.2	5–25	IM	7.5 mg/kg	12	1
Ketamine	2.3 (1.8–2.7)	0.3	2.1	0.04	0.16	35	B: 7.5	0.7–3	IV,PO,IM	0.5 mg/kg	4–6	1.5
Ketoconazole	8 (6.5–9)	0.0866	0.36	0.03	0.76	99	B: 6.51	1–10	PO	200–400	24	1–2
Ketoprofen	2.5	0.28	0.1	0.8	0.9	99	A: 5.94	0.4–6	PO	50	6	1.5 (0.5–2)
Ketorolac	5.5	0.126	0.2	0.91	1	99	—	—	IV, IM / PO	30 / 10	6 / 4–6	2 (IM) / 2–3
Labetalol	4.0 (3–5)	0.173	11.2	0.05	0.4	50	B: 7.38	0.025–0.2	PO	200–400	24	1.5
Lacidipine	7.5	0.09	8	0.01	0.2	90	—	0.0002–0.006	PO	4	24	1.5
Lamivudine	6	0.1	1.3 (0.9–1.7)	0.7	0.9	36	—	0.6–2	PO,IV	150	12	0.9
Lamotrigine	28	0.025	1.1	0.1	1	0.5	B: 5.7	40–100	PO	50–400	12–24	3 (1.5–4.5)
Lanatoside C	41	0.0169	4.4	0.2	0.6	25	NA	0.001–0.0015	PO	0.5–1.5	24	—
Lansoprazole	1.5	0.462	—	0.3	0.8	33	—	—	PO	30	12	1.7
Latamoxef	2.3 (1.8–2.9)	0.3	0.35	0.8	1	50	—	5–200	IM,IV	1000–2000	8–12	1 (IM)
Leflunomide	9 (6–12)	0.077	0.13	0	0.8	99	—	—	PO	20	24	6–12
Levamisole	3.5	0.2	2.3	0.05	0.65	—	—	0.03–0.15	PO	50	8	1.5
Levetiracetam	7	1	0.6	0.66	0.95	10	—	6–20	PO	500–1500	12	1.3
Levodopa	0.44	1.575	12.7	0.01	0.9	5	A: 2.3	0.2–4	PO	500–800	24	1.5
Levofloxacin	6.6	0.315	0.2	0.87	0.99	30	—	5–16	PO	500	24	1.1

(Continued)

Pharmacokinetic Parameters of Important Drugs (*Continued*)

DRUG	$t_{1/2}$ [h]	k_{el} or β [h⁻¹]	V_d [l/kg]	F_{el}	f	EPB [%]	pk_a	Ther. Range or MEC [µg/ml]	URA	D [mg]	τ [h]	t_{max} [h]
Levosimendan	1.26	0.55	0.39	–	NA	–	–	–	IV	0.2 µg/kg/ min for 24 h	NA	N/A
Lidocaine	1.8	0.39	1.5	0.1	0.35	66	B: 7.86	1.5–7	IV	20–50 mg/ kg/min	Infusion	NA
Lincomycin	5.4	0.128	0.4	0.15	0.4	72	B: 7.5	0.09–3	PO,IM	500	6–8	2–4
Linezolid	5	0.139	0.7	0.3	1	31	–	0.5–4	IV Inf PO	10 mg/kg 600	8–12 12	0.5 1–2
Lisinopril	12	0.058	1.8	1	0.3	–	B: 2.5,4, 6.7,10.1	0.03–0.04	PO	20–40	24	7 (6–8)
Lithium	19.2	0.036	0.8	1.0	1.0	0	NA	0.6–1.4 mEq/l	PO	300	6	–
Lomefloxacin	8	0.09	1.75	0.8	1	10	–	0.03–4	PO	400–1000	12–24	1.5
Loperamide	11 (7–15)	0.063	–	0.4	0.5	97	–	–	PO	2	after defecation	4–5
Lopinavir/Ritonavir	5.5	0.126	0.74[a]	0.02	–	99	–	9.6[b]	PO	400/100	12	4
Loracarbef	1	0.7	0.6	>0.9	0.9	25	–	8[b] (200 mg) 14[b] (400 mg)	PO	200–400	12	1.25
Lorazepam	13 (8–25)	0.053	1.5	0.01	0.85	90	11.5	0.02–0.05	PO	1–3	8	0.5–3
Losartan (active metabolite)	2 7.5	0.347 0.092	0.49 0.17	0.03 –	0.33 –	99 99.8	– –	0.280[b]	PO	50	24	1
Lovastatin	2.9	0.24	75	0.1	0.05	95	A: 5.5	0.015–3 ng/ml	PO	10–80	24	3
Maprotiline	43 (27–58)	0.0161	51.7	0.02	0.8	88	B: 10.2	0.2–0.3	PO	75–150	24	8–24
Mebendazole	5.5	0.126	2.0	0	0.17	95	–	–	PO	100	12	0.5–7
Meclofenamate	1.3	0.533	0.33	0.7	1	99	–	–	PO	50 100	4–6 8	0.5–2 0.5–2

Drug						%	pKa		Route	Dose	Interval	Peak
Mefenamic Acid	2	0.347	1.06	0.52	—	90	—	—	PO	250	6	2–4
Mefloquine	504 (312–576)	0.0013	20	0.1	0.9	98	B: 8.6	0.02–1	PO	250–1250	168	15 (8–21)
Melatonin	0.76	0.94	2.15	0	0.3	—	—	—	PO	2–50	24	1
Meloxicam	17 (15–20)	0.041	0.14	0.5	0.89	99.4	—	—	PO	7.5–15	24	4–5
Melphalan	1.1	0.6	—	0.0	0.5	87	—	0.1–0.3	IV,PO	0.2 mg/kg	8 for 6 days	—
Memantine	70 (53–97)	0.01	—	0.8	1.0	45	—	—	PO	10	12	5 (3–8)
Meperidine	3.5 (2–4)	0.2	4.7	0.1	0.52	64	B: 8.65	0.2–0.6	PO,IM,SC,IV	50–150	3–4	1.25
Mepindolol	4	0.17	5.4	0.7	0.7	50	—	0.01–0.04	PO	2.5–10	24	1.5
Meprobamate	12	0.058	0.7	0.1	0.9	0	B: 14	5–15	PO	400	8	1.5
Meropenem	1	0.7	0.25	0.7	NA	2	—	4–20	IV	250–1000	8	NA
Metamizol	6.9 (5–8)	0.01 4	0.01	0.95	1.0	20	A: 12.5	5–20	IV,PO,IM,R	7–15 mg/kg	4	1–1.5
Metformin	6.2	0.112	9.3[a]	1.0	0.55	0	B: 2.8	0.75[b]	PO	500	12	3.5
Methacycline	13 (10–16)	0.053	1.8	0.4	0.7	79	B: 3.02, 7.49, 9.3	1–10	PO	125	6	5
Methadone	25 (13–47)	0.0277	3.9	0.3	0.8	85	B: 8.62	0.3–1.1	PO,IM,SC	2.5–10	6–8	3
Methaqualone	19	0.0364	2.8	0.02	0.8	81	B: 2.4	1–4	PO	300	24	—
Methenamine	20	0.3465	0.6	0.9	0.8	—	B: 4.6	20	PO	1000	6	—
Methicillin	1	0.693	0.3	0.75	0	40	A: 3.01	1–6	IM,IV	1000	4	—
Methocarbamol	1.2	0.578	0.5	0	1	—	—	—	PO,IV	500–1000	6	1–2
Methotrexate	8.4	0.082	0.4	0.95	0.65	25	A: 4.3	—	IV,IM,PO	12–18 mg/m²	24 for 5 days	1–4
Low Dose Therapy								0.005				
High Dose Therapy	24	h	p.a.					2.2				
Methotrimeprazine	21	0.0346	29.8	0.01	0.5	—	B: 9.15	—	IM	10–30	4–6	—

(Continued)

388

Pharmacokinetic Parameters of Important Drugs (*Continued*)

DRUG	t$_{1/2}$ [h]	k$_{el}$ or β [h^{-1}]	V$_d$ [l/kg]	F$_{el}$	f	EPB [%]	pk$_a$	Ther. Range or MEC [µg/ml]	URA	D [mg]	τ [h]	t$_{max}$ [h]
Methyldigoxin	36	0.019	4.5	0.8 after demethylation	0.85	27	NA	—	PO	0.2–0.25	24	0.25–1.5
Methyldopa	1.7	0.4	0.5	0.7	0.4	20	—	0.03–4	PO,IV	500–2000	6–12	5 (4–6)
Methylphenidate												
d-form	6	0.12	2.6	0	0.22	—	—	—	PO,IV	10–40	12–24	2.3
l-form	3.6	0.19	1.8	0	0.22	—	—	—	PO,IV	10–40	12–24	3.2
6α-Methylprednisolone	1.5 (1.3–3.1)	0.46	0.41	0.1	1.0	85	2.6	—	PO	4–48	24	2.5
Metoclopramide	2.7	0.257	2.4	0.17	0.4	30	B: 7.32	—	IV,IM,PO	10	8	0.75
Metoprolol	3.2 (3–3.4)	0.2165	4.2	0.1	0.45	13	B: 9.7	0.025–0.1	PO	100–200	12	1.5
Metronidazole	8.0 (8–14)	0.087	0.75	0.08	0.8	15	B: 2.5	1–8	PO,IV	IV 7.5 mg/kg PO 250	6 8	1–3 1
Mexiletine	15 (9–20)	0.046	5.3	0.1	0.9	70	B: 9.05	0.5–2	PO,IV	200–300	8	2
Mezlocillin	0.8 (0.6–1.6)	0.866	0.38	0.5	0	50	A: 2.72	5–500	IV,IM	1500–4000	6	—
Mianserin	23	0.03	40	—	0.3	90	—	0.02–0.07	PO	30–200	24	—
Mibefradil	21 (17–25)	0.033	2.2 (1.8–2.7)	0.03	0.9	99	—	—	PO	50–100	24	1.5
Miconazole	22.5 (20–25)	0.0308	21	0.01	0.3–0.6	92	B: 6.65	0.001–10	IV PO	100–1200 100–500	6 12–24	NA 2.5
Midazolam	1.2	0.24	3.3 (0.9–6.6)	0.75	NA	95	B: 6.15	0.04–0.12	IM,IV	2–5	1 h before surgery	0.75 (IM)
Miglitol	2	0.347	0.18	0.95	0.7–1	4	—	—	PO	50–100	8	2–3
Minocycline	12 (10–16)	0.058	0.43	0.1	0.9	76	B: 2.8.5, 7.8	0.5–10	PO,IV	100	12	2
Miocamycin	1	0.7	4	0.05	—	47	—	0.0004–1.8	PO	600–1200	12	0.75

Mirtazapine	21.5	0.032	10.3	0.04	0.5	85	—	—	PO	15-30	24	2.5
Misoprostol	0.45 (0.3-0.6)	1.5	3.5	0.01	0.8	85	—	0.1-1000	PO	0.2	6	0.25
Moclobemide	1	0.7	1	0.005	0.4	50	B: 6.3	0.0006-0.28	PO,IV	300-600	8-12	1
Modafinil	11.3	0.061	0.79[a]	0.05	—	60	—	4.8-7[b] 1.3[c]	PO	200	24	1-2
Moexipril	5.5	0.24	0.7	0.01	0.13	50	—	0.015-0.25	PO	7.5-30	12-24	1.5
Mometasone Furoate	4.45	0.156	4.7	—	0.01	—	—	—	Inhal	0.4	—	2
Montelukast	4.6	0.151	0.14	0	0.64	99	—	0.3[b]	PO	10	24	2-4
Moricizine	2.5 (1.5-3.5)	0.3	4	0.01	0.4	95	B: 6.4	0.0006-0.8	PO	250	8	1 (0.5-2)
Morphine	2.3 (1.5-4)	0.3	1.0	0.1	0.4	35	B: 8.05	0.07-0.1	IV,IM,SC	10	4	3
Moxalactam	2.4	0.289	1.3	0.55	0	50	2.5,7.7, 10.2	20-100	IV,IM	700-2000	8	—
Moxifloxacin	12	0.058	1.85	0.2	0.9	50	—	4.5[b]	PO	400	24	1-3
Nabumetone	22.5	0.03	0.15	0.8	0.8	99	—	—	PO	1000-2000	24	9-12
Nadolol	14.1	0.049	2.1	0.7	0.4	30	B: 9.67	0.025-0.275	PO	80-240	24	3
Nafcillin	0.5 (0.5-1)	1.386	0.3	0.38	0.5	90	A: 2.65	0.03-1	IV,IM,PO	500	4-6	1
Nalidixic Acid	1.6	0.433	0.26-0.45	0.14	—	93	A: 1.6	5-50	PO	1000	6	1-2
Nalmefene	10.8	0.064	3.9	0.05	NA	45	76	—	IV,IM,SC	0.5-2	single dose	IM 2.3 SC 1.5
Naloxone	0.8 (0.7-0.9)	0.866	2.8	0	0.2	—	B: 7.94	0.01-0.03	IV	0.4-2	as needed	NA
Naproxen	17.1 (12-26)	0.039	0.12	0.1	1	99	A: 5	30-50	PO	275	6-8	2.5
Naratriptan	4.9	0.14	2.3	—	0.7	30	—	—	PO	2.5	24	2.5 (1.5-4)
Nateglinide	2.0 (1.6-3)	0.35	0.14	0.05	0.73	98	—	5.6[b]	PO	120	8	0.8
Nefazodone	3.5 (2-5)	0.2	0.5	0.55	0.2	99	—	0.05-0.18	PO	200-300	12	1
Nelfinavir	4.3 (3.5-5)	0.161	2.6[a]	0.02	—	98	—	3.4[b]	PO	750	8	2-4
Neomycin	2.5	0.277	0.2	0.5	0.03	—	—	5-10	PO	1000-2000	6	1-4

(Continued)

Pharmacokinetic Parameters of Important Drugs (*Continued*)

DRUG	$t_{1/2}$ [h]	k_{el} or β [h⁻¹]	V_d [l/kg]	F_{el}	f	EPB [%]	pk_a	Ther. Range or MEC [µg/ml]	URA	D [mg]	τ [h]	t_{max} [h]
Neostigmine	0.5 (0.25–1)	1.38	1.1	0.5	0.02	0	NA	—	IM SC PO	0.5 0.5 15–375	3 — within 1 day	— — —
Nesiritide	0.3	2.31	0.19	—	NA	—	—	—	IV Inf	0.01 µg/kg/min for < 48 h	NA	NA
Netilmicin	2.2	0.315	0.25	0.45	0	10	—	1–8	IV,IM	1–2 mg/kg	8–12	NA
Nifedipine	1.7 (1.5–4)	0.407	1.1	0.02	0.56	98	B: 6	0.015	PO	10–20	4–8	0.5
Nimodipine	9	0.08	1.5 (0.9–2.3)	0.01	0.2	95	—	0.08–0.1	PO	60	4	1
Nisoldipine	10 (7–12)	0.07	5.8	0	0.05	99	—	0.015–4.4	PO	10–60	24	8 (6–12)
Nitrazepam	22 (21–28)	0.0315	2.1	0.01	0.8	85	B: 3.2, 10.8	0.03–0.06	PO	5–10	24	—
Nitrofurantoin	0.33	2.1	0.3–0.7	0.4	0.5	40	A: 7.2	5–200	PO,IV	50–100	6	—
Nizatidine	1.5	0.5	1.2 (0.8–1.5)	0.65	0.7	35	B: 2.1, 6.8	0.01–2.5	PO	150	12	1.5 (0.5–3)
Nomifensine	4 (3–5)	0.1735	6.5	0	—	70	—	0.025–0.075	PO	50–150	24	—
Norepinephrine	0.04	16.9	0.1–0.5	0.02	NA	50	B: 9.78	NA	IV	0.1 µg/kg/min	—	NA
Norethindrone Acetate	10.4	0.071	6.46ᵃ	—	—	—	—	0.013ᵇ	PO	2	24	1.5
Norfloxacin	3–4	0.2	9.62	0.30	0.40	5–15	A: 6.34 A: 8.75	0.8–2.5	PO	400	12	1–2
Nortriptyline	27 (14–90)	0.0257	20	0.02	0.6	95	B: 9.73	0.05–0.8	PO	25	6	7–8.5
Ofloxacin	6.25 (3–9)	0.12	1–2.5	0.80	0.98	6.3	—	0.05–4.00	PO	200–400	6–8	1.5
Olanzapine	45 (20–70)	0.0154	15 (10–20)	—	—	93	—	—	PO	10	24	5–6
Olmesartan	13	0.053	0.24	0.42	0.26	99	—	—	PO	20	24	1–2
Omapatrilat	16 (14–19)	0.043	25.7	0.3	0.3	80	—	0.023ᵇ	PO	25	24	2

Drug	t½ (h)					%	pKa		Route	Dose	Interval	Tmax
Omeprazole	0.75 (0.5–1)	0.92	0.27	0.01	0.35–0.6	95	—	—	PO	20–40	24	1 (0.5–3)
Ondansetron	3	0.2	2	0.05	0.6	75	B: 7.4	0.003–0.03	PO,IV	8	12	2
Oseltamivir (active: Oseltamivir Carboxylate)	1.4 / 8 (6–10)	0.495 / 0.087	— / 0.36	— / 1.0	— / 0.75	42 / 3	— / —	0.045[b] / 0.35[b]	PO / —	75 / —	12 / —	1 / 4
Ouabain	22 (18–25)	0.0315	15.7	0.37	1	42	NA	0.0002	IV	0.25–0.5	24	NA
Oxacillin	1	0.693	0.33	0.55	0.7	90	A: 2.88	5–6	IM,IV,PO	500	6	1
Oxaprozin	46 (42–50)	0.015	0.178	0.65	0.95	99	—	—	PO	1200–1800	24	3–5
Oxazepam	12 (5–15)	0.058	1.2	0.02	1	96	B: 1.8, 11.1	1–2	PO	10–30	8	2
Oxcarbazepine	9 (5–14)	0.077	0.7	0.01	1	40	—	—	PO	300–600	24	—
Oxprenolol	1.9	0.365	1.2	0.05	0.45	—	B: 9.5	0.04–0.1	PO	20–80	8–12	2
Oxtriphylline	4.7 (2.7–7)	0.147	0.45	0.1	0.75	60	B: 8.79	8–20	PO	400	4	2.5
Oxybate Sodium	0.65	1.066	0.3[a]	0.03	—	—	—	—	PO	1500–4500	at bedtime & 2 h later	1
Oxybutynin	9	0.077	11.4[a]	—	0.06	—	6.96	0.014[b]	PO	5	8–12	5
Oxycodone	5.7	0.1	2.5	0.05	0.5	38	—	0.04–0.07	PO,IV	10–30	4	1.5
Oxytetracycliae	9.2 (6–10)	0.075	1.9	0.25	0.77	35	B: 3.5, 7.6	0.5–10	PO,IV,IM	250	6	2
Paclitaxel	14 (6–29)	0.05	2.3	0.1	NA	>95	—	—	IV Inf	175–225 mg/m²	3 wks	NA
Pancuronium	2.8 (1.4–4.2)	0.25	0.13–0.28	0.8	NA / NA	30	—	0.025–0.1	IV	0.01 mg/kg 0.02 mg/kg	48	NA
Pantoprazole	1	0.7	0.22	0.01	0.77	98	—	—	PO	10–40	24	2.4
Papaverine	1.6 (1.5–2)	0.433	0.2	0.01	0.53	87	B: 8.07	0.1–0.2	PO,IV	100–200	6	—
Pefloxacin	8.5 (7.5–10)	0.08	0.16	0.6	0.95	25	—	0.1–10	PO	400–1000	12–24	1.3

(Continued)

Pharmacokinetic Parameters of Important Drugs (*Continued*)

DRUG	t½ [h]	kel or β [h⁻¹]	Vd [l/kg]	Fel	f	EPB [%]	pka	Ther. Range or MEC [µg/ml]	URA	D [mg]	τ [h]	tmax [h]
Peginterferon Alfa-2a	80 (50–140)	0.0087	0.16	—	—	—	—	16 ng/ml[c] @week 48 8 ng/ml @week 1	SC	0.18	168	72–96
Peginterferon Alfa-2b	40 (22–60)	0.017	1.3[a]	0.3	—	—	—	320 pg/ml[c] @week 48 94 pg/ml[c] @week 4	SC	1 mg/kg	168	15–44
Peldesine	3.7	0.187	2.29	0.88	0.5	—	—	0.6[b] 0.9[b]	IV PO	18 mg/m² 40 mg/m²	— 6	NA 1.6
Penbutolol	27	0.0257	10.4	0.07	0.9	—	—	0.1–0.3	PO	40–60	24	—
Penicillamine	82 (75–90)	0.0084	2.9	0.02	0.65	40	A: 1.8, 7.9,10.5	2.5–4	PO	1000–2000	24	1.5
Penicillin G	0.7	0.99	0.5	0.8	0.3	65	A: 2.78	1.5–3	PO,IM	600	6	0.5
Penicillin V	0.6	1.155	0.4	0.26	0.6	80	A: 2.73	3–5	PO	250–500	6	0.5
Pentazocine	2.5	0.28	4.0	0.05	0.5	61	B: 9.5	0.03–0.1	IV,IM, SC,PO	30–50	3–4	1
Pentobarbital	22.3 (20–35)	0.031	1.0	0.01	1	45	A: 8.0	1–4	PO,IV,IM	30	8	0.6
Pentoxifylline	0.6	1.16	6.7	0	1	—	B: 0.28	0.4–1.2	PO	400	8	1
Perphenazine	10	0.07	20	0.01	—	85 (75–99)	—	0.001–0.02	PO	4–8	8	3.5 (2–5)
Phenacetin	1.0	0.693	1.6	0.002	0.13	33	B: 2.2	1–20	PO	300	4	—
Phenethicillin K	1.3	0.533	0.35	—	—	82	A: 2.73	0.1–0.8	PO	250–500	8	—
Phenobarbital	90 (72–100)	0.0077	0.7	0.35	0.9	51	A: 7.52, 11.77	10–50	PO	50–100	12	0.5
Phenprocoumon	151	0.00458	0.13	—	1	99	—	0.15–3.5	PO	1–4	24	—
Phenylbutazone	72 (48–110)	0.009	0.25	0	1	99	A: 4.5	40–150	PO	100–400	24	2.5
Phenylpropanolamine	3.5	0.2	1.8	0.85	0.65	—	B: 9	0.08–0.2	PO	25–75	4	1.5

Drug												
Phenytoin	22 (6–60)	0.0315	0.65	0.05	0.9	89	A: 8.31	10–20	IV,IM,PO	100–200	6	2
Pilocarpine	0.75	0.92	1.79	—	—	—	—	0.02	PO	5	—	1.25
Pimozide	18	0.039	0.21	0.01	0.45	—	—	0.18–0.2	PO	6	24	4
Pindolol	2.2 (2–3.6)	0.315	2.0	0.37	0.95	57	B: 8.8	0.05–0.15	PO	5–20	8	1.5
Pioglitazone	20 (16–24)	0.035	0.63	0.3	0.81–0.94	99	—	—	PO	15–30	24	2
Pirenzepine	10.0	0.07	0.25	0.3	0.3	10	—	0.02–0.05	PO	25–50	8–12	2.5–3
Piroxicam	40.8	0.017	0.13	0.05	1.0	99	A: 5.1	1.5–3.5	PO	20–40	24	3–5
Pleconaril	26.4	0.026	12.3[a]	—	—	—	—	0.3–6	PO	50–1000	24	3
Polymyxin B	4.4	0.157	—	0.6	—	—	B: 8.9	0.5–4	IM,IV,PO PO	0.5–0.8 mg/kg 100	8–12 6	— 2
Porfimer Sodium	250	0.0028	0.49	—	NA	90	—	2.6	IV	2 mg/kg	30 days	NA
Practolol	10.5 (5–15)	0.066	1.6	0.9	0.95	32	B: 9.5	1.5–5	PO	100–400	12	2
Pravastatin	1.4	0.495	9.4[a]	0.05	0.17	64	A: 5.5	—	PO	40–80	24	1.3
Prazosin	2.9 (2–5)	0.239	0.6	0·01	0.57	97	B: 6.5	0.001–0.075	PO	0.5–10	8–24	2
Prednisolone	2.3–2.8	0.28	0.33	0.05–0.2	0.73–1.00	80–96	—	0.1–0.4	PO,IM,IV	5–60	6,12,24	0.5–1.5
Prednisone	2.5	0.28	3.1	0.05–0.2	1	80–90	—	0.1–0.4	IV,IM,PO	5–50	6	3
Pregabalin	7.4 (4–12)	0.094	0.6[a]	0.9	—	0	—	1.9[b]	PO	300	8	1.3
Primidone	6.5 (3–12)	0.107	0.8	0.1	0.8	19	—	5–12	PO	250–500	8	4
Probenecid	5 (4–12)	0.139	0.15	0.05	1	90	A: 3.4	100–200	PO	250	12	3
Procainamide	3 (2.5–4.5)	0.23	2	0.5	0.85	15	B: 9.23	4–12	PO,IV,IM	500–1000	4–6	1
Promethazine HCl	4.4	0.16	2.4	0.02	0.25	93	B: 9.1	0.01–0.02	IV,IM,PO	6–50	4–6	2 (1–4)
Propantheline	3	0.231	2.1	0.1	0.1	—	—	—	PO,IV,IM	15–30	6	4
Propofol	19.6	0.035	40	—	NA	—	—	—	IV	1–2 mg/kg until anesthesia then 0.1–0.2 mg/kg/min	NA	NA

(Continued)

Pharmacokinetic Parameters of Important Drugs (*Continued*)

DRUG	$t_{1/2}$ [h]	k_{el} or β [h⁻¹]	V_d [l/kg]	F_{el}	f	EPB [%]	pk_a	Ther. Range or MEC [µg/ml]	URA	D [mg]	τ [h]	t_{max} [h]
Propoxyphene	6.5	0.107	5.4	0.015	0.2	76	A: 6.3	0.2–0.8	PO	65	4	2
Propranolol	3.8 (3.5–6)	0.182	5.5	0.01	0.35	93	B: 9.45	0.05–0.1	PO,IV	10–40	6	1.25
Propylthiouracil	1.4 (1–2)	0.495	0.36	0	0.8	75	B: 8.3	2–6	PO	50–100	8	1.5
Protriptyline	78	0.0089	0.3	—	1	—	—	0.05–0.3	PO	5–10	6–8	24–30
Pseudoephedrine	6.9	0.1	2.8	0.96	1	—	B: 9.86	—	PO	60	6	—
Pyrazinamide	9.5	0.073	—	—	0.8	10	—	30–50	PO	15–30 mg/kg	24	2
Pyrimethamine	96	0.00722	2.2	0.25	1	27	B: 7.2	0.07	PO	25	168	1.5–8
Quetiapine	7	0.099	10	—	—	83	—	—	PO	25–400	12	1–2
Quinapril	2.3	0.3	1.1	0.01	0.6	97	—	0.06–0.6	PO	10–40	12–24	1.6
Quinidine	6.3 (4–7)	0.11	3	0.2	0.75	82	B: 5.4,10	1–8	PO,IM	300–600	6	1.25
Quinine	16.4	0.0422	1.2	0.15	1	70	B: 4.3,8.7	17.0	PO	600	8	1–3
Quinupristin Dalfopristin	0.75 0.45	0.92 1.54	1.0 0.56	0 0	NA NA	— —	— —	2.4–3.2b 6.2–8b	IV Inf	7.5 mg/kg	8–12	NA
Rabeprazole	0.82	0.845	0.55a	0.01	0.52	96	—	0.3b	PO	20	24	3.5
Ramipril	5.1	0.14	1.3	0.02	0.28	73	—	0.004–0.013	PO	2.5–20	24	1
Ranitidine	2.3	0.301	1.6	0.8	0.6	15	—	0.1–0.2	PO	150	12	2.5
Reboxetine	12.5	0.055	31.4a	0.09	—	95	—	0.111b	PO	4	12	2
Remifentanil	0.2	3.46	0.1	0.015	NA	70	B: 7.07	0.001–0.003	IV Inf	1–5	as needed	NA
Repaglinide	0.8	0.87	0.44	0.01	0.56	98	—	0.046b	PO	0.5–4	6,8,12	0.8
Reserpine	110 (50–170)	0.0063	6	0.1	>0.5	96	B: 6.6	0.001–0.007	PO	0.1–0.5	24	3.5
Retigabine	7	0.1	6a	—	—	—	—	0.5–1.5	PO	100–300	12	1.5

Drug									Route			
Ribavirin	150 (120–170)	0.0046	—	0.17	0.64	—	—	2–10	PO	400–600	12	2
Ribozyme	0.55	1.26	0.035	0.14	NA	—	—	1.5–3.75[b]	IV Inf	10–30 mg/m²	—	NA
Rifabutin	3.50	0.2	0.4	0.07	0.69	—	—	0.9[b]	SC	20 mg/m²	—	3.25
Rifampin	45	0.015	9.3	0.05	0.2	85	—	0.35	PO	300	24	2.5
	3 (2–5)	0.231	0.6	0.15	1	87	B: 7.1, 7.9	0.5–10	PO	600	24	2
Rifapentine	13.2	0.053	1.0	0.17	—	98	—	15	PO	600	72	5–6
Riluzole	46 (42–49)	0.015	26.5	0.02	0.5	96	—	0.2[b]	PO	50	12	0.75
Risedronate	210	0.0033	95[a]	0.01	<0.01	—	—	0.001–0.005[b]	PO	5 / 35	24 / 168	1 / 1
Risperidone	3 fast met. 20 slow met.	0.23 / 0.035	1.1	0.3	0.7	90	—	NA no correl.	PO	4–16	12	1.5
Ritonavir	2.2	0.314	0.4[a]	0.04	—	99	—	3–12	PO	600	12	2
Rivastigmine Tartrate	1.5	0.462	2.2 (1.8–2.7)	0	0.4	40	—	—	PO	1.5–6	12	0.5–2
Rizatriptan	2.5	0.277	3.6	—	0.45	14	—	0.037[b]	PO	5–10	d	1.25
Rofecoxib	17	0.041	1.3	0.72	0.93	87	—	0.2[b]	PO	12.5–25	24	2–3
Rolitetracycline	10	0.0693	0.6	0.6	0.7	50	A: 7.4	1–10	IV,IM	150–350	8–12	1.5
Rosiglitazone	3.5	0.198	0.25	0.64	0.99	99.8	—	0.1–0.3	PO	4	12	1
Rosuvastatin	20	0.035	—	0.1	0.2	88	—	0.02[b] (40 mg)	PO	5–80	24	3–5
Roxifiban (active XV459)	120	0.058	6.7 (D 0.75 mg) 10.4 (D 1.5 mg)	—	—	—	—	0.025[b], 0.03[b] (0.75 mg) 0.03[c], 0.046[b] (1.5 mg)	PO	0.75–1.5	24	4.5 (3–6)
Roxithromycin	10	0.07	20	0.07	0.75	98	—	6–14	PO	150	12	2 (1–3)
Salicylate	4 (2–19)	0.173	0.14	0.15	1	70	A: 3.0	20–300	PO	325–650	4	0.6
Scopolamine	1.76	0.39	4.78	—	0.57 (IM)	—	—	—	SC,IM, IV Inf PO	0.5 0.5 0.32–0.65	—	0.25 (IM)

(Continued)

Pharmacokinetic Parameters of Important Drugs (Continued)

DRUG	$t_{1/2}$ [h]	k_{el} or β [h⁻¹]	V_d [l/kg]	F_{el}	f	EPB [%]	pk_a	Ther. Range or MEC [µg/ml]	URA	D [mg]	τ [h]	t_{max} [h]
Secobarbital	28 (15–40)	0.0247	1.52	0.05	0.9	35	A: 7.74	1–15	PO,IV,IM	50–250	once	—
Sertraline	26	0.027	20	0.02	—	98	—	0.02–0.05	PO	50–200	—	5–8
Sibrafiban (active metabolite: R₀ 44-3888)	2.2	0.315	0.6ᵃ	—	—	—	—	0.0024–0.075	PO	10	12	1–2
Sildenafil	4	0.173	1.5	0	0.4	96	—	—	PO	25–100	NA	1 (0.5–2)
Simvastatin	2.5	0.28	—	0.13	0.05	95	—	—	PO	5–80	24	2
Sirolimus	68	0.01	12	0.02	0.18	92	—	0.06ᵇ	PO	5	24	1.5
Sisomicin	3.0	0.231	0.19	0.5	0	10	—	1–8	IV,IM	1 mg/kg	8	NA
Sotalol	14	0.0495	1.85	0.75	1	54	B: 9.8	0.5–4	PO	100–200	8–12	—
Sparfloxacin	17.5 (15–20)	0.04	5.5	0.12	0.9	37	A: 6.27	0.4–1	PO	200–300	24	4 (3–5)
Spectinomycin	1	0.693	0.12	0.75	1	—	B: 6.95, 8.7	7.5–20	IM	2000–4000	12	1
Stavudine	1.3	0.5	0.8	0.4	0.85	0	—	0.002–1.4	PO	30–40	12	1
Streptomycin	2.4 (2–3)	0.289	0.26	0.5	0	34	B: 7 8.7	20–25	IM,IV	7.5–15 mg/kg	12	1–2
Sufentanil	2.5	0.28	2.5	0.01	1	92	—	0.002–0.003	IV	0.35	once	NA
Sulfadiazine	17 (10–24)	0.041	0.9	0.6	0.9	45	A: 6.48	100–150	PO,IV	1000–1500	4–6	1.5
Sulfadimethoxine	69	0.01	0.65	0.6	1	99	A: 6.1	1–50	PO	500	24	2
Sulfaethidole	7.7	0.09	0.18	—	0.9	99	A: 5.6	0.5–1	PO	650–2000	12	2
Sulfamerazine	22 (15–30)	0.0315	0.35	—	0.9	75	A: 7	50–200	PO	1000	8	1.5
Sulfamethazine	9 (8–10)	0.077	0.5	0.3	0.9	80	A: 7.4	50–200	PO	1000	6	1.5
Sulfamethizole	1.5 (1–2)	0.462	0.35	0.75	0.9	90	A: 5.4	50–200	—	—	—	2
Sulfamethoxazole	10 (8–12)	0.0693	0.3	0.35	0.9	68	A: 6	50–200	PO	1000	8–12	2

Sulfamethoxypyrimidine	37	0.0187	0.28	—	1	87	A: 6.54	1–20	PO	500	24	2
Sulfasalazine	3.5	0.2	0.9	0.05	0.3	95	A: 2.4	10–20	PO	1000	6–8	1.5–6
Sulfinpyrazone	10 (3.8–13)	0.0693	0.74	0.35	0.95	99	A: 2.8	5–20	PO	100–200	12	2
Sulfisomidine	7.5	0.092	0.31	0.09	0.8	86	A: 7.4	10–50	PO	1000	4–8	2
Sulfisoxazole Acetyl	10.5	0.066	1.2	—	—	85	A: 5	1–20	PO	1000–2000	4–6	2
Sulfisoxazole	6	0.1155	0.16	0.5	1	86	A: 4.9	90–150	PO,IM,IV	1000–2000	4–6	2
Sulindac	7.8	0.888	0.05	0.5	0.9	93	—	—	PO	150–200	12	3
Sumatriptan	2.5	0.277	2.4	—	0.15	21	—	0.05[b]	PO	25–100	[d]	2
Tacrine	2.5	0.27	6	0.03	0.17	55	—	0.7–35	PO,IV	40–80	6	1.5 (0.5–3)
Tacrolimus	34	0.02	1.91	0.01	NA	99	—	0.01[c] 0.03[b]	IV	0.03–0.05 mg/kg	24	NA
*in kidney transplant pt.	18.8*	0.037*	1.4*	—	0.17–0.22	—	—	0.02*	PO	0.1–0.2 mg/kg	24	1.5
**in liver transplant pt.	11.7**	0.059**	0.85**	—	0.17–0.22	—	—	0.04**				
Tadalafil	17.5	0.039	—	—	—	—	—	—	PO	10–25	NA	2
Tamoxifen	168	0.004	—	0.01	1.0	99	8.85	—	PO	20–40	24	4–5
Tamsulosin	12 (9–15)	0.078	0.23	—	0.9	99	—	—	PO	0.4	24	1
Tegaserod Maleate	11	0.063	5.25	0.03	0.1	98	—	0.004[b]	PO	6	12	NA
Teicoplanin	47 (32–62)	0.0147	0.85	0.75	1	—	—	0.01–4	IV	400	24	0.5–1
Telmisartan	24	0.029	7.1	0.01	0.5	99.5	—	—	PO	40	24	NA
Tenecteplase	1.8 (1.5–2.2)	0.385	0.043	0	NA	—	—	—	IV	50	NA	
Tenofovir Disoproxil Fumarate	17.5	0.040	1.3	0.8	0.35	0.07	—	0.3	PO	300	24	1
Terazosin	12	0.05	0.5	0.1	0.85	92	B: 7.04	0.01–0.04	PO	1–5	12–24	1
Terbinafine	36	0.0193	13.5	0	0.4	99	—	1–1.5	PO	250	24	2
Tetracycline	6.8 (6–10)	0.102	1.3	0.6	0.8	55	B: 8.3	0.5–10	PO,IM,IV	250	6	3
Tetrazepam	15	0.05	3.3	0.5	0.9	—	—	0.3–0.8	PO	50	24	2

Pharmacokinetic Parameters of Important Drugs (Continued)

DRUG	$t_{1/2}$ [h]	k_{el} or β [h⁻¹]	V_d [l/kg]	F_{el}	f	EPB [%]	pk_a	Ther. Range or MEC [µg/ml]	URA	D [mg]	τ [h]	t_{max} [h]
Thalidomide	5.4	0.128	1.2ᵃ	<0.01	—	—	—	1–2	PO	100–300	24	3.5
Theophylline	5.5 (3–9)	0.126	0.45	0.08	1	59	A: 8.75	10–20	PO,IV,IM,R	100–200	6	2.5
Thiocolchicoside	2.8	0.25	1.13ᵃ	0.17	—	13	—	0.06ᵇ	IM	4	12	1
Thymol	10.2	0.068	0.25ᵃ	0	—	—	—	0.09ᵇ	PO	1	NA	2
Thyroxine	110 (96–168)	0.0063	0.15	0	0.7	99.95	A: 2.2,6.7	0.04–0.13	PO	0.05–0.3	24	2–6
Tiagabine	8	0.087	2.4	0.02	0.9	96	—	>0.2	PO	4–56	24	0.75
Ticarcillin	1.2	0.578	0.21	0.86	0	60	A: 2.5,3.4	>50	IV,IM	1000	6	—
Ticlopidine	7.9	0.088	11.8	0	0.8	98	—	1–2	PO	250	12	2
Timolol	4.9	0.141	3.14	0.2	0.75	10	—	0.005–0.01	PO	10–300	8–12	1
Tinzaparin	3.75	0.185	0.07	—	86.7	—	—	—	SC	50 Xa IU/kg	24	4–6
Tiopronin	18	0.04	6.5	0.5	0.6	90	—	2.5–6	PO	800–1000	24	5 (4–6)
Toborinone	2.5	0.28	1.65	0.2	NA	0.06 (98 platelet bound)	—	0.1ᵇ	IV Inf	1 mg/kg/min for 4 h	NA	—
Tobramycin	2	0.347	0.25	0.9	1	<10	B: 6.2, 7.4,7.6	2–10	IV	1–2 mg/kg	8	NA
Tocainide	12.5 (11–14)	0.055	1.6	0.4	0.95	50	—	5–10	PO	300–600	8	1–2
Tolamolol	2.5	0.277	3.1	0.05	0.3	91	B: 9.2	—	PO	100–300	8–12	—
Tolazamide	7.0 (4.7–8)	0.099	—	0.15	0.05	—	A: 3.5, 5.17	—	PO	250	12–24	4–8
Tolbutamide	7 (4–8)	0.099	0.12	0	1	87	A: 5.5	50–250	PO	500	12	3.5
Tolmetin	5	0.14	0.12	>0.5	1.0	99	A: 3.5	20–40	PO	400	8	0.5–1
Topiramate	21	0.033	0.7	0.7	0.8	17	—	—	PO	200	12	2

Torsemide	3.2 (2–4.1)	0.22	0.2	0.28	0.85	98	A: 7.1	1–3	PO,IV	20–100	24	1
Tramadol	6.5	0.107	2.7	0.3	1	20	—	—	IV	50–100	—	NA
					0.99			—	IM	50–100	6–8	0.75
					0.75			0.3b (100 mg PO)	PO	50–100	6–8	2
					0.8			0.6b (100 mg, q6hr)	R	50–100	6–8	2
Trandolapril	1	0.7	0.25	0.005	0.01	80	—	—	PO	2–4	24	1
Trandolaprilat measured	20	0.03	3	0.15	0.5	94	—	2.5–5	—	—	—	5
Tranexamic Acid	2	0.3	0.15	0.95	0.4	3	—	0.06–1	PO,IV	1750	8	3
Treprostinil	3 (2–4)	0.231	0.2	0.04	1	91	—	—	SC Inf	1.25 ng/kg/min	—	NA
Triacetyloleandomycin	4.5	0.154	2.3	0.36	—	—	B: 6.6	1.25	PO	250–500	6	2
Triamcinolone Acetonide	2.5	0.28	1.96	0.4	0.25 (Inhal) 0.1 (PO)	68	—	—	Nasal Inhal	0.22–0.44	24	0.5
							—	—	IM	40	168	3
							—	—	IV	0.4	—	NA
							—	—	PO	4–60	24	1
Trimethoprim	8.8	0.0787	2.0	0.6	1	70	B: 7.2	0.5–12	PO	160	12	2–4
Troglitazone	24	0.029	0.21	0.03	0.55	99	—	0.2–3	PO	200–600	24	2–3
Trovafloxacin	9	0.077	1.2	0.06	0.88	76	—	1–2	PO	200	24	1–2
Tubocurarine	2.0	0.347	0.3	0.43	0 (IV only)	40	B: 8,9.3	0.6	IV	6–12	as required	NA
Tyramine	0.533	1.32	87.7a	—	—	—	—	0.038b	PO	200	NA	0.5
Valacyclovir (active: Acyclovir)	3 (2.5–3.3)	0.231	2.12	0.36	0.54	15	—	5b	PO	1000	8	1
Valdecoxib	9.5 (8–11)	0.073	1.23	0.9	0.83	98	—	—	PO	10–20	12,24	3
Valganciclovir (active: Ganciclovir)	4.1	0.169	1.06	0.9	0.6	2	—	5b	PO	900	24	1–3
Valproate	12.2 (9–18)	0.0568	0.14	0.05	0.9	90	A: 4.95	20–100	PO	250–1000	8	2
Valsartan	6	0.116	0.24	0.13	0.25	95	—	—	PO	80–160	24	3

(Continued)

Pharmacokinetic Parameters of Important Drugs (*Continued*)

DRUG	$t_{1/2}$ [h]	k_{el} or β [h⁻¹]	V_d [l/kg]	F_{el}	f	EPB [%]	pk_a	Ther. Range or MEC [µg/ml]	URA	D [mg]	τ [h]	t_{max} [h]
Vancomycin	6 (5–6.5)	0.116	0.47	0.95	0	10	—	5–40	IV,PO	500	6	—
Vardenafil	3.5	0.198	4.71	0	0.2	95	3.4	0.015[b]	PO	NA	1 (0.5–2)	2
Venlafaxine	3.5	0.2	6.5	0.05	0.92	30	—	0.05–0.4	PO	75–375	8–12	2
Verapamil	2.9 (2.5–7)	0.239	5.3	0.7	0.22	90	—	0.1–0.7	IV,PO	IV: 0.075–0.15 mg/kg PO: 80–160	8	1.5
Verteporfin	5.2	0.133	0.63	0.01	NA	—	—	1.3[b]	IV Inf	6 mg/m²	NA	1–2
Vesnarinone	44.7	0.0155	0.23	0.18	—	—	—	3.4[b]	PO	30	24	2.5–8.5
Vigabatrin	7	0.099	0.8	0.7	0.80	—	—	—	PO	1000–4000	24	2
Vinblastine	25	0.027	27.3	0.2	NA	90	B: 5.4	—	IV	0.1–0.2 mg/kg	1–2 weeks	—
Vincamine	2.0 (1.6–2.5)	0.3465	0.58	0.06	0.3	64	B: 6.17	—	PO	20–60	12	1
Vincristine	85 (19–155)	0.008	8.4	0.12	NA	75	B: 5	—	IV	0.05 mg/kg	1 week	NA
Vinorelbine	37 (27–44)	0.019	33	0.11	0.4	13.5 (80 to platelets, lymphocytes)	—	—	IV PO	30 mg/m² 60 mg/m²	168 168	NA 1.5–3
Vlomycin	2	0.346	0.24	0.8	—	5	B: 2.8, 5.87	25–100	IM	500	12	—
Voriconazole	12.9 Dose dependent	0.053	4.6	0.02	0.96	58	—	0.5–5	PO IV Inf	50–200 3 mg/kg/hr in 1–2 hr	12 12	1–2
Warfarin	46	0.015	0.11	0	0.9	99.5	A: 5.05	1–10	PO,IM,IV	5–10	24	—
Zafirlukast	10	0.07	1	0	1	99	—	—	PO	20	12	3
Zalcitabine	2.2	0.315	0.94[a]	0.78	—	—	—	0.011[b]	PO	0.75	8	1
Zaleplon	1	0.7	1.7	0.01	0.3	60	—	—	PO	10	24	1

Zanamivir	3 (2.5–5.1)	0.23	2.4	1.0	0.17	10	—	0.14[b]	Inhal	10	12	1–2
Ziconotide	4.6 (2.9–6.5)	0.15	0.0018 in CSF	—	NA	—	—	—	Intrathecal	0.01–0.1	—	NA
Zileuton	2.5	0.277	1.2	0.005	1	93	—	5[b]	PO	600	6	1–2
Zimelidine	5 (4.3–6)	0.1386	3	0	0.3	90	—	—	PO	50–300	24	—
Ziprasidone	7 (4–10)	0.099	2	—	—	99	—	—	PO	20–80	12	4–5
Zoledronic Acid	4526	1.5×10^{-4}	100	0.6	NA	—	—	0.4–2.25[b]	IV Inf	4–16	3–4 weeks	NA
Zolmitriptan	2.8	0.25	7.4[a]	—	0.39	25	—	3.3[b]	PO	2.5	d	1.75
Zolpidem	2.3	0.301	0.54	0.01	0.7	92	—	0.19[b]	—	10	24	0.5–2
Zomepirac	4.3	0.161	0.98	0.22	0.95	99	A: 4.5	0.1–10	PO	50–100	4–6	0.5–1
Zonisamide	63	0.011	1.45	0.22	—	40	—	2–5[b]	PO	100–200	24	2–6

Index

In this index, page numbers in *italics* designate figures; page numbers followed by the letter "t" designate tabular material.